Inflammation in the 21st Century

Edited by Vijay Kumar, Alexandro Aguilera Salgado and Seyyed Shamsadin Athari

Published in London, United Kingdom

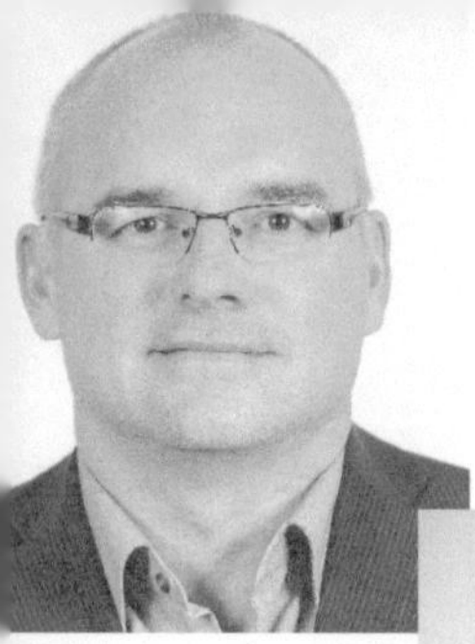
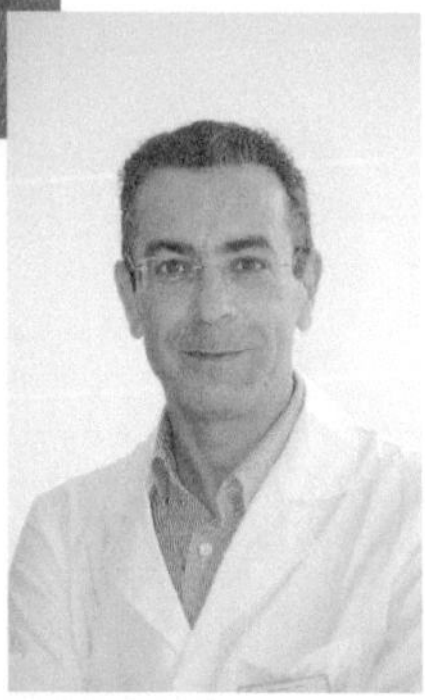
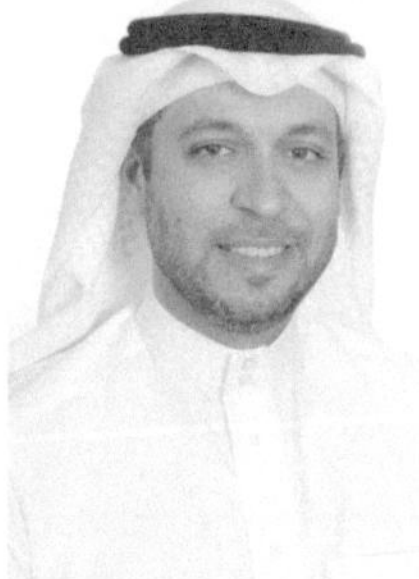
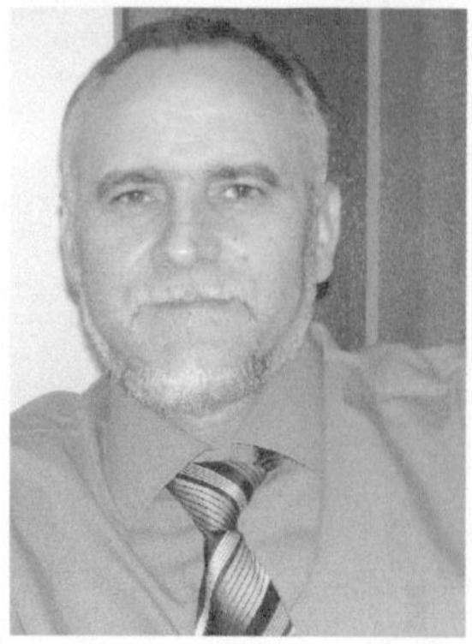
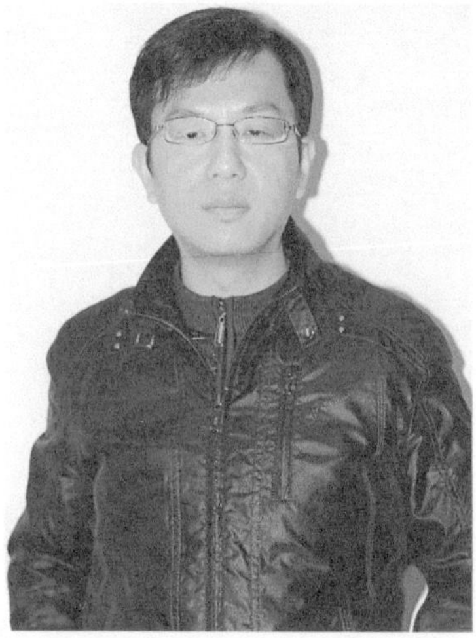
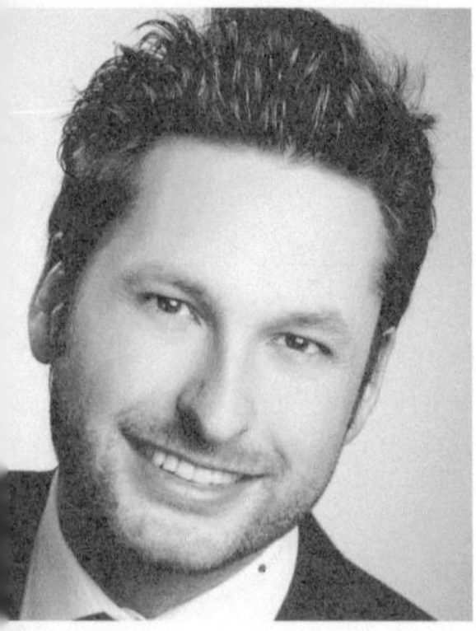
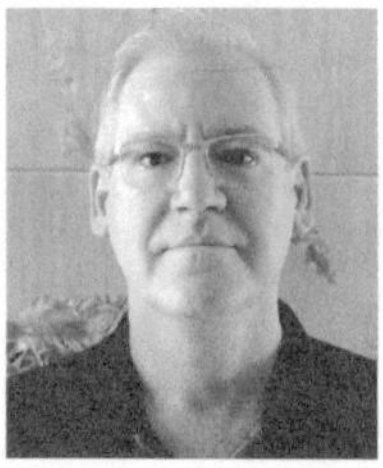

IntechOpen

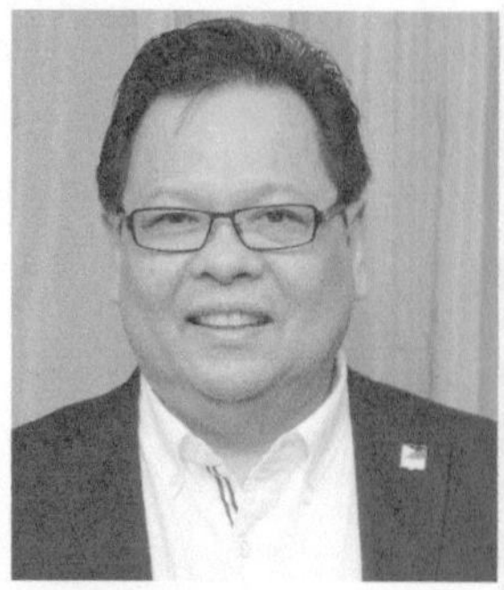
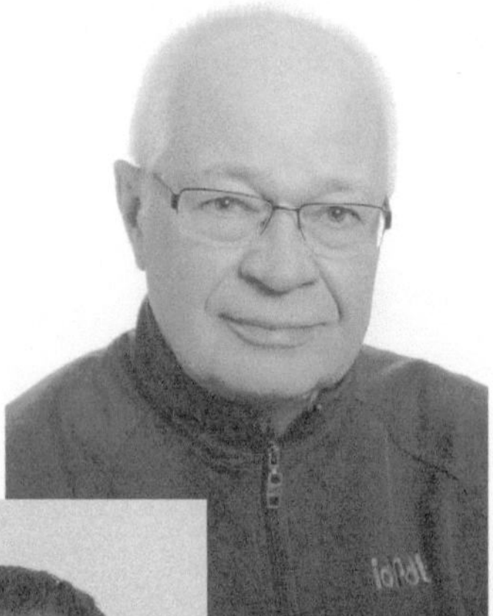
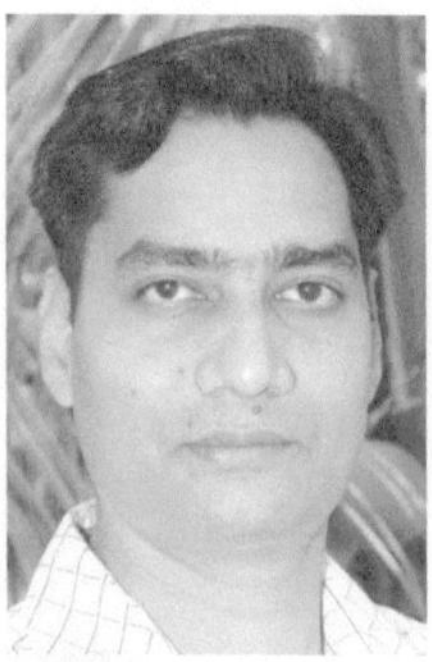
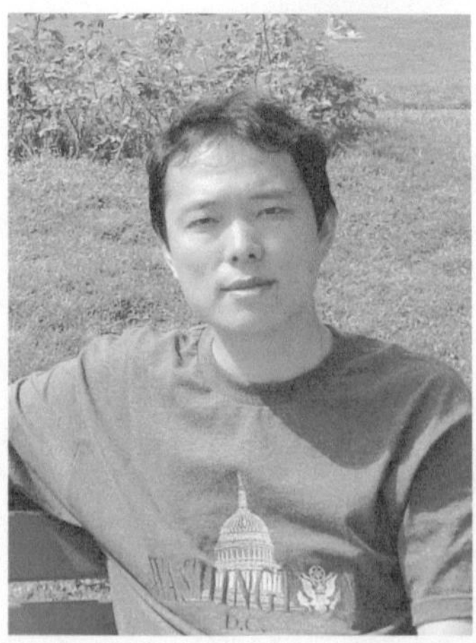
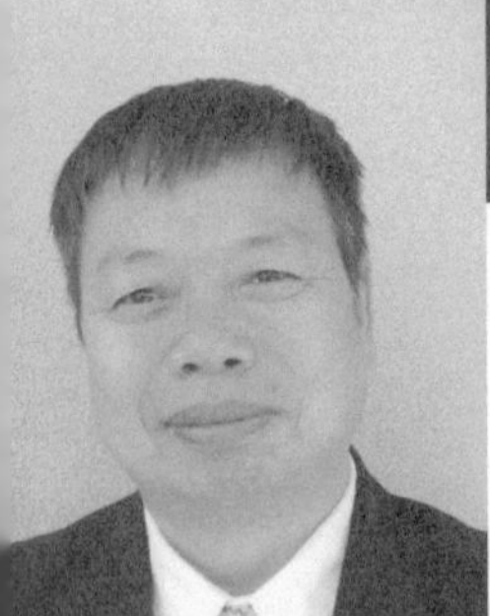
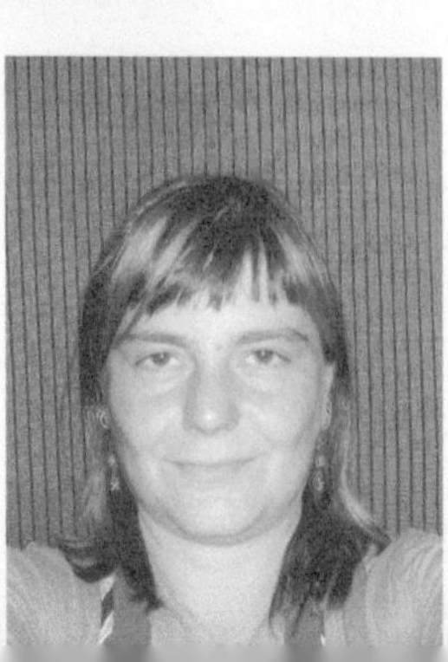

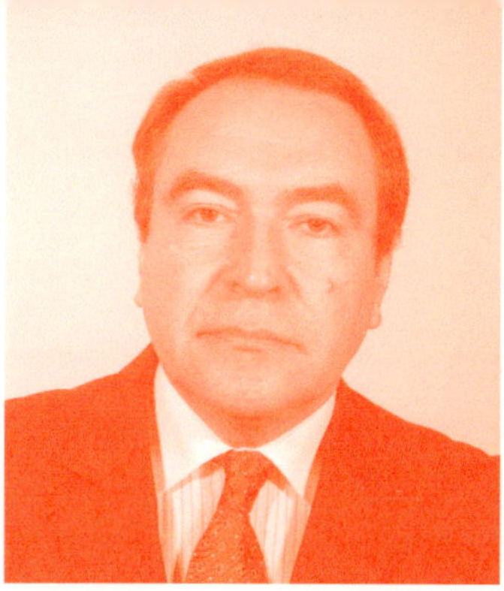
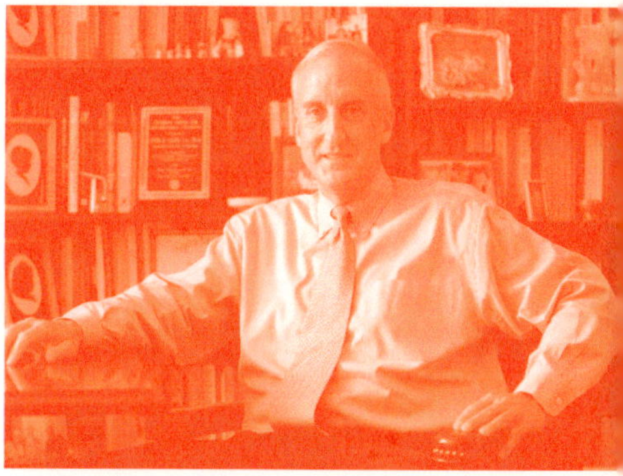
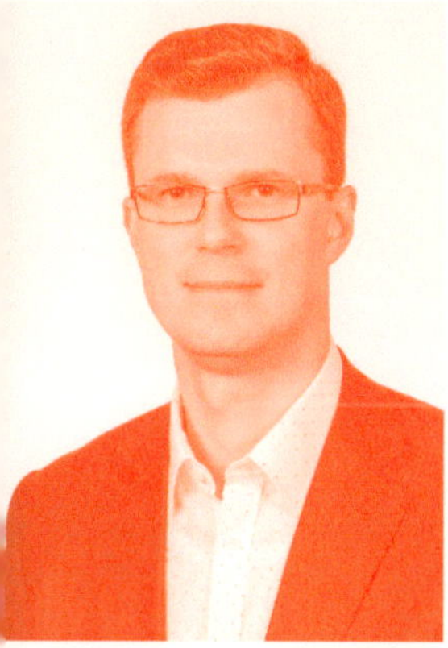
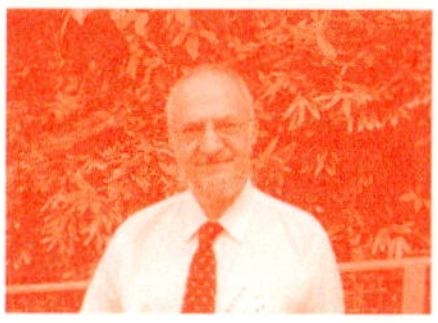
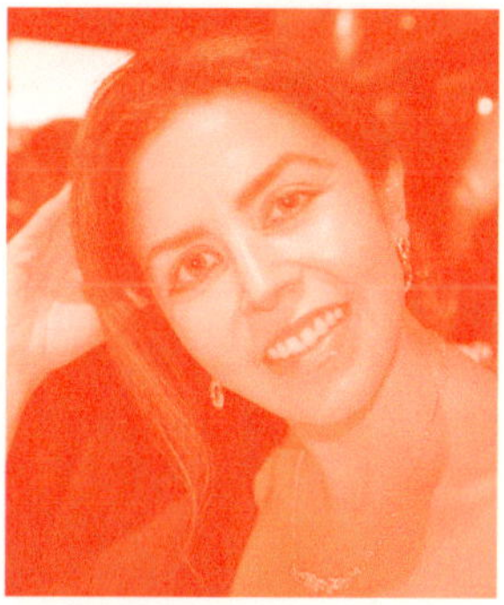

Supporting open minds since 2005

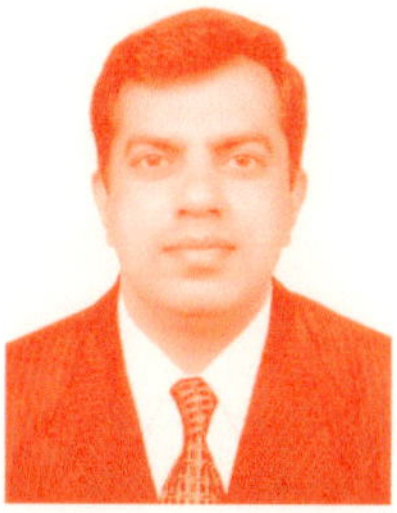
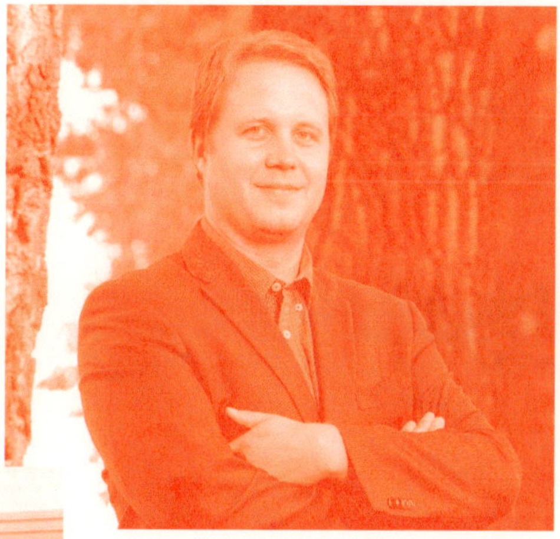
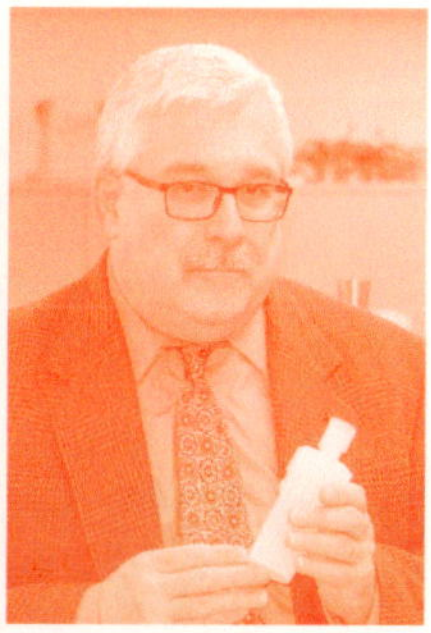
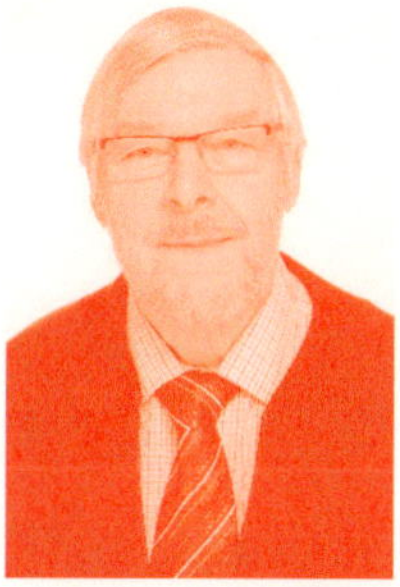
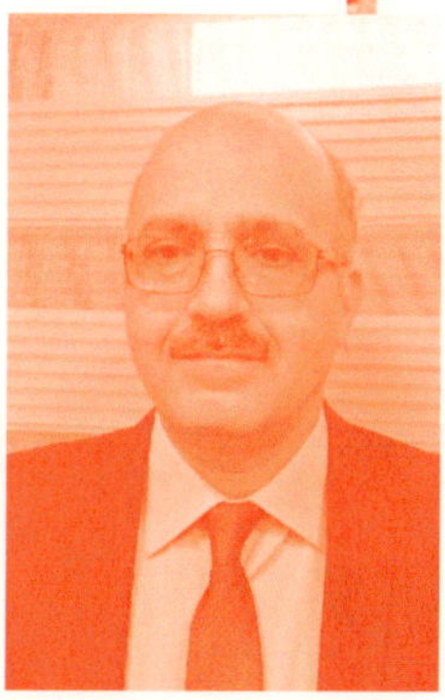
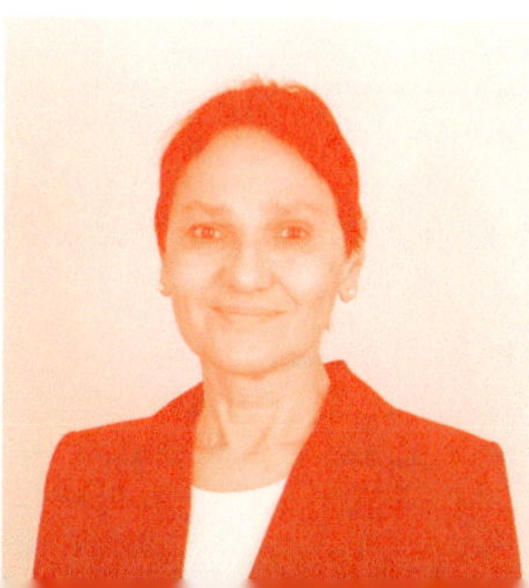
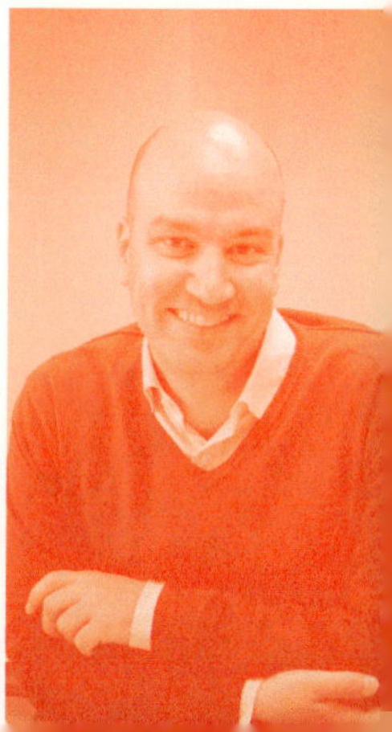

Inflammation in the 21st Century
http://dx.doi.org/10.5772/intechopen.91647
Edited by Vijay Kumar, Alexandro Aguilera Salgado and Seyyed Shamsadin Athari

Contributors
Marcos H. Toyama, Renato Yassutaka Faria Yaedú, Ana Carolina Bonetti Valente, Marina De Almeida Barbosa Mello, Juliana Specian Zabotini Da Silveira, Sandro Michelini, Cardone Marco, Alessandro Fiorentino, Failla Alessandro, Giovanni Moneta, Alexandro Aguilera Salgado, Brigida Iorio, Gianpaolo Tartaro, Roberto De Luca, Giuseppe Colella, Sheniz Yuzeir, Liana Todorova Gercheva, Erkan Yıldız, Camila Lima, Etienne Macedo, Maria De Fatima Vattimo, Begum Rokeya, Mohammad Asrafuzzaman, Maliha Tabassum Rashid, Shaeri Nawar, Alpana Mukhuty, Vivekanandhan Aravindhan, Sibi Joy Manohar, Katarína Bauerova, Silvester Poništ, Katarina Pruzinska, Behzad Dalvand, Panagiotis Tsikouras, Nikolaos Nikolettos, Anastasia Bothou, Anna Chalkidou, Xanthoula Anthoulaki, Stefanos Zervoudis, Aggeliki Gerede, Ifigenia Apostolou, Fotini Gaitatzi, Spyridon Michalopoulos, Georgios Dragoutsos, Ioannis Tsirkas, Theopi Nalbanti, Natalia Sachnova, Alexios Alexiou, Christina Tsiggalou, Eirini Bampageorgaka, Konstantinos Nikolettos, Christos Tsalikidis, Panagiotis Petsidis, Nour Amin Elsahoryi, Vijay Kumar, Caroline R.C. Costa, Mariana N. Belchor, Danielle P. Novaes, Marcos A. de Oliveira, Rolando Ie, Henrique Hessel Gaeta, Daniela de O. Toyama

First published in London, United Kingdom, 2022 by IntechOpen
IntechOpen is the global imprint of INTECHOPEN LIMITED, registered in England and Wales, registration number: 11086078, 5 Princes Gate Court, London, SW7 2QJ, United Kingdom
Printed in Croatia

British Library Cataloguing-in-Publication Data
A catalogue record for this book is available from the British Library

Additional hard and PDF copies can be obtained from orders@intechopen.com

Inflammation in the 21st Century
Edited by Vijay Kumar, Alexandro Aguilera Salgado and Seyyed Shamsadin Athari
p. cm.
Print ISBN 978-1-83968-641-2
Online ISBN 978-1-83968-642-9
eBook (PDF) ISBN 978-1-83968-643-6

For EU product safety concerns:
IN TECH d.o.o., Prolaz Marije Krucifikse Kozulić 3, 51000 Rijeka, Croatia, info@intechopen.com or visit our website at intechopen.com.

Meet the editors

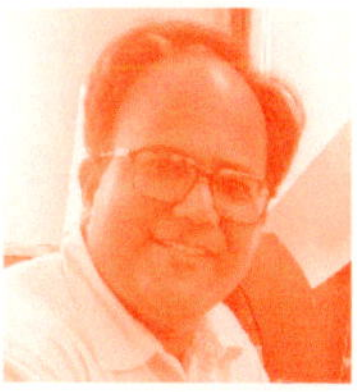

Dr. Vijay Kumar Ph.D. has more than 16 years of research experience in the field of bacterial infections, including sepsis and pneumonia, innate immunity, immunopharmacology, immunomodulation, and inflammation. He obtained his Ph.D. in June 2009 from the Department of Microbiology, Panjab University, Chandigarh, India. Dr. Kumar is the recipient of the prestigious Piero Periti review article award for 2008, awarded by the Journal of Chemotherapy in the field of immunomodulation and antimicrobials for the article titled Innate Immunity in Sepsis Pathogenesis and Its Modulation: New Immunomodulatory Targets Revealed. He was the recipient of junior research and senior research fellowship (2004–2009) offered by the Indian Council of Medical Research (ICMR), New Delhi, India. He has been awarded 17 international travel awards to attend various international conferences in the field of infection and immunity. So far, he has published 70 publications in peer-reviewed international journals in this field. To date, he has achieved more than 2 100 citations and h-index 21 (Google scholar). He has contributed several articles on inflammation and immunity as invited contribution as well as in special issues of the journals, including the Journal of Leukocyte Biology, EXCLI Journal, and Frontiers in Immunology. He is serving as an associate editor for Frontiers in Immunology (Inflammation section), executive guest editor for the journal called Coronaviruses, and editorial board member of Frontiers in Biosciences along with other journals. He is also serving as an invited reviewer for several immunology journals, such as Scientific Reports, British Journal of Pharmacology, Pharmacological Reports, Frontiers in Immunology, Frontiers in Medicine, Journal of Inflammation Research, Cellular and Molecular Immunology, Immunology, Innate Immunity, etc.

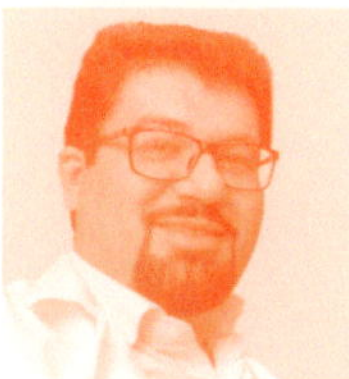

Dr. Seyyed Shamsadin Athari is an assistant professor of immunology at the Department of Immunology, School of Medicine, Zanjan University of Medical Sciences, Zanjan, Iran. He has an allergy and asthma toxicology postdoctoral degree and asthma management and controlling network fellowship. He has published more than 90 manuscripts in international journals on immunology, allergy, and asthma and more than 28 books. He is also on the editorial board of more than 65 international journals in medical sciences and has more than 12 inventions in medical sciences and has recorded 12 gene sequences in the gene bank. Dr. Athari has been invited as a top speaker for more than 40 international congresses and symposiums and has received several scientific awards from different scientific societies as a young top researcher and young scientist.

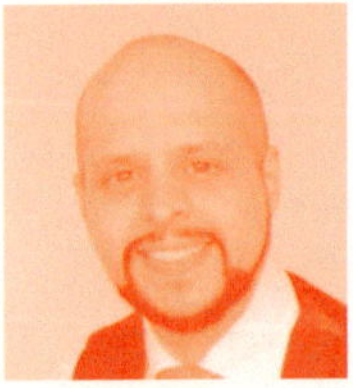

Dr. Alexandro Aguilera Salgado is a 36-year-old certified plastic and reconstructive surgeon from Mexico City. He started his plastic surgery residency in 2011 at Hospital General Dr. Manuel Gea González, followed by two full-time fellowship programs: one in hand surgery, mentored by Dr. Carlos Gargollo at Hospital Angeles Pedregal, and the other one in facial palsy and peripheral nerve, mentored by Dr. Alexander Cardenas at Hospital General Dr. Manuel Gea González. After completing his fellowships, he started working as an attending physician at the National Institute of Pediatrics, which is a national reference center in Mexico for patients with complex congenital, traumatic and acquired upper extremity diseases, where he is the chief of the Hand and Peripheral Nerve Department. He is also part of the Continuing Medical Education Program of the Mexican Association of Plastic Surgery.

Contents

Preface

As mentioned in the ancient textbooks of Ayurvedic medicine, inflammation was known to Ayurvedic physicians of the Indian Peninsula already back in 1 500 BCE and in 600 CE as a manifestation of a disease. They characterized inflammation as an elevation, swelling or edema, heaviness, and pain. After this, in 5 CE, a Greek physician introduced the term edema for inflammation. Later on, Aulus Cornelius Celsus (30 BCE–38 CE) described inflammation with four cardinal signs, that is, redness (*rubor*), elevated heat (*calor*), swelling (*tumor*), and pain (*dolor*), as occurring during acute inflammation in response to the localized acute infection or trauma. These four signs are known as Celsus tetrad of inflammation. Galen and later on Virchow (1871), with a more precise definition, introduced the fifth sign of inflammation called loss of function (*functio lasea*) of the affected organ or tissue. The modern term inflammation is derived from the Greek word *inflammare,* meaning to set on fire.

The present book aims to discuss in detail the pathogenesis of inflammation, in a sterile context and infection-induced inflammation along with advances in its management. The 1st chapter "*Introductory Chapter: The Journey of Inflammation and Inflammatory Disease Research - Past, Present, and Future*" discusses the history, present studies and future directions of research focused on inflammation and inflammatory diseases. The 2nd chapter titled "*Prolouge: Initial Approach to Edema*" introduces the topic of edema. The 3rd chapter titled "*Peripheral Edema: Differential Diagnosis*" describes the pathogenesis of peripheral edema, including the lower limb edema in different conditions, differential diagnosis, and management. The 4th chapter "*Edema Induced by sPLA2 from* Crotalus durissus terrificus *Involves PLC and PKC Signaling, Activation of cPLA2, and Oxidative Stress*" discusses the pathogenesis of edema induced by *Crotalus durissus terrificus* involving phospholipase C (PLC) and protein kinase C (PKC) as signaling molecules. The 5th chapter "*Edema Management in Oral and Maxillofacial Surgery*" discusses the management of edema observed during oral and maxillofacial surgery. This chapter is crucial as edema is seen in patients who underwent surgery. The 6th chapter "*Neutrophil Counts and Rates in Otorhinolaryngology*" discusses the importance of neutrophils (potent innate immune cells playing a crucial role in the inflammatory process) in otorhinolaryngology. The 7th chapter "*Neutrophil Gelatinase-Associated Lipocalin as a Promising Biomarker in Acute Kidney Injury*" discusses the use of neutrophil gelatinase-associated lipocalin (NGAL) as a potential marker for acute kidney injury (AKI). The 8th chapter "*The Role of Neutrophil Extracellular Traps (NETs) in the Pathogenesis and Complications of Malignant Diseases*" discusses the importance of neutrophil extracellular traps (NETs) in the pathogenesis and complications of malignant diseases. NETs are large, extracellular web-like structures comprised of cytosolic and granule proteins assembled on the scaffold of decondensed chromatin, having both nuclear and mitochondrial DNA, which trap circulating pathogens during microbial infections. The 9th chapter "*The Role of Introns for the Development of Inflammation-Mediated Cancer Cell*" is of importance and discusses the role of introns in the transformation of normal cell into cancer cell during inflammation. This chapter is intended to discuss the genetic changes involved in the transformation of normal cell into cancer cell during chronic inflammation, as chronic inflammation is one of the causal factors for cancer development. The 10th chapter "*Celiac Disease*" discusses celiac disease (a chronic inflammatory disease of the gut) which incidence is increasing due to modern lifestyle. The 11th chapter "*Sialoendoscopy in Juvenile Recurrent Parotitis That Could Be Primary Pediatric Sjogren's Syndrome*" discusses the use of sialoendoscopy in juvenile recurrent parotitis that may be a primary pediatric Sjögren's syndrome (an autoimmune disease). The 12th chapter "*Inflammation in the Pathogenesis of Rheumatoid Arthritis and in Experimental Arthritis: Evaluation of Combinations of Carnosic Acid and Extract of* Rhodiola rosea *L. with Methotrexate*" discusses the use of carnosic acid and extract of *Rhodiola rosea* L. with methotrexate in rheumatoid arthritis (RA), an autoimmune disease primarily affecting small joints, and the involvement of inflammation as the major disease mechanism. The 13th chapter "*Antiphospholipid Syndrome and Pregnancy-Diagnosis, Complications and Management: An Overview*" discusses the impact of antiphospholipid syndrome (another autoimmune disease) in the pregnancy outcome. The 14th chapter "*Non-Allergic Rhinitis*" discusses nonallergic rhinitis that occurs independently of allergen exposure and the diagnosis and treatment options. The 15th chapter "*Islet Inflammation: The Link between Type 2 Diabetes and Pancreatic Cancer*" discusses the islet inflammation (inflammation of pancreatic cells involved in the insulin secretion) that plays a crucial role in the pathogenesis of type 2 diabetes mellitus (T2DM). This chapter links T2DM and pancreatic cancer as results of chronic pancreatic inflammation. The 16th chapter "*Hypomelanosis Secondary to Cutaneous Inflammation*" discusses hypomelanosis and the disease links to the different cutaneous inflammatory conditions. The 17th chapter "*Helminth Induced Immunomodulation against Metainflammation and Insulin Resistance*" discusses the suppression of chronic inflammation associated with meta-inflammation and T2DM via helminthic infections through inducing immunomodulation. Hence, the current book will prove beneficial to audience interested in the wide aspect of inflammation and inflammatory diseases.

Vijay Kumar
Department of Pharmaceutical Sciences,
College of Pharmacy,
University of Tennessee Health Science Center (UTHSC),
Memphis, TN, USA

Alexandro Aguilera Salgado
National Institute of Pediatrics,
Mexico

Seyyed Shamsadin Athari
Zanjan University of Medical Sciences,
Iran

Section 1

Introduction

Chapter 1

Introductory Chapter: The Journey of Inflammation and Inflammatory Disease Research - Past, Present, and Future

Vijay Kumar

1. Introduction

Inflammation is known to ancient Indian Ayurvedic physicians dating back to 1500 BC that is well described in ancient Ayurvedic medicine textbooks (*Charaka Samhita*, *Susruta Samhita,* and *Astanga Samgraha)* [1]. Inflammation and the associated edema have gotten attention in Ayurveda as a pathological manifestation of the disease [2, 3]. Ayurvedic medicine mentioned inflammation in different ways, which include *Shotha and Shopha, and* many other terms *(Svayathu, Utsedha,* and *Samhata)* [2]. Ancient Ayurvedic medicine practitioners characterized inflammation in different ways, including elevation, edema, heaviness, and pain. The Greek physician, Hippocrates in the 5th century BC coined the term edema. Furthermore, Later on, Aulus Celsus (30 BC-38 AD) described the four major signs of inflammation, which include *Rubor*, *Calor*, *Tumor*, and *Dolor* [4]. Galen, the Roman physician introduced the fifth sign of inflammation as *loss of function*. However, *Virchow* in 1871 more precisely described the *function laesa* (loss of function) sign of inflammation [5, 6].

The modern terminology of inflammation has been derived from the Latin word *inflammare* (to set on fire) [6]. Now inflammation is considered as a host-generated protective host immune response in response to acute trauma or pathogens or their PAMPs (pathogen-derived molecular patterns) to contain the damage or to remove/kill the pathogen [7]. The inflammation pathogenesis is a complex process involving the network of cellular and molecular signaling to restore homeostasis and induce tissue/organ repair and regeneration. However, any dysregulation of the inflammatory process may lead to the development of severe inflammatory conditions, including systemic inflammation and sepsis (during infection). Furthermore, any persistent inflammation (staying for months and years) may cause chronic inflammatory disorders (cancer and autoimmune diseases) [8–10]. The cellular components of the immune system (macrophages, neutrophils, mast cells, dendritic cells (DCs), T cells, and B cells etc.) play a central role in the process of both acute and chronic inflammation involve (**Figure 1**) [11–14].

IntechOpen

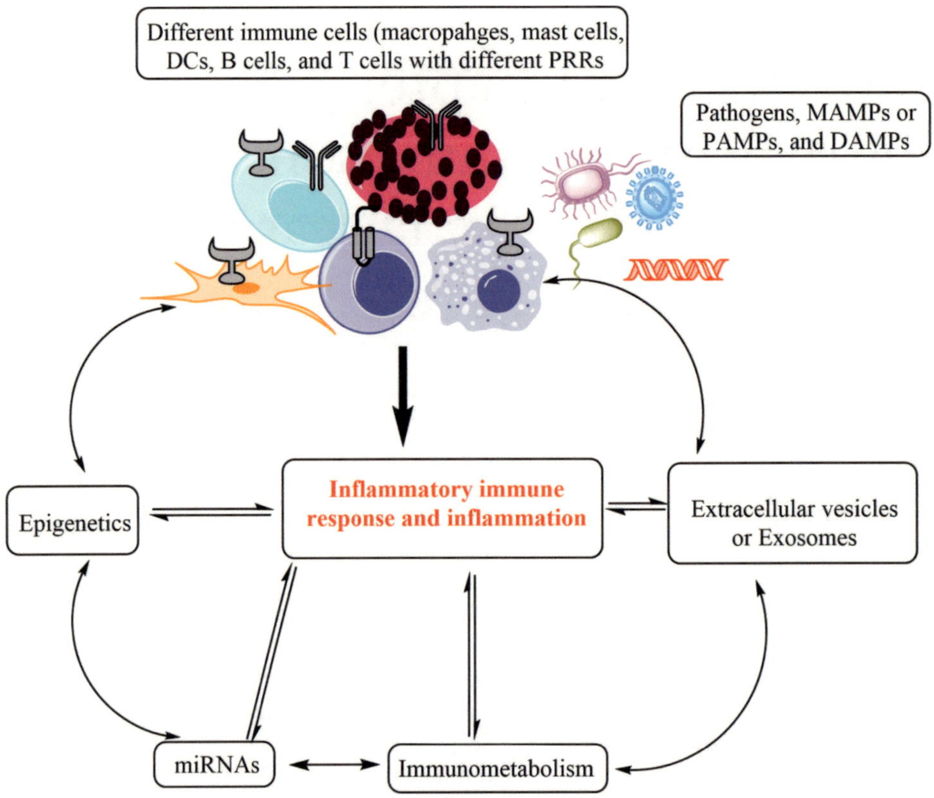

Figure 1.
Schematic representation of immune cell activation in response to different pathogens, PAMPs, MAMPs through interacting with different PRRs (mentioned in the text) to generate inflammatory immune response. This immune response is governed by immunometabolic reprograming, epigenetics, miRNAs, and the release of extracellular vesicles or exosomes, which directly or indirectly interact and affect each other.

2. Pattern recognition receptors (PRRs) in inflammation and inflammatory diseases

The receptors expressed by these immune cells called **pattern recognition receptors** (PRRs) (**Figure 1**) are present on the outer surface of the cell membrane as well as in the cytosol, including different toll-like receptors (TLR1-TLR13 in mammals, including humans), intracellular PRRs (NOD [Nucleotide-binding and oligomerization domain])-like receptors (NLRs; NOD1 and NOD2), absent in melanoma-like receptors (ALRs, AIM2), and many more mentioned somewhere else recognize the potential pathogen and/or inflammogen to mount a protective inflammatory immune response [1, 15–17]. The intracellular proteins (NLRC1 or NLPR1, NLRP3, NLRC4, pyrin, and AIM2 or absent in melanoma 2 that recognizes cytosolic DNA) form an inflammatory complex called inflammasome upon recognition of intracellular threat (damage-associated molecular patterns or DAMPs). The inflammasome also becomes activated upon the recognition of external danger called pathogen or microbe-associated molecular patterns (PAMPs or MAMPs) and DAMPs by cell surface PRRs, which signal these inflammasome proteins to activate and stimulate another cascade of inflammation resulting in the release of pro-inflammatory cytokines (IL-1β, IL-18, and IL-33) and the cell death called pyroptosis that further aggravates the inflammatory process [18]. The details of inflammasomes in inflammation and inflammatory disease are mentioned somewhere else [18, 19]. The activation of cell surface PRRs, including TLRs (TLR2 and TLR4), may activate the inflammasome or TLRs and inflammasomes work in cooperation to control the inflammatory process [20, 21]. Another, cytosolic PRR system called cGAS (cyclic GMP-AMP synthase, recognizes cytosolic dsDNA)-stimulator of interferon genes (STING) pathway recognizes cytosolic dsDNA and induces the synthesis of type 1 interferons (IFNs) [22, 23]. The over-activation of this pathway is involved in different autoimmune and auto-inflammatory diseases, along with other inflammatory conditions discussed in detail somewhere else [22–24]. The details of inflammatory pathways mediated by TLRs, inflammasomes, cGAS, and other PRRs have been discussed by the author somewhere else in detail [1, 18, 21, 22, 24–27].

3. Immunometabolism in inflammation and inflammatory diseases

Like, other non-immune cells, immune cells also have their energy demand that plays a crucial role in the maintenance of immune homeostasis and the mounting of the immune response to protect against invading foreign agents, including the pathogen and allergen. The metabolic changes occurring in immune cells from their normal/control stage (absence of inflammogen, pathogen, PAMPs, MAMPs, or DAMPs) to their activation or activated stage is called immunometabolic reprogramming [28]. Hence, the metabolic pathways governing or regulating the energy demand of immune cells to maintain immune homeostasis is called **immunometabolism** [28]. The metabolic demand of immune cells increases during the inflammatory process and reprogramming of different metabolic pathways governing the immune function takes place that depends on the immune cell type and the inflammatory conditions (**Figure 1**) [29]. The author has described immunometabolism of different immune cells and their immunometabolic reprogramming and its therapeutic targeting during inflammation and inflammatory diseases elsewhere [1, 30–35].

4. Epigenetics in inflammation and inflammatory diseases

Epigenetics (deals with the reversible impact of behavior and environmental factors on our genetic machinery without changing the DNA sequence. However, it may change the way of reading the genetic information coded by the DNA) also plays a crucial role in the inflammatory process and inflammatory diseases. The most frequent epigenetic changes involve aberrant DNA methylation and histone acetylation and deacetylation. The enzymes (arginine and lysine methyltransferases, DNA methyltransferase, histone acetyltransferases (HAT), and histone deacetylases or HDAC) involved in the process of epigenetics also control the inflammatory process, including airway inflammation, atopic dermatitis, and autoimmune diseases [36–41]. The histone modifications, DNA methylation, and noncoding RNAs (ncRNAs) have emerged as master regulators of gene expression, including the inflammatory genes [42]. The targeting of these enzymes, including HAT and HDAC, has shown great anti-inflammatory potential in diverse inflammatory diseases. However, advances in the biological sciences have shown the interaction between epigenetics and immunometabolism converges at inflammation and regulates different inflammatory diseases, including cancer (**Figure 1**) [42–45]. Hence, epigenetics-based immunotherapies are emerging for targeting chronic inflammatory diseases, including cancer and autoimmunity [46].

5. Extracellular vesicles in inflammation and inflammatory diseases

Extracellular vesicles (EVs) are generated by different cell types, including the immune cells to remove cellular waste and communicate with adjacent as well as distant cells [47]. These EVs may contain protein, DNA, RNA, micro RNA (miRNA or miRs), and cytokines depending on the cell type and cell/tissue microenvironment. The microvesicles (MVs), a kind of EVs released from apoptotic cells are less-inflammatory than those released from viable cells [48]. These MVs have different miRs (miR-155, miR-34b, and miR-34a), which get dysregulated in autoimmune diseases, including systemic lupus erythematosus (SLE) in comparison to normal individuals. EVs play a crucial role in cell–cell communication in pulmonary inflammation upon exposure to toxicants [49]. EVs also affect immunometabolism during diverse inflammatory conditions, including autoimmunity (**Figure 1**) [50, 51]. The different types of EVs, their contents (miRs), and their role in inflammation and therapeutic potential, including in sepsis and coronavirus disease-2019 (COVID-19) have been discussed somewhere else [47, 52–56].

6. MicroRNAs (miRNA) in inflammation and inflammatory diseases

MicroRNAs (miRNAs) are small non-coding RNAs (typical length, 18–24 nucleotide long), which are crucial in regulating protein-coding genes via post-transcriptional repression [57]. They play an important role in regulating innate and adaptive immunity from their developmental stages to function during diverse inflammation conditions, including cancer and autoimmunity as fine-tuners of the system [57–60]. For example, miR-181a and miR-223 are crucial in the establishment and maintenance of immune cell fate [58]. The miR-146 also regulates innate immunity through controlling TLR signaling and ensuing cytokine response. They (miR-155 and miR-181a) regulate central elements of the adaptive immune response such as antigen presentation and T cell receptor (TCR) signaling [58]. Chronic inflammatory diseases exhibit altered miR (miR-203 and miR-146) levels, indicating their crucial role in immunological pathologies/diseases. The details of miRs in immunity and inflammation are discussed somewhere else [59, 61]. The emerging evidences have shown the regulation of immune cell metabolism or immunometabolism by miRs [62, 63]. The non-coding RNAs (ncRNAs) also regulate inflammasome activity controlling the inflammatory immune response [64]. More recently an atlas of miR expression in 63 different mouse immune cell populations has been generated and connected with an assay for transposase-accessible chromatin using sequencing (ATAC–seq), chromatin immunoprecipitation followed by sequencing (ChIP–seq), and nascent RNA profiles to establish a map of miRNA promoter and enhancer usage in immune cells [65]. This will help to delineate the *cis*-regulatory elements controlling miRNA signatures of the immune system.

7. Conclusion

The story of inflammation had started from the Ancient Indian peninsula through the Ayurvedic medicine that further developed into its four peculiar signs (*rubor, tumor, calor, and dolor*) and fifth end-stage sign indicating the loss of function. The development in biomedical sciences, including immunology, cell signaling, pharmacology, epigenetics, and molecular biology or medicine has helped to understand the pathogenesis of inflammation (both, acute, and chronic) and associated inflammatory disease, varying from autoimmunity to cancer to severe infectious diseases, including the current COVID-19 pandemic. Thus, the long journey of inflammation that started dating back to 1500 BC and 600 AD has seen significant development in understanding its pathogenesis under diverse conditions and therapeutic advancement. Further studies in the 21st century will open new avenues to control and prevent inflammatory diseases responsible for human morbidity and mortality.

Author details

Vijay Kumar
Department of Pharmaceutical Sciences, College of Pharmacy, University of Tennessee Health Science Center (UTHSC), Memphis, TN, USA

*Address all correspondence to: vij_tox@yahoo.com; vkumar7@uthsc.edu

References

[1] Kumar V. Inflammation research sails through the sea of immunology to reach immunometabolism. International Immunopharmacology. 2019;**73**:128-145

[2] Ballakur V. Inflammation in ayurveda and modern medicine. International Ayurvedic Medical Journal. 2013;**1**(4):1-7

[3] Rao KVS. Immunology in India: An emerging story. Nature Immunology. 2008;**9**:1319

[4] Rocha e Silva, M. A brief survey of the history of inflammation. 1978. Agents and Actions. 1994;**43**:86-90

[5] Ley K. History of Inflammation Research. In: Ley K, editor. Physiology of Inflammation. New York, New York, NY: Springer; 2001. pp. 1-10

[6] Scott A, Khan KM, Cook JL, Duronio V. What is "inflammation"? Are we ready to move beyond Celsus? British Journal of Sports Medicine. 2004;**38**: 248-249

[7] Fullerton JN, Gilroy DW. Resolution of inflammation: a new therapeutic frontier. Nature Reviews Drug Discovery. 2016;**15**:551

[8] Shalapour S, Karin M. Immunity, inflammation, and cancer: an eternal fight between good and evil. The Journal of Clinical Investigation. 2015;**125**: 3347-3355

[9] Chen Z, Bozec A, Ramming A, Schett G. Anti-inflammatory and immune-regulatory cytokines in rheumatoid arthritis. Nature Reviews Rheumatology. 2019;**15**:9-17

[10] Shen HH, Yang YX, Meng X, Luo XY, Li XM, Shuai ZW, et al. NLRP3: A promising therapeutic target for autoimmune diseases. Autoimmunity Reviews. 2018;**17**:694-702

[11] Kumar V, Ahmad A. Role of MAIT cells in the immunopathogenesis of inflammatory diseases: New players in old game. International Reviews of Immunology. 2017:1-21

[12] Kumar V. Innate lymphoid cells: new paradigm in immunology of inflammation. Immunology Letters. 2014;**157**:23-37

[13] Kumar V, Sharma A. Neutrophils: Cinderella of innate immune system. International Immunopharmacology. 2010;**10**:1325-1334

[14] Kumar V, Sharma A. Mast cells: emerging sentinel innate immune cells with diverse role in immunity. Molecular Immunology. 2010;**48**:14-25

[15] Weiss E, Kretschmer D. Formyl-peptide receptors in infection, inflammation, and cancer. Trends in Immunology. 2018;**39**:815-829

[16] Kawai T, Akira S. The roles of TLRs, RLRs and NLRs in pathogen recognitionInt Immunol. 21:313. International Immunology. 2009;**21**: 317-337

[17] Kanneganti T-D, Lamkanfi M, Núñez G. Intracellular NOD-like receptors in host defense and disease. Immunity. 2007;**27**:549-559

[18] Kumar V. Inflammasomes: Pandora's box for sepsis. Journal of Inflammation Research. 2018;**11**:477-502

[19] Guo H, Callaway JB, Ting JPY. Inflammasomes: mechanism of action, role in disease, and therapeutics. Nature Medicine. 2015;**21**:677-687

[20] Hanamsagar R, Hanke ML, Kielian T. Toll-like receptor (TLR) and inflammasome actions in the central nervous system. Trends in Immunology. 2012;**33**:333-342

[21] Kumar V. The complement system, toll-like receptors and inflammasomes in host defense: Three musketeers' one target. International Reviews of Immunology. 2019;**38**:131-156

[22] Kumar V. A STING to inflammation and autoimmunity. Journal of Leukocyte Biology. 2019;**106**:171-185

[23] Decout A, Katz JD, Venkatraman S, Ablasser A. The cGAS–STING pathway as a therapeutic target in inflammatory diseases. Nature Reviews Immunology. 2021;**21**:548-569

[24] Kumar V. The Trinity of cGAS, TLR9, and ALRs Guardians of the Cellular Galaxy Against Host-Derived Self-DNA. Frontiers in Immunology. 2020;**11**:624597

[25] Kumar V. Toll-like receptors in immunity and inflammatory diseases: Past, present, and future. International Immunopharmacology. 2018;**59**:391-412

[26] Kumar V. Toll-like receptors in the pathogenesis of neuroinflammation. Journal of Neuroimmunology. 2019;**332**:16-30

[27] Kumar V. Toll-like receptors in sepsis-associated cytokine storm and their endogenous negative regulators as future immunomodulatory targets. International Immunopharmacology. 2020;**89**:107087

[28] O'Neill LAJ, Kishton RJ, Rathmell J. A guide to immunometabolism for immunologists. Nature Reviews Immunology. 2016;**16**:553-565

[29] Voss K, Hong HS, Bader JE, Sugiura A, Lyssiotis CA, Rathmell JC. A guide to interrogating immunometabolism. Nature Reviews Immunology. 2021;**21**:637-652

[30] Kumar V. T cells and their immunometabolism: A novel way to understanding sepsis immunopathogenesis and future therapeutics. European Journal of Cell Biology. 2018;**97**:379-392

[31] Kumar V. Targeting macrophage immunometabolism: Dawn in the darkness of sepsis. International Immunopharmacology. 2018;**58**:173-185

[32] Kumar V. How could we forget immunometabolism in SARS-CoV2 infection or COVID-19? International Reviews of Immunology. 2021;**40**:72-107

[33] Kumar V. Immunometabolism: Another Road to Sepsis and Its Therapeutic Targeting. Inflammation. 2019;**42**:765-788

[34] Kumar V. Dendritic cells in sepsis: Potential immunoregulatory cells with therapeutic potential. Molecular Immunology. 2018;**101**:615-626

[35] Kumar V. Natural killer cells in sepsis: Underprivileged innate immune cells. European Journal of Cell Biology. 2019;**98**:81-93

[36] Shanmugam MK, Sethi G. Role of epigenetics in inflammation-associated diseases. Sub-Cellular Biochemistry. 2013;**61**:627-657

[37] Adcock IM, Tsaprouni L, Bhavsar P, Ito K. Epigenetic regulation of airway inflammation. Current Opinion in Immunology. 2007;**19**:694-700

[38] Schmidt AD, de Guzman Strong C. Current understanding of epigenetics in atopic dermatitis. Experimental Dermatology. 2021;**30**:1150-1155

[39] Nielsen HM, Tost J. Epigenetic changes in inflammatory and autoimmune diseases. Sub-Cellular Biochemistry. 2013;**61**:455-478

[40] Stylianou E. Epigenetics of chronic inflammatory diseases. Journal of Inflammation Research. 2018;**12**:1-14

[41] Surace AEA, Hedrich CM. The Role of Epigenetics in Autoimmune/ Inflammatory Disease. Frontiers in Immunology. 2019;**10**:1-16

[42] Karin M, Shalapour S. Regulation of antitumor immunity by inflammation-induced epigenetic alterations. Cellular & Molecular Immunology. 2021:1-8

[43] Guzik TJ, Cosentino F. Epigenetics and Immunometabolism in Diabetes and Aging. Antioxidants & Redox Signaling. 2018;**29**:257-274

[44] Raghuraman S, Donkin I, Versteyhe S, Barrès R, Simar D. The emerging role of epigenetics in inflammation and immunometabolism. Trends in Endocrinology and Metabolism. 2016;**27**:782-795

[45] Verberk SGS, de Goede KE, Van den Bossche J. Metabolic–epigenetic crosstalk in macrophage activation: an updated view. Epigenomics. 2019;**11**: 719-721

[46] Dunn J, Rao S. Epigenetics and immunotherapy: The current state of play. Molecular Immunology. 2017;**87**: 227-239

[47] Kumar V, Kiran S, Kumar S, Singh UP. Extracellular vesicles in obesity and its associated inflammation. International Reviews of Immunology. 2021:1-15

[48] Claßen L, Tykocinski LO, Wiedmann F, Birr C, Schiller P, Tucher C, et al. Extracellular vesicles mediate intercellular communication: Transfer of functionally active microRNAs by microvesicles into phagocytes. European Journal of Immunology. 2017;**47**:1535-1549

[49] Andres J, Smith LC, Murray A, Jin Y, Businaro R, Laskin JD, et al. Role of extracellular vesicles in cell-cell communication and inflammation following exposure to pulmonary toxicants. Cytokine & Growth Factor Reviews. 2020;**51**:12-18

[50] de Candia P, De Rosa V, Gigantino V, Botti G, Ceriello A, Matarese G. Immunometabolism of human autoimmune diseases: from metabolites to extracellular vesicles. FEBS Letters. 2017;**591**:3119-3134

[51] Zhou Z, Tao Y, Zhao H, Wang Q. Adipose extracellular vesicles: Messengers from and to macrophages in regulating immunometabolic homeostasis or disorders. Frontiers in Immunology. 2021;**12**:666344-666344

[52] Buzas EI, György B, Nagy G, Falus A, Gay S. Emerging role of extracellular vesicles in inflammatory diseases. Nature Reviews Rheumatology. 2014;**10**:356-364

[53] Li Y, Tan J, Miao Y, Zhang Q. MicroRNA in extracellular vesicles regulates inflammation through macrophages under hypoxia. Cell Death Discovery. 2021;**7**:285

[54] Burgelman M, Vandendriessche C, Vandenbroucke RE. Extracellular vesicles: A double-edged sword in sepsis. Pharmaceuticals (Basel). 2021;**14**(8):1-40

[55] Kronstadt SM, Pottash AE, Levy D, Wang S, Chao W, Jay SM. Therapeutic potential of extracellular vesicles for sepsis treatment. Advanced Therapeutics (Weinh). 2021;**4**(7):1-29

[56] Xia X, Yuan P, Liu Y, Wang Y, Cao W, Zheng JC. Emerging roles of extracellular vesicles in COVID-19, a double-edged sword? Immunology. 2021;**163**:416-430

[57] Sonkoly E, Pivarcsi A. microRNAs in inflammation. International Reviews of Immunology. 2009;**28**:535-561

[58] Sonkoly E, Ståhle M, Pivarcsi A. MicroRNAs and immunity: Novel players

in the regulation of normal immune function and inflammation. Seminars in Cancer Biology. 2008;**18**:131-140

[59] Tahamtan A, Teymoori-Rad M, Nakstad B, Salimi V. Anti-inflammatory microRNAs and their potential for inflammatory diseases treatment. Frontiers in Immunology. 2018;**9**:1-4

[60] Mehta A, Baltimore D. MicroRNAs as regulatory elements in immune system logic. Nature Reviews Immunology. 2016;**16**:279-294

[61] Zhou X, Li X, Wu M. miRNAs reshape immunity and inflammatory responses in bacterial infection. Signal Transduction and Targeted Therapy. 2018;**3**:14

[62] Yao Q, Song Z, Wang B, Zhang JA. Emerging roles of microRNAs in the metabolic control of immune cells. Cancer Letters. 2018;**433**:10-17

[63] Nelson MC, O'Connell RM. MicroRNAs: At the Interface of Metabolic Pathways and Inflammatory Responses by Macrophages. Frontiers in Immunology. 2020;**11**:1797

[64] Wang W, Yang N, Yang YH, Wen R, Liu CF, Zhang TN. Non-coding RNAs: Master regulators of inflammasomes in inflammatory diseases. Journal of Inflammation Research. 2021;**14**: 5023-5050

[65] Rose SA, Wroblewska A, Dhainaut M, Yoshida H, Shaffer JM, Bektesevic A, et al. A microRNA expression and regulatory element activity atlas of the mouse immune system. Nature Immunology. 2021;**22**:914-927

Section 2

Edema

Chapter 2

Prolouge: Initial Approach to Edema

Alexandro Aguilera Salgado

1. Introduction

Edema is one of the most underrated signs that can be found in many patients. The first step is to understand what edema is in order to give this sign the importance we should. It can be caused by many different situations, so once we find it, we must study our patient completely in order to reach an adequate diagnosis and start treating our patient correctly.

Edema is the swelling from fluid accumulation at the intercellular tissue originated from the abnormal expansion of the interstitial fluid volume. Fluid at the interstitial and intravascular space is regulated by the gradient between the hydrostatic and the oncotic capillary pressures, so when this balance is altered by local or systemic situations, this fluid begins to accumulate [1].

2. Patient history

The approach to edema must begin with a complete interrogation of the patient's background. The history must include the date of the first symptoms, if edema is altered by position, if it is unilateral or bilateral, history of previous chronic diseases, substance abuse, drugs used by the patient, and any other symptoms related to the appearance of edema. With these simple questions, we can get an initial idea of the diagnosis.

The acute onset of edema of less than 72 hours is more characteristic of deep venous thrombosis, cellulitis, popliteal cyst rupture, acute compartmental syndrome, or the use of calcium channel blockers. Also, stasis can play an important role in this acute setting as in venous insufficiency, venous obstruction, or lymphatic obstruction. On the other hand, the chronic onset of edema can be seen with the appearance or as a complication of chronic diseases like chronic cardiac insufficiency, pulmonary hypertension, and thyroid, renal, or hepatic disease.

3. Physical exam

We must include a complete physical exam in every patient, in order to investigate and rule out every possible cause of edema. For example, if we are thinking the cause of edema in our patient to be cardiac insufficiency, we must look for rales or crackles, dyspnea, cyanosis, or any other sign or symptom. Our efforts should always be focused on investigating each new sign we can find, so we can further investigate them until we have the correct diagnosis.

4. Diagnosis

Once we have an idea of the possible cause of edema, we can complete our investigation with some specific studies, like complete blood count, electrolytes, hepatic enzymes, albumin, creatinine, urine analysis, glucose, and thyroid stimulating hormone [2]. Other additional and specific tests should be indicated depending on the clinical presentation, for example, if we are thinking in a cardiac etiology, we should order an electrocardiogram, echocardiogram, and chest radiograph. Another common study in certain cases when we are thinking of a lymphatic origin is a lymphoscintigraphy which can be helpful to distinguish lymphedema from venous edema and determine the cause of lymphedema. We have to keep in mind every possible situation causing edema as we can see in **Figure 1** [3].

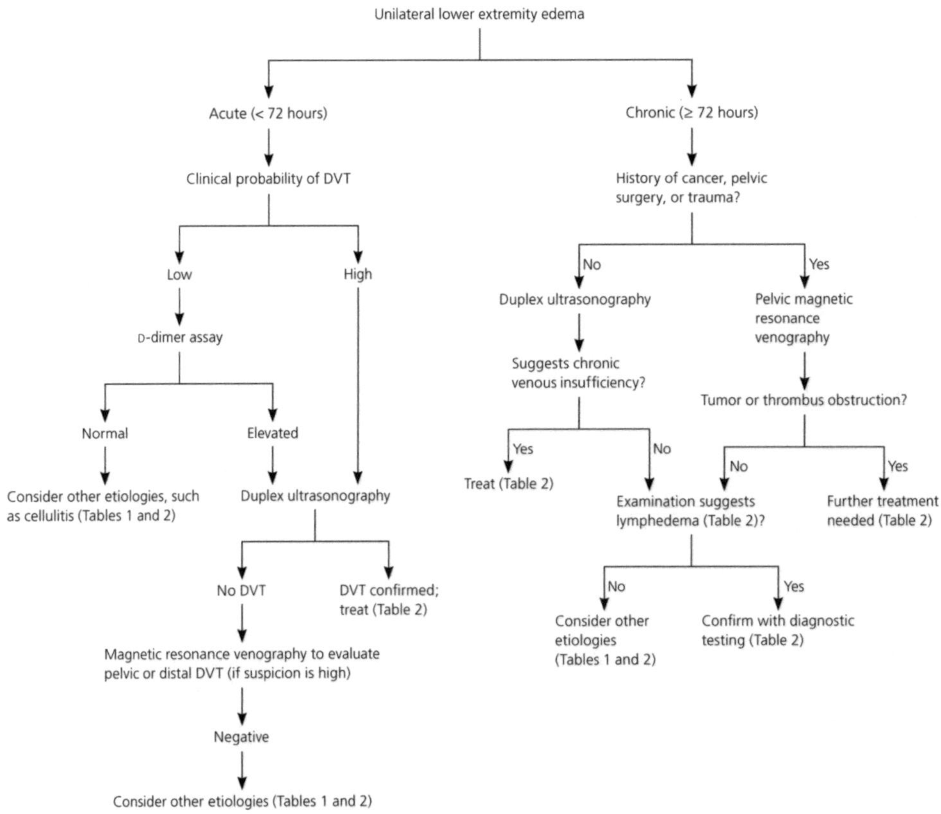

Figure 1.
Algorithm for the diagnosis of edema.

5. Treatment

The treatment plan is set once we have an accurate diagnosis [4].

6. Conclusions

As any other signs or symptoms we can think of, edema should be thoroughly investigated. In this book, we will find a comprehensive overview of the mechanisms and pathophysiology of edema formation and the signs and symptoms which can be seen in the different types of edema so we can reach an accurate diagnosis in order to establish the adequate treatment of this specific situation.

Author details

Alexandro Aguilera Salgado
Hand and Peripheral Nerve Department, National Institute of Pediatrics, Mexico City, Mexico

*Address all correspondence to: alexandruss@hotmail.com

References

[1] Cho S, Atwood JE. Peripheral edema. The American Journal of Medicine. 2002;**113**(7):580-586

[2] Yale SH, Mazza JJ. Approach to diagnosing lower extremity edema. Comprehensive Therapy. 2001;**27**(3):242-252

[3] Trayes KP, Studdiford JS, Pickle S, Tully AS. Edema: Diagnosis and management. American Family Physician. 2013 Jul 15;**88**(2):102-110

[4] O'Brien JG, Chennubhotla SA, Chennubhotla RV. Treatment of edema. American Family Physician. 2005;**71**(11):2111-2117

Chapter 3

Peripheral Edema: Differential Diagnosis

Sandro Michelini, Alessandro Failla, Giovanni Moneta, Alessandro Fiorentino and Cardone Marco

Abstract

Peripheral edemas can be generated by multiple causes, local and/or systemic. The difficulties in recognizing the exact nature of the edema and the cause that originates it often lead to erroneous considerations that determine an inappropriate therapeutic approach. In this chapter the various causes that generate peripheral edema are analyzed (systemic: cardiac diastolic dysfunction, kidney failure, liver failure, myxedema, from drugs, and idiopathic; and local: venous and/or lymphatic transport insufficiency). They are also described, according to the diagnosis made and the clinical and instrumental criteria to attain a correct and early diagnosis and to proceed to the most appropriate therapeutic measures (drugs, surgery, physical rehabilitative by means of manual and mechanical techniques) in individual cases.

Keywords: peripheral edema diagnosis, edema diagnosis, peripheral edema of limbs differential diagnosis

1. Introduction

Lower limb edema recognizes more etiological factors that are frequently confused during differential diagnosis. Sometimes there are more causes with preponderance of one over the other, either local or systemic.

The doubts in the diagnostic definition derive from an insufficient evaluation of clinical symptomatological aspects and of any instrumental and hemato-chemical tests performed in individual cases.

From a correct clinical and consequently ethiopathogenetic classification derives the most appropriate therapeutic option. Pharmacological, physical rehabilitative, or surgical therapies not inspired by edema correction principles based on its ethiopathogenesis may result in therapeutic failure or even in the worsening of local or systemic clinical status.

1.1 Description

The causes of edema of the lower limbs are various (local and/or systemic), sometimes multiple, and are to be found on the basis of a series of anamnestic and semeiological elements that, if properly considered and identified, allow better management of the clinical picture [1].

Too often, in fact, even today we are witnessing the diagnosis of lymphostatic edemas of lower limbs, ignoring that in many cases the loco-regional lymphatic system is normally developed and adequately functional.

The same monolaterality of edema, by itself alone, allows to address the diagnostic suspicions towards a local and non-systemic cause. A systemic cause of edema of lower limbs, in fact, always determines bilateral edema (albeit with relative prevalence in one of the two limbs), never being unilateral [1].

Therefore, on the one hand, it is necessary to have a clear presence of the systemic causes of edema and of the loco-regional ones and, on the other hand, the clinical and instrumental criteria which, together, allow to formulate the correct diagnosis and to prepare the most indicated therapeutic measures.

2. Causes of edema of the lower limbs

2.1 Local

- Insufficiency of the superficial lymphatic system (the deep one does not assume the importance that it has as in the venous system); it can be unilateral or bilateral [2–7].

- Insufficiency of the deep venous system (the insufficiency of the superficial one is not able to autonomously generate edema, as many subjects with varicose veins of the lower limbs do not have localized or widespread edema and, above all, clinically present the feet 'dry'). In these cases the edema is unilateral (post-thrombotic syndrome) [8, 9].

- Lipedema which is normally bilateral and frequently associated with a similar clinical aspect of the upper limbs [10–12].

- Inflammatory/infectious states of the soft tissues (joints, tendons, muscles) or bones.

- Benign or malignant neoplasms (primitive or metastatic).

2.2 Systemic

- Heart failure (from diastolic dysfunction) [13]

- Hepatic insufficiency [14]

- Acute and chronic renal failure

- Myxedema [15]

- Drugs edema

- Idiopathic edema

Among the **loco-regional** causes, the most important and frequent is represented by lymphedema (primary and secondary).

2.3 Lymphedema

Lymphedema derives from an altered (qualitative or quantitative) development of the loco-regional system. In primary forms (which may occur at birth or, more frequently, in the second, third, fourth, fifth decade of life), an altered development of the lymphatic pathways, an altered lymph-node architectural code (lymphadenodysplasia), or an insufficient number of them (often on a genetic basis in the development of lymph glandular stations) causes a slowing of the lymphatic return that can go as far as the stop of the flow at the loco-regional level. In some cases the familiarity for the affection is documented, in others (the so-called sporadic forms, because we do not know their existence in other family members), the lymphedema appears in the only subject clinically affected without affecting other members of the same family nucleus; then there is a third type of primary lymphedema in which the edema constitutes only one (and not always the "determinant") of the various clinical aspects of a syndrome (Prader-Willi, Noonan, Proteus, Hennekam, Gorham-Stout).

The secondary forms are sometimes considered primary for the predisposition in some subjects to develop secondary edema following certain clinical conditions (one example is the "post-mastectomy lymphedema", which develops in one in four woman, while the others remain with the same limb, in volume and consistency, throughout their lives, even if they are of the same age and in the same physical condition, and undergo the same surgery by the same operator); the genesis and the ethiopathogenetic evolution, in these cases, are the same as in the primary forms; in these cases, as a result of inflammatory processes, traumas, or, more frequently, surgical lymphadenectomy for neoplasms or radiotherapy, the anatomical continuity of the local lymphatic circulation is lost in an acquired manner so that the clinical picture of the lymphostasis is observed. One of the clinical peculiarities of lymphedema of the lower limbs is the different progression of stasis along the limb: from the more distal portions towards the proximal ones in the primary forms and from the proximal ones to the distal ones in the secondary forms (**Figure 1a** and **b**).

Lymphedema is characterized by being the only edema with high interstitial protein concentration, distinguishing itself for this from all other types of edema [16, 17]. The presence of a high rate of proteins in the interstitium determines the activation of fibroblasts that increase their production of collagen fibers, inducing more or less early and more or less marked tissue sclerosis. Lymphatic edema, therefore, is characterized by an early increase in the consistency of the tissues in which it is located and that, in the most advanced clinical stages, can reach the wooden consistency. Under these conditions the compression of the skin generates a depression (or "pitting test") that can be "fleeting" or even absent [18–23].

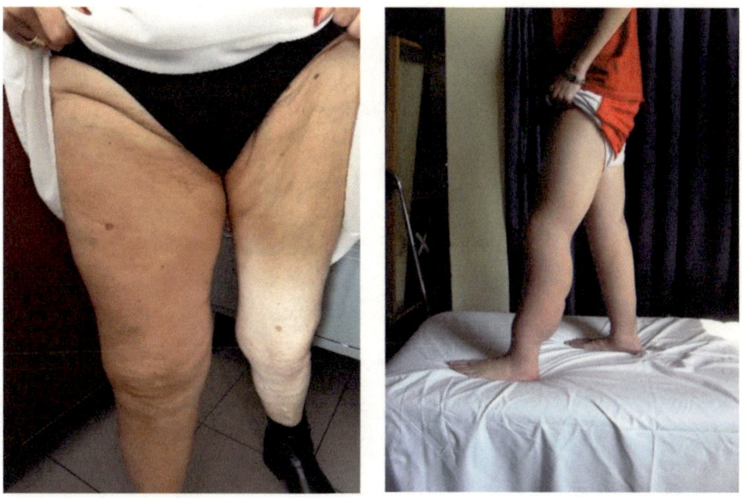

(a) **(b)**

Figure 1.
Lymphedema of the lower limb: primary (a) and secondary (b).

For the rarefaction of the arteriolar capillaries which, with the same volumetric unit, is carried out in the cutaneous and subcutaneous tissues, the skin color is not "rosy" as in the skin of normal limbs but pale. For the same ethiopathogenetic reason, the limb skin with lymphedema is colder than of a normal limb [24–28].

The lymphatic system presents some well-recognizable outward signs. The lymphatic system communicates us, but often the examiner does not recognize the messages sent. An example of this is the location of the primary or metastatic cancer in the lymphatic system itself. Sometimes a monolateral edema of the upper limb, sent for decongestive complex therapy with the prescription of a manual lymphatic drainage cycle for forearm edema and a recent onset, may be the expression of a symptomatic edema of a metastatic cancer (**Figure 2a** and **b**). In these cases, an aprioristic therapeutic approach, without the most opportune clinical considerations, can fatally delay the care that the patient really needs.

The commonly recognized four clinical stages of the disease are:

- **First stage:** It is the pre-clinical stage in which there is an undoubted predisposition to the possible onset of lymphedema (a consanguinity of a patient with primary lymphedema, mastectomized with limbs coincident in terms of volume and consistency of the two limbs).

- **Second stage:** The edema is present and regresses partially with nighttime rest and decongestive physical treatments.

- **Third stage:** Elephantiasis with disappearance of the bony and tendon saliencies normally present in the affected limb.

- **Fourth stage:** Elephantiasis complicated by verrucosis, pachydermia, ulcer, or tissue changes in the lymphosarcomatosis sense.

In primary forms of lower limbs, there is also a pathognomonic sign that takes its name from the person who first described it: the Stemmer sign. Its positivity consists in the impossibility to "pinch" with the fingers of the examiner the skin of the patient's toe; you cannot lift it from the underlying bone phalanx due to the

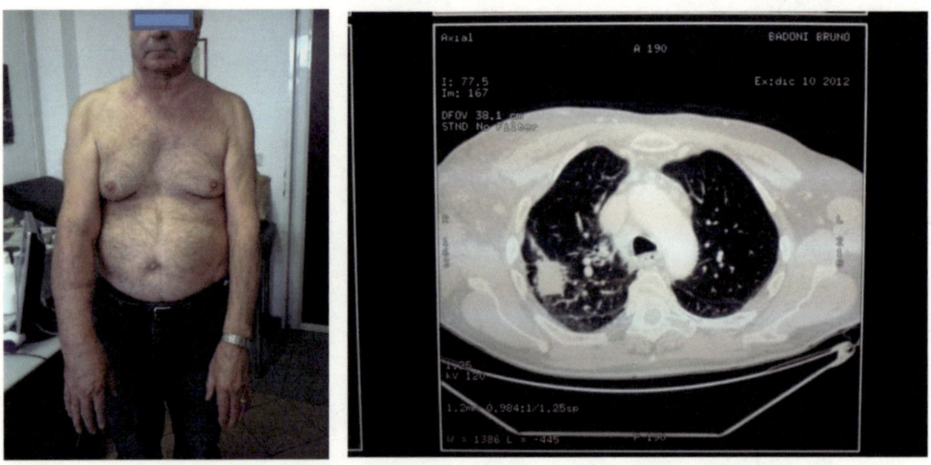

(a) (b)

Figure 2.
Forearm and hand edema, determined by the presence of metastases of the supraclavicular lymph nodes from unknown primitive pulmonary cancer (first clinical manifestation of neoplasia).

early fibrosis that is generated in the over-factory layers of the tissue itself. The diagnosis of lymphedema is clinical (fundamental is the anamnesis and a correct objective examination); however, there are some instrumental exams that complete the picture, allowing a better definition of the therapeutic approach and the prognostic one. In the primary forms, the lymphoscintigraphy is essential which consists of subcutaneous inoculation, at the root of the toes, of some drops of radioactive tracer (nanocolloids of albumin labeled with technetium 99) which has a particular tropism for the lymphatic system. After inoculation, the patient practices physical exercise to allow the tracer to "gain" more quickly the lymphatic pathways. After 30′, and after 90′, a gamma-chamber performs that uptake of the tracer which, in the meantime, is distributed in the lymphatic vessels and lymph nodes of the whole lower limb and in the iliac chains. The resulting image provides important morphological indications on the normal/pathological development of the lymphatic system allowing better orienting the therapeutic intervention and being able to conceive also a prognosis.

The high-resolution ultrasound examination also highlights the thickening of the epidermis on the affected side, the increase in thickness of the over-fascial layer, and the tissue compressibility that is a function of the more or less developed fibrosis.

The ultrasound also allows the monitoring of pharmacological, physical rehabilitative, and surgical treatment by comparing the pre- and posttreatment over-fascial thicknesses.

Videofluoroscopy is more complex and difficult to access because it is not widely practiced at a territorial level. It consists of the study of the anatomy physio-lymphatic pathology by injection of a dye, the indocyanine green, which flows into the lymphatic vessels and allows to visualize the flow in real time (on videoscope) both basal and during manual or mechanical stimulation; the lymphangio-MR, even less widespread as practiced in very few centers at the international level, allows, in more detail, to highlight the entire local lymphatic system and its possible anatomical defects.

2.4 Venous edema

It is very rare, in contrast to the lymphatic stasis edema, to observe a venous edema deriving from the supra-fascial venous compartment. In this sense the lymphatic system and the venous system behave in a completely opposite way from the clinical point of view. Lymphedema never develops in deep tissues, unless congenital dysplasia is located in the deep tissues; it is always located at the supra-fascial level.

Venous edema, on the other hand, never develops in the supra-fascial compartment (in the clinical practice, it is common to find patients who have large varicose veins of the lower limbs, but their feet are "dry", with no signs of edema.). Venous edema is an edema that is located at a deep level (for this reason, it is difficult to manage, from the therapeutic point of view, with conventional manual or mechanical drainage techniques). It is located at the sub-fascial level and, in the overwhelming majority of cases, represents the most striking aspect of the permanent clinical picture of a so-called "post-thrombotic syndrome" (**Figure 3**).

In deep venous thrombosis of the lower limbs, in fact, after thrombotic occlusion of the deep veins, follows more or less precociously a "compensatory" dilatation of the deep collateral and often superficial circle in correspondence of the same anatomical district (secondary or symptomatic varices). This muscular imbibition (therefore deep) assumes the characters of chronicity and corresponds to the permanent edema in which it is not possible to observe alterations of skin color or

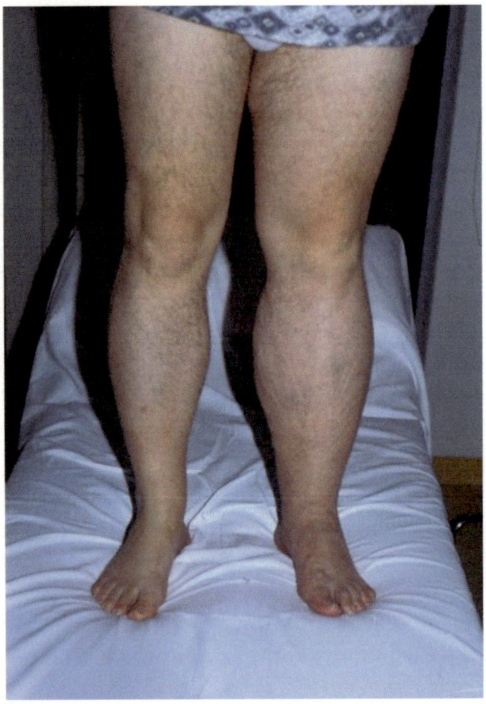

Figure 3.
Post-thrombotic oedema of the lower limb.

skin temperature in its correspondence, and the pitting sign is absent and does not appreciate changes in tissue texture. In doubtful cases (previous venous thrombosis passed "unobserved" from a clinical point of view due to lack of characteristic signs and symptoms), a key examination is represented by the computerized tomography.

According to the "CT cuts" of the two limbs in comparison with the lymphatic edema it is possible to observe an increase in supra-fascial thickness, over-folded with the sub-fascial compartment coinciding in the two limbs, in venous edema (from deep vein thrombosis); on the contrary, the supra-fascial thicknesses appears coincident, while the sub-fascial thickness is considerably increased in the affected side.

Symptoms in the post-thrombotic syndrome of the lower limb (in the one-sided form) are generally non specific; patients often show paresthesia, rarely pain, mostly vague, hardly epicritic, and often associated with protopathic sensitivity.

The so-called venous claudication which consists in pain during walking but with a variable free-range of motion (unlike "arterial claudication"), is rare and appears in the worsening of the deep venous circulation due to incomplete recanalization of the deep venous axis when the acute phase is past.

Obviously, the high-resolution ultrasound examination in these cases shows a relative increase of the sub-fascial layers, and the echo color Doppler of the examined districts confirms the outcomes of deep vein thrombosis with frequent evidence of parietal sclerosis and partial or total disappeared endoluminal valvular structures.

2.5 Phlebolymphedema

Phlebolymphedema represents a particular type of peripheral edema that is determined by the contemporary ethiopathogenetic association of venous and lymphatic insufficiency. It is generally present in cancer, due to the simultaneous macroscopic and microscopic anatomical involvement of the two venous and lymphatic drainage systems of a certain anatomical district[8].

The most striking manifestation is a secondary lymphedema of the lower limb determined by inguinal or pelvic lymphadenectomy (necessary for compliance with surgical criteria of "radical cancer therapy") associated with a partial or complete occlusion of a deep venous vessel of the limb same. In these cases the increase in interstitial oncotic pressure determined by the mechanical lymphatic stasis (removal of lymphoglandular stations) is associated with a venous hypertension (increase of the intravascular hydrostatic pressure in the venous side of the microvascular tissue unit) caused by the occlusion of the main venous axis of outflow from the lower limb itself (**Figure 4**).

2.6 Lipedema

Lipedema is a very common disease in the female population consisting predominantly of lipid cells that is established in certain specific anatomical districts. It has a familiar character with the male that results (as found in several pedigrees) in "healthy carrier." In the lower limbs, the localization can be variable but always bilateral; it can be limited to the thighs, but it can also affect the gluteal regions, affecting only the legs, affecting the thighs and legs, or involving, in addition to these, the buttocks (**Figure 5**). The feet are always spared. Sometimes the arms and forearms are also affected, and hands are always spared. The edema is associated with constant pain, which becomes acute with the passing of the hours of the day and during the summer, and ease of spontaneous bruising [10–12, 29].

Edema, generally, appears at puberty and is exacerbated at some particular moments in a woman's life (breastfeeding more than pregnancy and menopause). The edema appears simultaneously in all the regions of the affected limbs, and there is never a progression along the limbs (neither in the distal-proximal or proximal-distal sense) but only a possible simultaneous increase of the edematous zones. It is an edema that does not respond to hypocaloric dietary treatments or physical exercise.

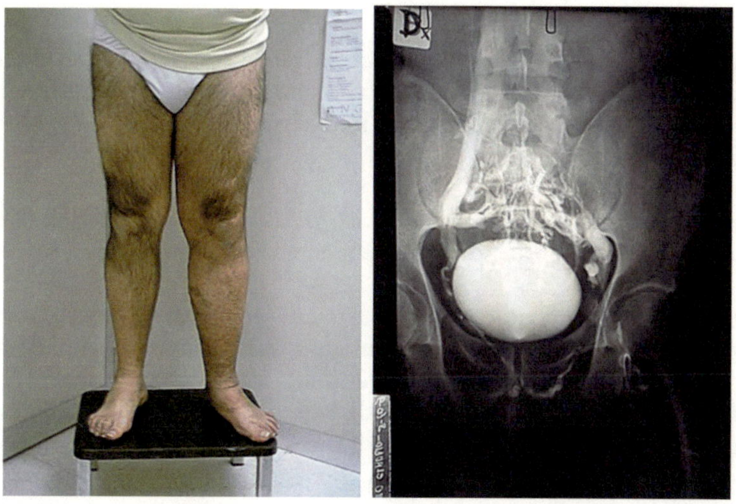

(a) (b)

Figure 4.
(a and b) Phlebolymphedema: a case of prostate cancer with pelvic lymphadenectomy associated with venous left iliac thrombosis. (a) Clinical case and (b) phlebography of the lower limb.

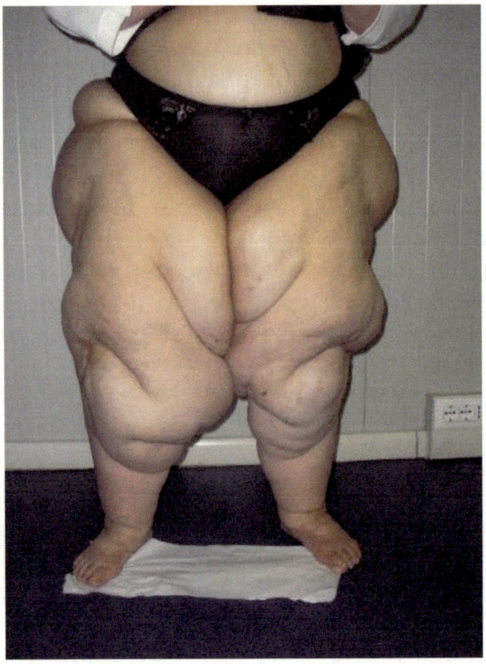

Figure 5.
Lipedema of the lower limbs.

We recognize four clinical stages of the disease:

- **First stage:** Mild edema located in the sites already described in the possible combinations with conserved limb conformation. The skin presents slight and widespread increase in consistency.

- **Second stage:** Important edema involving the sites described in the possible combinations, with pain and gross deformations of some regions of the limbs. Increased skin of consistency.

- **Third stage:** Painful elephantiasis with extremely gross plication, alteration of the gait pattern, and possible cutaneous lesions, prevalent on the inner surfaces of the thighs. Occurrence of serotine foot edema or after prolonged standing station.

- **Fourth stage:** Painful elephantiasis with gross plication, alteration of the gait pattern, trophic lesions, and permanent edema of the feet (lipolymphedema).

The lymphoscintigraphy of lower limbs, in the early stages, shows a normal development and draining lymphatic circulation. In the advanced clinical stages of the disease, it is possible to underline bilateral sub-rotuleous stagnation of the tracer (dermal back flow) and lymph node stop that corresponds, from the clinical point of view, to the so-called lipolymphedema of the lower limbs.

High-resolution ultrasound allows to highlight a constant echogenic pattern of the supra-fascial compartment (skin-fascia). It is an extremely useful test for the differential diagnosis with lymphedema of the lower limbs. In lipedema, in fact, the compression of tissues with a linear probe shows a reduction in the sub-fascial thicknesses with the supra-fascial which remained unchanged; in the case of lymphedema, on the contrary, the compression with linear probe shows a decrease in the over-fascial thicknesses, while the sub-fascial remain unchanged. This testifies that in lipedema the volumetric increase is given by an increased cellular component (hypertrophic and hyperplastic lipid cells) while in the lymphedema the volumetric increase is given by more or less copious presence of extracellular interstitial fluids that the pressure of the probe can move.

The BMI is variable in the two pathologies. In lipedema it is generally within the limits of the norm and is not minimally influenced by physical treatments nor by the overall weight loss. In lymphedema it can be equally variable even if it is higher on average than in patients with lipedema.

The differential diagnosis with obesity is quite simple. In the obese patients, the collection of fatty deposits is widespread in all the body regions with a particular preference for the anatomical areas typical of each sex (gynoid type and android type).

Obesity responds positively to physical exercises and diet, in all body districts, while lipedema is not affected at all by these factors.

2.7 Inflammatory or infectious states

The edema of the lower limb can be determined by inflammatory and/or infectious diseases. In these cases the localization is generally monolateral and is secondary to an inflammatory/infectious process of the soft tissues (cellulitis, myositis, myofascitis, necrotizing fasciitis). The localization may involve only one area of the limb (thigh, leg, foot) assuming the topographic configuration of the "suspended edema." Besides the edema, all the other characters of inflammation are generally present (increase in skin temperature, hyperemia, pain, and reduction of functional capacity (*functio laesa*). The resolution of edema is due, in these cases, to anti-inflammatory and pharmacological treatment and, if necessary, to antibiotics. A special case of edema that can induce doubts of differential diagnosis with deep vein thrombosis and that is determined by the presence of serous cyst of the popliteal cable is known as Baker's cyst. Particularly developed, it can compress the surrounding venous and lymphatic vessels, inducing a distal edema (generally subpatellar) also extended to the whole leg and to the foot. With the treatment of cystic formation (puncture with evacuation, surgical excision, simple anti-inflammatory therapy), we are witnessing the resolution of the edema.

2.8 Benign or malignant neoplasms

Benign or malignant tumoral formations may develop in the lower limbs, especially the soft tissues (mainly muscles). Their localization, particularly in the leg muscles, occupying space, also due to the compressive phenomena exerted on the surrounding vessels, can determine circumscribed or diffused edema which, for the differential diagnosis, must make use of more discriminating investigations, such as CT or MR. Obviously, the edema, in these cases, recedes only after surgical removal of the mass.

2.9 Systemic causes

2.9.1 Edema in heart failure (from diastolic dysfunction)

In the case of heart failure, the echocardiographic examination may be apparently normal (the ventricular ejection fraction, in these cases, provides normal indications, and no particular problems are highlighted). In these conditions, however, a careful clinical examination is required which highlights a bilateral and symmetrical lower limb edema (often confused with lymphedema); the sign of the fovea is particularly evocable and persistent over time. The Stemmer sign is negative (**Figure 6**). The edema is established by an important increase in venous pressure in the microvascular tissue units, whereby the normal pressure gradient at the micro-tissutal level which, from the hydrostatic point of view, under normal conditions, would help the return of fluids from the interstitium towards the venous capillaries is gone and many water molecules remain in the interstitium. The thoracic auscultation demonstrates the presence of bilateral basal crackles. The liver may appear increased in volume and with rounded margins[13]. The subject refers to dyspnea for slight efforts or even at rest. During nocturnal rest the patient needs to observe a decubitus which raises the thorax and head with respect to the other bodily districts. In these cases, the dosage of the inactive form of the Brain Natriuretic Peptide (BNP, substance produced by the cardiac endothelium, whose serum concentration increases in the case of inability of filling by the cardiac chambers) results elevated, suggesting that the heart has difficulty in receiving fluids returning from the periphery (second- or third-degree diastolic dysfunction); this dysfunctions are relatively frequent in women above 65 years. In these cases conventional draining physical therapies risk aggravating subjective and objective symptoms, and the same elastic garment to be worn in the morning should be prescribed only after the clinical compensation obtained with the appropriate dosage of diuretics and positive inotropic drugs (e.g., digoxin) indicated for each individual case.

2.9.2 Hepatic insufficiency

The edema of hepatic insufficiency can be defined as "gravitational"; it is collected mainly in the sloping body areas. It is essentially localized in the toes and feet when the subject is standing or sitting with the legs "dangling." When the subject is lying on the bed, the most gravitational area is the presacral region[14]. It is not uncommon in these cases, if the patient holds a higher limb outside the bed, observe the edema at the level of the elbow of the arm itself. The conventional physical therapies, even in this case, do not solve the problem that benefits only from the administration of intravenous albumin. It is hypo-albumin, which in fact generates edema: since each protein molecule behaves like a kind of magnet to water molecules (it attracts them); in the case of hypo-albuminemia, liquids are no longer held within the intra-vascular compartment and tend to flee to intertial space, following the gravity.

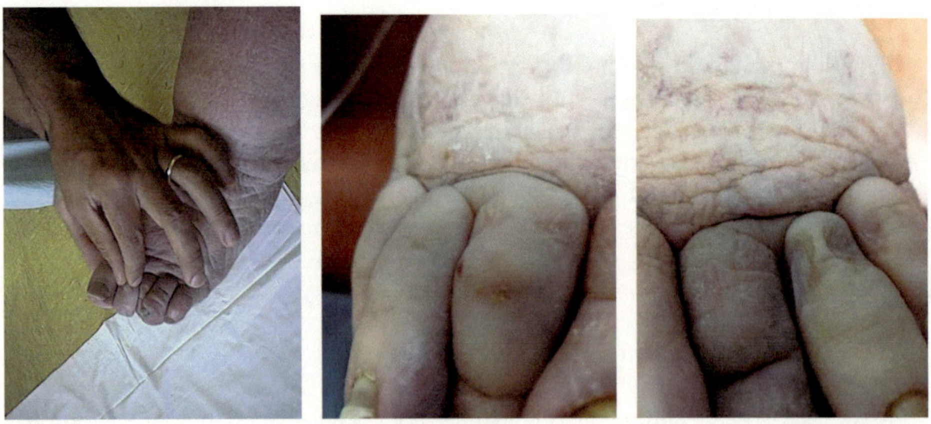

(a) (b) (c)

Figure 6.
Stemmer sign: positive in lymphedema (a), negative in cardiac failure (b) before compression and (c) after compression.

2.9.3 Acute and chronic renal failure

In chronic renal failure at third or fourth stage, the relative inability of the nephron to produce "pre-urine" inevitably leads to a generalized "water retention" affecting all body districts. The subject, frequently, in the morning wakes up with the edematous eyelids and only an adequate dosage of diuretics, respecting the values of the electrolytes and, above all, of the renal function (azotemia, creatinine). Decongestive physical treatments cannot find an elective indication even in this form.

2.9.4 Myxedema

Myxedema is a particular form of edema affecting the lower limbs (generally bilaterally, symmetrically, and localized to the pretibial surfaces) determined by accumulation of mucopolysaccharides in the derma. In these cases, the pretibial edema is also accompanied by ocular edema (exophthalmos), with generalized dryness of the skin and, sometimes, psychic hypo-evolution [15]. It is determined by serious conditions of hypothyroidism (congenital or acquired), in which TSH (which, for various reasons, does not respond to the thyroid parenchyma) would stimulate tissue fibroblasts and adipocytes to replicate and produce mucopolysaccharide complexes, with local deposition inside the dermis, or, on the contrary, in cases of hyperthyroidism (as in Flaiani-Basedow's disease). This type of edema is reversible and recognizes as a fundamental therapeutic treatment the correction of thyroid defect (in defect or excess of glandular function). It is presented as a "suspended edema," not painful, and without local typical signs of inflammatory processes.

2.9.5 Drug edema

Drug edema occurs, in most cases, by a particular idiosyncrasy of the subject to certain molecules. The drugs most commonly called into question in these forms are some molecules with antihypertensive effect (especially amlodipine and other calcium antagonists, in which the edema is localized mainly in the two ankles—bilateral edema—and in the back of the feet, and the sartanics that can induce generalized edemas, up to anasarca) and the corticosteroids which cause a generalized water retention. In all these forms, physical treatment is not conclusive, and the therapy consists in the simple suspension of the drug (with substitution with different molecules). In almost all the cases, the complete resolution of the clinical picture is achieved within a maximum of 7 days from the suspension of the drug.

2.9.6 Idiopathic edema

Many authors are reminded of the possible presence of "idiopathic edema," or an edema (generally distal and bilateral) that arises at certain times of the day (especially after prolonged standing) or in the summer season. It regresses with the wearing of the definitive elastic garment for a variable period of time.

2.9.7 Differential diagnosis of edema of the lower limbs

The differential diagnosis of edema of the lower limbs can be easily formulated through simple observations concerning skin color, skin temperature, mono- or bilaterality localization, the presence of the sign of pitting, the presence of the Stemmer sign, the sense of progression of the edema along the limb, and the date of onset of edema, compared to the time of observation. From a combined analysis of these elements, it is possible to easily reach the diagnosis that can be further confirmed by other exams, already described in the individual-treated paragraphs [4, 12, 30–36].

In particular, in relation to:

- ***Skin color***: in the cardiac edema, it can appear bright pink up to taking on bluish-cyanotic nuances, in particular at the level of visible mucous. In the hepatic edema, it can assume a yellowish shade; in case of renal failure, it can appears "greenish." In superficial venous root edema (acute varicophlebitis), it can be red to cyanosis. In the deep vein thrombosis edema, it generally maintains the rosy color that coincides with that of the healthy limb. Lipedema, myxedema, idiopathic edema and the drugs-related one keep rosy the complexion; instead the skin remains pale in primary or secondary lymphedema, tending to whitish, due to the rarefaction of the arteriolar capillaries which occurs in the tissue volumetric unit [39].

- ***The cutaneous temperature*** remains normal in cardiac, hepatic, renal, and idiopathic edema, in myxedema, lipedema, and drug-related edema. It remains normal also in deep vein thrombosis edema (except in cases where there is an important lymphatic overload of the superficial circle—with vicarious goals—that can cause a slight reduction of skin temperature in the affected limb compared to the contralateral one). In superficial venous root edema (varicophlebitis), the local temperature increases, while in lymphedema, primary or secondary, for the same reason for which the skin is whitish (except for concomitant acute lymphangitis), it is also characterized by a decrease in local temperature [37, 38].

- ***Mono- or bilateral localization***: in all edemas of a "systemic" cause (cardiac, hepatic, renal, myxedema, drug-related), the localization is always bilateral and generally symmetrical. Also in lipedema it is bilateral. In lymphatic edema, both primary and secondary, localization can be both unilateral and bilateral. Idiopathic edema, superficial venous cause edema (varicophlebitis), and deep venous cause (deep venous thrombosis) are generally unilateral.

- ***Pain***: in the "systemic" causes of edema, pain is generally absent, unless concomitant algogenic irritating spines coexist. In the edema caused by superficial varicophlebitis, often cyclical exacerbations are present. In the deep vein thrombosis edema, pain is not acute; it is deaf, not well definable from the anatomical point of view, and not epicritic, diffused to the interested limb. Pain is one of the peculiar characteristics of the clinical picture in lipedema. It is variable in various hours of the day being described as particularly important in the evening hours and in the summer season (obviously also depending on the clinical stage of the disease).

- ***Pitting sign***: it is particularly present and persistent in the diastolic heart dysfunction edema, as in the typical edema of the hepatic insufficiency and in that of the renal insufficiency. It is present in myxedema, idiopathic edema, drug-related edema, and edema of superficial venous affections. It is generally absent in deep vein thrombosis. It is also fleeting and not very persistent in lymphatic edema, both primary and secondary, due to tissue fibrosis that more or less establishes in the tissues due to the persistence of interstitial protein component which induces fibrosis with consequent increase of tissue consistency itself. In lipedema, in the early clinical stages, the pitting sign is absent (the volumetric increase is determined by the exclusive presence of hyperplastic and hypertrophic adipose cells and not to fluids in the interstitium). It can appear in the most advanced clinical stages (lipolymphedema) [39].

- ***Stemmer's sign***: it is pathognomonic of lymphedema. It is in fact undetectable in all edemas that recognize a systemic cause, in idiopathic edema, and in lipedema (in which the feet are always spared from the edematous localization). In lymphedema, it is always present, and if it would be well-known by general practitioners and, unfortunately, also by many specialists, many unnecessary examinations (repeated echo color Doppler, Rx, high-resolution ultrasound, computed tomography, and MRI) would not be prescribed, looking for what is not recognized by simple clinical examination (it is of very frequent experience, even today). In the secondary forms of lymphedema of the lower limb, the Stemmer sign is initially negative and is only positively delayed [40].

- ***Progression of edema along the limb***: in systemic edema and idiopathic edema as well as in primary lymphedema, the progression of edema in the lower limbs takes place in a distal-proximal direction (first the toes and the foot are affected and then the leg and, lastly, the thigh). In secondary lymphedema, on the contrary, the progression takes place in the opposite direction, in the proximal-distal direction (first the thigh is affected and then the leg and lastly the foot and the toes with consequent "late" positivity of the Stemmer sign). In Lipedema and myxedema, there is no progressive development of the edema itself, but this originates and increases simultaneously in all the body regions involved [41, 42].

- ***Time of onset***: the time of onset of the edema is extremely variable. Cardiac edema occurs due to continuous pharmacological adjustments, especially diuretic therapy, generally given by months or years with alternating clinical intensity, as well as hepatic or renal edema. Drug-related edema appears after 1 to 3/4 days of taking the drug responsible for the side effect (an easily traced anamnestic data), and normally, as recalled, it reduces completely after the suspension of the drug. Lipedema generally appears at puberty (between 15 and 20 years of age) and may present clinical resurgence in particular moments of the woman's fertile life. Myxedema may arise at birth or develop in subsequent periods depending on thyroid glandular activity. Idiopathic edema generally occurs at puberty. Venous edema certainly occurs the most sudden, both in the superficial (varicophlebitis) and in the deep (deep vein thrombosis) form. In this last case, the edema appears absolutely fast and involves the whole limb from the level of localization of the thrombus in the deep vein. In these cases the appearance and evolution (proximal-distal) is almost immediate. From coincident arts we highlight the important edema within 6–12 h from the onset. The formation of the thrombus precedes the clinical evidence of the edema that only manifests when the dimensions of the thrombus hinders a large part of the habitual venous return [43–45].

3. Conclusions

The opinion that an edema of the lower limbs, regardless of the patient's age, of the general clinical conditions and symptoms and signs that accompany the picture, is of a lymphostatic nature is still widespread today. So it happens that many cardiologists send to the angiologist or to the vascular surgeon patients over 70 years, with a fairly delineated symptom complex, albeit unidentified, with the diagnosis of "recent-onset limb lymphedema"; clinical cases that, if properly considered, are of strict cardiological relevance and not of physical rehabilitative medicine. Just as Lipedema is still unknown, as a pathology, by over 50% of the same vascular surgeons and of the angiology and by the overwhelming majority of family doctors [46].

The hemato-chemical and instrumental examinations are undoubtedly useful for a better definition of individual cases, both for the purposes of the therapeutic approach and the prognosis and monitoring.

However, the diagnosis must be essentially clinical and is based on the considerations described, simply by analyzing the individual objective and subjective parameters, between them, and crossing the information. Clinical experience can accelerate the diagnosis and the accuracy of the subsequent therapeutic approach, but it is fundamental, in any case, that before a definitive diagnosis, we consider the "semeiological picture" which, combined with an accurate clinical history, allows to reach the certainty of differential diagnosis.

Even today there are diagnostic mistakes in evaluation of many edema of the lower limbs. The lack of specific clinical experience and the underestimation of important anamnestic elements, supported by clinical evidence that often are not sought in the various details or, the misinterpretation of instrumental investigations can lead to inaccurate ethiopathogenetic diagnoses with negative consequences from the point of view of treatment that is undertaken in the individual clinical case.

The proposed analysis aims at avoiding reckless or "discounted" clinical judgments, but not responding to the real needs of the individual patient, and helping the medical doctor, the physiotherapist, and the nurse to follow the most appropriate diagnostic and therapeutic procedures in line with the current principle prevention, early diagnosis, and treatment.

Conflict of interest

The authors declare no conflict of interest.

Author details

Sandro Michelini*, Alessandro Failla, Giovanni Moneta, Alessandro Fiorentino and Cardone Marco
Department of Rehabilitation, S. Giovanni Battista Hospital, Rome, Italy

*Address all correspondence to: s.michelini@acismom.it

References

[1] Tiwari A, Cheng KS, Button M, Myint F, Hamilton G. Differential diagnosis, investigation, and current treatment of lower limb lymphedema. Archives of Surgery. 2003;**138**(2):152-161

[2] Michelini S. Phlebolymphoedema. From Diagnosis to Therapy. Bologna: Edizioni P.R.; 1998

[3] Badini A, Fulcheri E, Campisi C, Boccardo F. A new approach in histopathological diagnosis of lymphedema: Pathophysiological and therapeutic implications. Lymphology. 1996;**29**(S):190-198

[4] Gasbarro V, Michelini S, Antignani PL, Tsolaki E, Ricci M, Allegra C. The CEAP-L classification for lymphedemas of the limbs: The Italian experience. International Angiology. 2009;**28**(4):315-324

[5] Lee B, Andrade M, Bergan J, Boccardo F, Campisi C, Damstra R, Flour M, Gloviczki P, Laredo J, Piller N, Michelini S, Mortimer P, Villavicencio JL. Diagnosis and treatment of primary lymphedema. Consensus Document of the International Union of Phlebology (IUP)-2009. International Angiology. 2010;29(5):454-470

[6] International Lymph Framework. Best Practice for the Management of Lymphoedema. 2nd ed. 2012. Available at: www.lympho.org

[7] The diagnosis and treatment of peripheral lymphedema: 2013 consensus document of the international society of lymphology. Lymphology;**46**(2013):1-11

[8] Michelini S, Cardone M. Veno-lymphatic vascular malformations: Medical therapy. In: Mattassi R, Loose DA, Vaghi M, editors. Hemangiomas and Vascular Malformations. Italia: Springer; 2015. pp. 445-450

[9] Michelini S, Pissas A, Olszewski W, Dimakakos E, Cordero IF, Caldirola R, et al. Linforoll: A new device for lymphoedema treatment: Preliminary experience. Lymphology. 2015;**47**(Suppl):218-221

[10] Mariani G, Campisi C, Taddei G, Boccardo F, Martini F, Rahimi Mansour A, et al. The current role of lymphoscintigraphy in the diagnostic evaluation of patients with peripheral lymphedema. Lymphology. 1998;**31**(Suppl):316-319

[11] Cavezzi A, Michelini S. PHlebolymphoedema. Bologna: Edizioni P.R; 1998

[12] Nicolaides AN. Therapeutic outcome and quality of life in patients with chronic venous and lymphatic disorders. Phlebolymphology. 2008;**20**:2-3

[13] Schmeller W, Hueppe M, Meier-Vollrath I. Tumescent liposuction in lipoedema yields good long-term results. The British Journal of Dermatology. 2012;**166**:161-168

[14] Schmeller W, Meier-Vollrath. Lipödem: Ein update (Lipedema: an update). Lymphol Forsch Prax. 2005;**9**(1):10-20

[15] Forner-Cordero I, Szolnoky G, Forner-Cordero A, Kemény L. Lipedema: An overview of its clinical manifestations, diagnosis and treatment of the disproportional fatty deposition syndrome—Systematic review. Clinical Obesity. 2012;**2**:86-95

[16] Pascual-Figal DA, Domingo M, Casas T, Gich I, Ordoñez-Llanos J, Martínez P, et al. Usefulness of clinical and NT-proBNP monitoring for

prognostic guidance in destabilized heart failure outpatients. European Heart Journal. 2008;**29**(8):1011-1018

[17] Younossi ZM, Guyatt G, Kiwi M, Boparai N, King D. Development of a disease specific questionnaire to measure health related quality of life in patients with chronic liver disease. Gut. 1999;**45**:295-300

[18] Schwartz KM, Fatourechi V, Ahmed DDF, Pond GR. Dermopathy of Graves' disease (pretibial myxedema): Long-term outcome. The Journal of Clinical Endocrinology & Metabolism. 2002;**87**(2):438-446

[19] Bellini C, Arioni C, Mazzella M, Campisi C, Taddei G, Boccardo F, et al. Lymphoscintigraphic evaluation of congenital lymphedema of the newborn. Clinical Nuclear Medicine. 2002;**27**(5):383-384

[20] Boccardo F, Michelini S, Zilli A, Campisi C. Epidemiology of lymphedema. Phlebolymphology. 1999;**26**:24-28

[21] Werngren-Elgstrom M, Lidman D. Lymphoedema of the lower extremities after surgery and radiotherapy for cancer of the cervix. Scandinavian Journal of Plastic and Reconstructive Surgery and Hand Surgery. 1994;**28**(4):289-293

[22] Campisi C, Michelini S, Boccardo F, Zilli A. Lymphedema epidemiology in Italy. Lymphology. 1998;**31**(Suppl):243-244

[23] Casley-Smith J. Modern Treatment for Lymphoedema. Adelaide: The Lymphoedema Association of Australia, Inc.; 1994

[24] Dellachà A, Fulcheri E, Boccardo F, Campisi C. Post-surgical lymphedema: Iatrogenic or pre-existing disease? Lymphology. 1998;**31**:562-565

[25] Földi E, Földi M. Physiothérapie Complete Décongestive. Paris: Editions Frison-Roche; 1993

[26] Leduc A. Le drainage lymphatique. Paris, Masson: Théorie et pratique; 1980

[27] Michelini S, Failla A, Moneta G, Campisi C, Boccardo F. Clinical staging of lymphedema and therapeutical implications. Lymphology. 2002;**35**:168-176

[28] Michelini S, Failla A. Linfedemi: Inquadramento diagnostico clinico e strumentale. Minerva Cardioangiologica. 1997;**45**(Suppl I): 11-15

[29] Tosatti E. Lymphatique profonds et lymphoedèmes chroniques des membres. Paris: Masson; 1974

[30] Vodder E. La méthode Vodder—Le drainage lymphatique manuel. DK-2880, Bagsvaer: Inst. For Lymph Drainage; 1969

[31] Olszewski W. Recurrent bacterial dermatolymphangioadenitis (DLA) is responsible for progression of lymphoedema. Lymphology. 1996;**29**(Suppl):331

[32] Michelini S, Campisi C, Failla A, Boccardo F. Proposal for stadiation of phlebolymphoedema. European Journal of Lymphology and Related Problems. 1995;**6**(20):I-14

[33] Campisi C. Lymphoedema: Modern diagnostic and therapeutic aspects. International Angiology. 1999;**18**(1):14-24

[34] Case TC, Witte CL, Witte MH, Unger EC, Williams WH. Magnetic resonance imaging in human lymphedema: Comparison with Lymphangioscintigraphy. Journal of Magnetic Resonance Imaging. 1992;**10**:549-558

[35] Ferrel RE, Levinson KL, Esman JH, Komak MA, Lawrence EC, Barmada MM, et al. Hereditary lymphedema evidence for linkage and

genetic heterogeneity. Human Molecular Genetics. 1998 Dec. 7;**13**:2073-2078

[36] Michelini S, Failla A, Moneta G. Lymphedema: Epidemiology, disability and social costs. Lymphology. 2002;**35**:169-171

[37] Michelini S, Failla A, Moneta G, Zinicola V, Romaldini PD. International classification of lymphedema functioning and disability evaluation. European Journal of Lymphology. 2007;**17**(51):16-19

[38] Michelini S, De Giorgio D, Cestari M, Corda D, Ricci M, Cardone M, et al. Clinical and genetic study of 46 Italian patients with primary lymphoedema. Lymphology. 2012;**45**:3-12

[39] Michelini S, Failla A, Moneta G, Cardone M, Michelotti L, Zinicola V, et al. Linee guida e protocolli diagnostico-terapeutici nel linfedema. Eur. Med. Phys. 2008;**44**(Suppl. 1-3)

[40] Michelini S, Failla A, Moneta G, Zinicola V, Macaluso B, Cardone M, et al. Treatment of lymphedema with shockwave therapy: Preliminary study. The European Journal of Lymphology and Related Problems. 2007;**17**(51):29

[41] Michelini S, Failla A, Moneta G, Cardone M, Fiorentino A. Immunestimulation and reduction of infective complications in patients with lymphoedema. European Journal of Lymphology and Related Problems. 2009;**20**(56):17-18

[42] Partsch H. Indirect lymphography in different kinds of leg oedema. In: Lymphology: Advances in Europe. Ecig: Genova; 1989. pp. 95-99

[43] Pecking AP, Cluzan RV. Assessment of lymphatic function: 15 years experience using radionuclide methods. Lymphology. 1994;**27**(Suppl):301-304

[44] Schingale FJ. Lipoedema. In: Schingale FJ, editor. Lymphoedema, Lipoedema: A Guide for those Effected. Hannover: Schlütersche; 2003. pp. 64-71

[45] Trévidic P, Marzelle J, Cormier JM. Apport de la microchirurgie au traitement des lymphoedèmes. In: Editions Techniques -Encycl. Méd. Chir. Paris, France: Techniques chirurgicales-Chirurgie vasculaire; 1994 F.a. 43-225

[46] Földi M. The therapy of lymphedema. European Society of Lymphology. 1993-1994;**14**:43-49

Chapter 4

Edema Induced by sPLA2 from *Crotalus durissus terrificus* Involves PLC and PKC Signaling, Activation of cPLA2, and Oxidative Stress

Marcos H. Toyama, Caroline R.C. Costa, Mariana N. Belchor, Danielle P. Novaes, Marcos A. de Oliveira, Rolando Ie, Henrique Hessel Gaeta and Daniela de O. Toyama

Abstract

sPLA2 from *Crotalus durissus terrificus* venom, free of crotapotin (Cdt sPLA2), purified and isolated sPLA2, was able to significantly increase lipid peroxidation, which occurred simultaneously with increased arachidonic acid (AA) metabolism. In addition, MDA and AA levels were elevated at 15 min after Cdt sPLA2 injection and after peak edema (negative control). Thus, oxidative stress and ROS play important roles in the inflammation induced by Cdt sPLA2. On the other hand, edema induced by sPLA2 involves the direct and indirect mobilization of arachidonic acid by the involvement of phosphokinase C (PKC) and phospholipase C (PLC), which indirectly stimulates cytosolic PLA2 (cPLA2). We also observed that the specific antivenin against Cdt venom had no significant effect on the neutralization of induced edema compared to the natural products 5-caffeine-linoleic acid (5CQA) and dexamethasone (AACOCF3). Our results also indicate that there was improvement in the inhibition of edema of natural polyphenolic compounds compared to antivenin or inhibition of the enzymatic activity of sPLA2 due to the fact that 5CQA is a potent antioxidant compound. Thus, our results show a clear correlation between increased arachidonic acid metabolism and oxidative stress.

Keywords: *Crotalus durissus terrificus* (Cdt), secretory snake venom phospholipase A2, edema, PKC, PLC, inflammation, oxidative stress

1. Introduction

1.1 Arachidonic acid "dogma"

Arachidonic acid (ARA) is a 20-carbon chain fatty acid with four methylene-interrupted *cis* double bonds; the first, with respect to the methyl end (omega, ω or n), is located between carbons 6 and 7. Arachidonic acid (AA) has three possible destinations: participating in the remodeling process of the cell membrane, release into the extracellular medium by diffusion, or its intracellular metabolism [1, 2]. In addition to AA, lysophosphatidic acid (lyso-platelet aggregation factor (PAF)) is another product of the enzymatic hydrolysis of membrane phospholipids, which, in the presence of lyso-PAF acyl transferase, is converted in PAF [3]. PAF is an extracellular lipid signaling molecule involved in a range of cellular activities, including survival, differentiation, cellular proliferation, morphological changes, and migration, among others [4]. Besides, its biological action is mediated by the presence of a cellular receptor (PAF-receptor (PAF-R)) (**Figure 1**). These physiological and pharmacological activities of PAF depend on the presence of its receptors, designated as PAF-R1 to PAF-R6. These receptors are G protein-coupled transmembrane receptors, and recent studies revealed that the PAF-R signaling pathway clearly affects different aspects of tumor progression [5, 6]. In the literature, it is well established that phospholipases A2 (PLA2s) are key enzymes involved in AA generation by hydrolytic digestion of membrane phospholipids. PLA2 is a superfamily

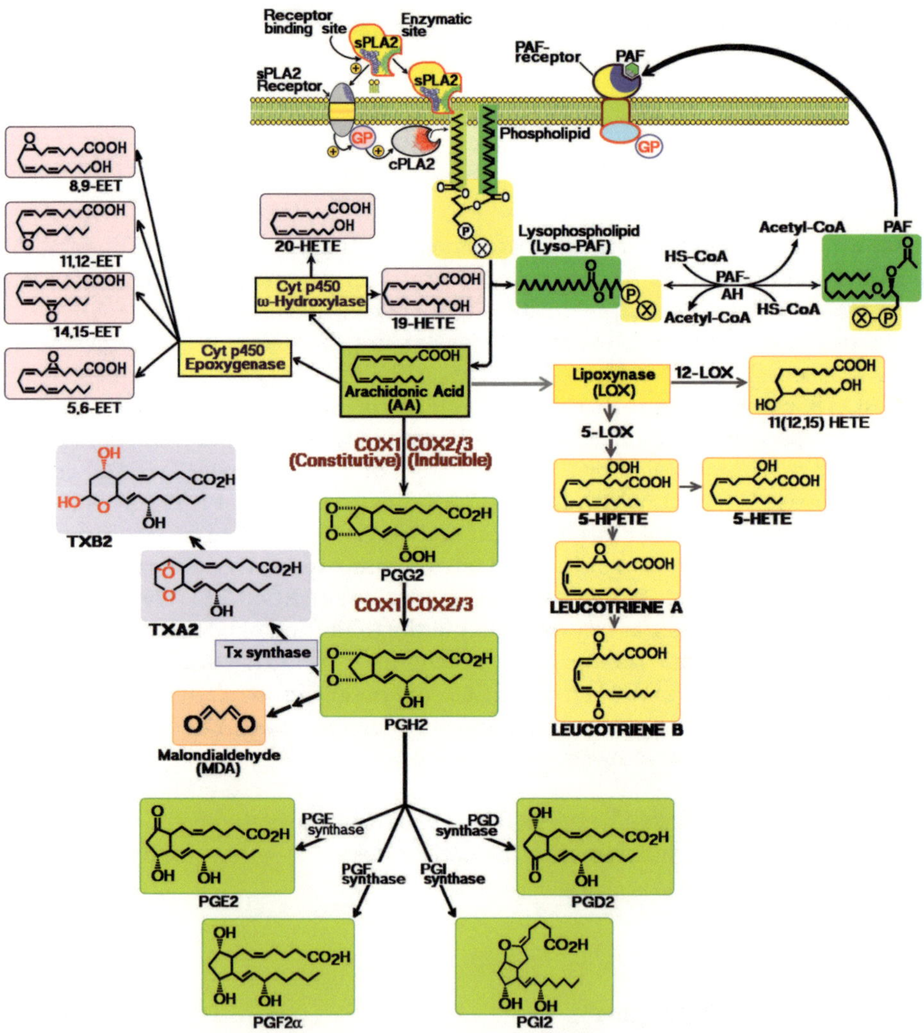

Figure 1.
Central dogma of arachidonic acid metabolism. AA cascade and its destination following three major oxidative pathways: (1) cyclooxygenase (COX), producing prostaglandins and related eicosanoids; (2) lipoxygenase (LOX), forming leukotrienes and related compounds; and (3) CYP450, forming arachidonic acid epoxides.

of enzymes distributed throughout six major classes: secretory PLA2 (sPLA2), calcium-dependent cytosolic PLA2 (cPLA2), calcium-independent cytosolic PLA2 (iPLA2), lysosomal PLA2 (lPLA2), mitochondrial PLA2 (mPLA2), and, more recently, PAF-acetyl hydrolases (PAF-AHs). PAF-AHs are a small family of phospholipases A2 with a high specificity for the hydrolysis of the unsaturated fatty acid residue located at the sn-2 position [7, 8]. sPLA2 is considered a simple and primitive enzyme, acting as an inducer of the inflammatory process, besides being able to act as a pseudohormone. In addition to generating AA directly, this enzyme can also increase the activity of cPLA2 [9]. Furthermore, the produced AA usually follows one of three distinct enzymatic pathways involving cyclooxygenase, lipoxygenase, and cytochrome P450. Several products of these routes can modulate the functions of ion channels, protein kinases, and ion pumps. In addition, newly formed eicosanoids are excreted and mediate various physiological functions, including insulin secretion and muscle contraction, and most of these actions involve protein G. Ultimately, the products of AA metabolism are rapidly degraded [1, 10]. Briefly, AA, as well as other polyunsaturated fatty acids (PUFAs) generated at the cellular level, can be mobilized through the hydrolytic activity of various enzymes. It is possible to highlight the action of PLA2 through a single reaction pathway that produces AA and lysophospholipid (LysP), which is considered the classical pathway of AA generation—it is the most widely known and studied. In addition, AA is metabolized by cyclooxygenase (COX) and 5-lipoxygenase, resulting in the synthesis of prostaglandins and leukotrienes, respectively. These intracellular messengers play an important role in the regulation of signal transduction, leading to pain and inflammatory responses. Recently, the literature has shown that AA can follow a third pathway, resulting in its metabolism by cytochrome P450 enzymes—Cyt450 epoxygenase and Cyt450 omega hydroxylase. P450s are typical monooxygenases, which enzymatically cleave molecular oxygen, followed by the insertion of a single atom of oxygen into the substrate, while the remainder is released as water [11–14]. Cytochrome P450s metabolize AA to produce the collectively designated hydroxyeicosatetraenoic acids and epoxyeicosatrienoic acids; these bioactive compounds are generated in a tissue- and cell-specific manner, and numerous biological functions have been revealed (**Figure 1**).

2. Secretory phospholipase A2

Phospholipase A2 (EC 3.1.1.4, PLA2) belongs to the group of enzymes, which catalyze the hydrolysis of the ester bond at the sn-2 position of glycerophospholipids and, consequently, are capable of generating free fatty acids, including arachidonic acid (AA). Under physiological conditions, PLA2s are crucial for membrane phospholipid homeostasis, ensuring membrane stability, fluidity, and permeability, and they are involved in the regulation of transport processes through the cell membrane. Phospholipases A2 are enzymes widely diffused in bacteria, plants, venom (of various animals), and mammal cells. Several studies suggest that these enzymes can be classified into 19 groups, which have been identified in mammalian tissues. Besides, many of these groups exhibit significant A2 phospholipase enzymatic activity. At a high level, PLA2s can be classified into two groups: cytosolic PLA2 (cPLA2), and a large and diverse group of secretory PLA2s (sPLA2). Cytosolic PLA2 comprises calcium-dependent cPLA2 (cPLA2), calcium-independent cytosolic PLA2 (iPLA2), lysosomal PLA2 (lPLA2), mitochondrial PLA2 (mPLA2), and, more recently, PAF-acetyl hydrolases (PAF-AHs), which display a small family of phospholipases A2 with high specificity for hydrolysis of the unsaturated fatty acid residue located at the sn-2 position [7, 8, 10]. Several studies suggest that the proinflammatory action induced by mammalian sPLA2 and even snake venom sPLA2 involve a significant increase of both oxidative activity and reactive oxygen species (ROS) in the cell. ROS are involved in processes such as lipid peroxidation and protein carbonylation, which, at certain levels, can lead to pathological events [15]. Studies conducted by Chiricozzi et al. (2010) [16] reveal that there is a relationship between the increased enzymatic activity of sPLA2, which belongs to the IIA family, and a significant cellular production of free radicals, which contribute strongly to the development of neurodegenerative diseases. Snake venom sPLA2 shares similar mechanisms of action and the same pathways of action with mammalian sPLA2. Experimental evidence in the literature demonstrates that both sPLA2 isoforms are able to induce inflammation and other similar biological activities [10, 17–19]. It is noteworthy that literature data demonstrate sPLA2 can activate signaling events that cannot be explained simply by its catalytic activity, and this fact emphasizes that sPLA2 could act essentially as a ligand of a receptor, rather than as an enzyme [20]. In contrast, studies suggest that products generated by sPLA2 may act as second intracellular messengers, and its enzymatic activity provides a crucial point in the biosynthesis pathways of several classes of inflammatory mediators [21]. In addition, studies performed with other sPLA2s suggest that, during the inflammatory process, leukocytes are recruited to the damaged site (via chemotaxis), where there are conditions necessary to produce a "respiratory explosion." This condition is characterized by high oxygen consumption and the production of reactive oxygen species (ROS), such as the superoxide anion radical ($O_2^{-\bullet}$) and hydrogen peroxide (H_2O_2), which can generate the hydroxyl radical (•OH) directly or indirectly through chemical reactions, such as Fenton and Harber Weiss [22].

Nucleic acids, proteins, and lipids are important targets of ROS, and their attack may lead to an increased risk of mutagenesis due to the modification of these molecules. Moreover, during the inflammatory process, they synthesize soluble mediators, such as arachidonic acid metabolites, cytokines, and chemokines, which lead to the recruitment of more cells that are involved in the inflammatory process to the injured site, thus increasing ROS production. These key mediators may activate signal transduction cascades and induce changes in transcription factors, such as nuclear transcription factor κ-β (NFκ-β) and signal transducer/transcriptional activator 3 (STAT 3), which mediate the response to cellular stress. In addition, induction of cyclooxygenase-2 (COX2) was reported to contribute to nitric oxide synthesis by the enzyme inducible nitric oxide synthetase (iNOS), besides the increased expression of tumor necrosis factor (TNF-α), interleukin-1 (IL-1), interleukin-6 (IL-6), and alterations in the expression of specific microRNAs [23, 24]. It should be noted that nitric oxide can form reactive nitrogen species (RNS) that are highly damaging to cells [25, 26]. Signaling of inflammation is recognized globally by IL-1, IL-6, and TNF-α through Toll-like receptors (TLRs), which belong to the IL-1R family. IL-1 and TNF-α represent the proinflammatory cytokine archetypes that are readily released in response to tissue injury or infection, and they represent a programmed recognition system to trigger inflammation [27–29]. It is important to note that although nitric oxide ($NO^{-\bullet}$), generated by iNOS, has been revealed to have an essential role as a cellular marker, in an environment with oxidative stress, it can react with $O_2^{-\bullet}$ to generate peroxynitrite (NOO^-) and other harmful RNS species [26, 30]. Some authors suggest that preventing the formation of NOO- or inducing its efficient decomposition in inflammatory processes may result in a new therapeutic strategy for the treatment of inflammatory processes [30]. In this context, enzymes such as glutathione peroxidase (Gpx) and peroxiredoxin (Prx) appear to have great importance, since they respond to NOO^- decomposition with high efficiency [30–33].

3. Edema induced by sPLA2 from *Crotalus durissus terrificus* involves oxidative stress signaling

There is no significant evidence that enzymatic toxins from snake venom are able to increase cellular oxidative stress during inflammation [34]; there has been neither a molecular nor a physiological connection shown between edema and other pharmacological activities induced by secretory phospholipase A2 from *Crotalus*

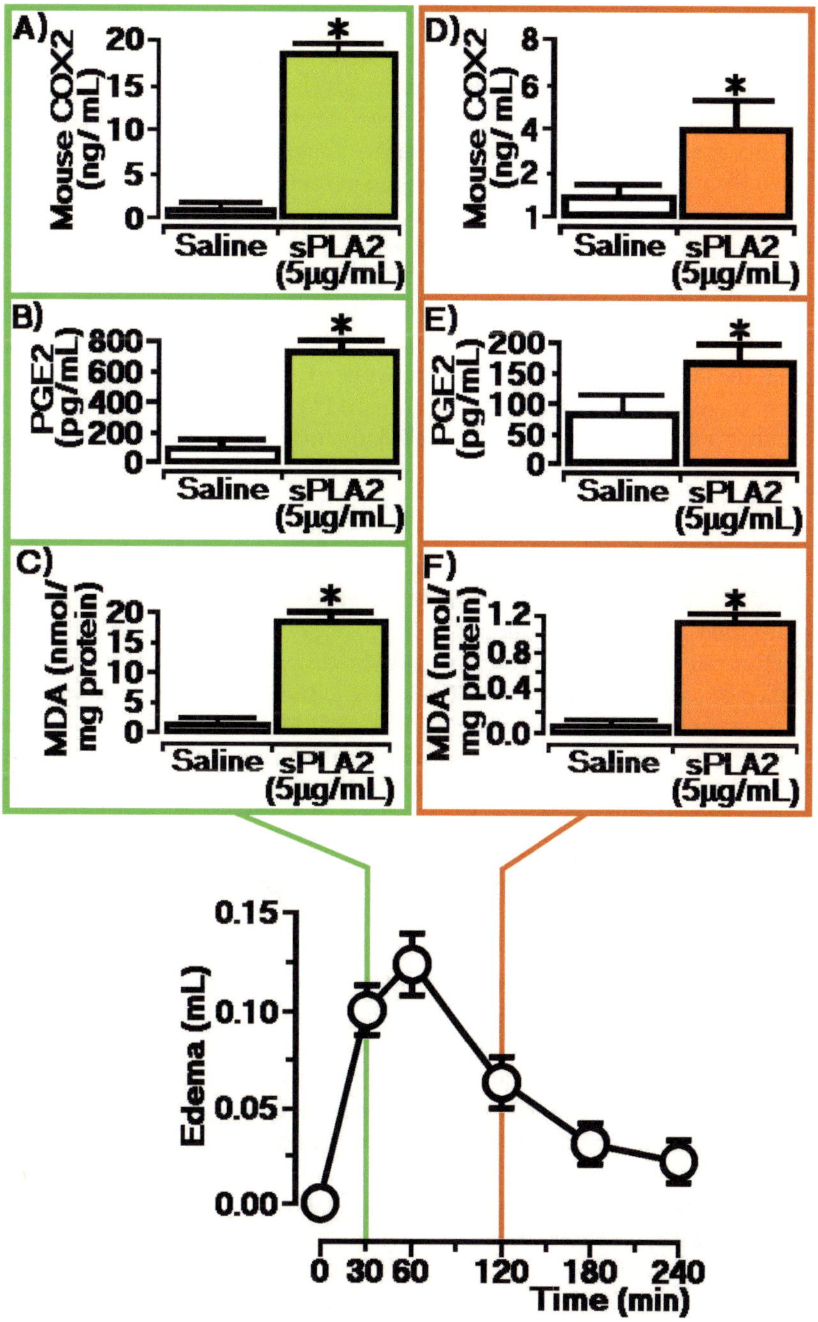

Figure 2.
Edema values induced by Cdt sPLA2 at the adjusted concentration of 10 µg/site (n = 5). Blood and tissue samples were collected from the animals in two phases: at 30 min (B–D) and 90 min (E–F). Measurements of COX2, PGE2, and MDA levels are representative of the analysis of five animals.

durissus terrificus (Cdt sPLA2). However, our results show there is a biochemical, physiological, and temporal connection between the AA metabolism induced by sPLA2, culminating in edema, and the increase of cellular oxidative stress, which was evaluated by measuring malondialdehyde (MDA) content. MDA is a highly reactive three-carbon dialdehyde produced as a byproduct of polyunsaturated fatty acid peroxidation and AA metabolism. This compound produced by oxidative stress can interact with several molecules, including proteins, lipoproteins, and DNA. The main source of MDA in biological samples is the peroxidation of polyunsaturated fatty acids with two or more methylene-interrupted double bonds [35, 36]. H_2O_2 represents a messenger capable of altering redox homeostasis, contributing, at various levels, to related inflammatory diseases. Although H_2O_2 is not an inherently reactive compound, it can be converted into highly reactive and deleterious products that kill cells. In this context, several studies have shown that plant phenolic compounds have great neutralization capacity toward hydrogen peroxide, because these compounds can donate electrons to hydrogen peroxide and neutralize it as water [37, 38].

The edema values plotted in **Figure 2A** were obtained by subtracting the edema values induced by saline (negative control). In this work, we evaluated the activity of COX2 and quantified PEG2 and MDA in blood and tissue samples collected at two different time points—30 and 90 min after sPLA2 administration. **Figure 2A** shows that the amount of COX2 present in swollen tissue after a 5 μg/site Cdt sPLA2 injection was 18.7 ± 1.23 ng/mL (n = 5), compared to values resulting from saline injection that were close to zero. In **Figure 2B**, quantification of PGE2 in the blood of animals collected after Cdt sPLA2 injection (5 μg/site) reveals a concentration of 783 ± 32.4 pg./mL (n = 5), while the saline treatment resulted in 65 ± 18.6 pg./mL (n = 5). Thus, the amount of PGE2 was 12-fold higher than the control values. MDA, produced during lipid peroxidation, is widely used for determining oxidative stress, and the results (shown in **Figure 2C**) indicate that the amount of MDA in plasma was 17.82 ± 8.65 nmol, whereas the amount of MDA released after the saline injection was 0.58 ± 0.22 nmol (n = 5). The results presented in **Figure 2A–C** were obtained before the edema peak, and they show that COX2, PGE2, and MDA levels were extremely high in comparison with the control. However, the samples from the material collected at 90 min or after the peak of edema showed that the COX2, PGE2, and MDA levels did not significantly vary from the control (saline), as shown in **Figure 2D–F**.

4. Edema induced by sPLA2 from *Crotalus durissus terrificus* involves PLC and PKC signaling

The metabolism of AA is a crucial point in the course of proinflammatory secretory phospholipase A2 (sPLA2). These enzymes basically have two distinct molecular domains, one involved in catalysis and the other responsible for receptor interaction, which allows sPLA2 to mobilize other enzymes involved in the production of proinflammatory mediators. In addition, studies indicate that sPLA2 receptors can mediate their activity through G-protein, and therefore, they can trigger the activation of phospholipase C (PLC), activating the phosphokinase C (PKC) signaling pathway and leading to potentialization of cytoplasmic PLA2 (cPLA2) and COX2. In **Figure 2A**, we show the effect of the different treatments on edema induced by sPLA2 of *Crotalus durissus terrificus* (Cdt sPLA2). In **Figure 2A**, the results clearly show that the edema peak induced by sPLA2 produces an increase of 0.278 ± 0.016 mL (5 μg/site; n = 5). About 20 μL of PKC inhibitor (GF109203X; Tocris 30 mg/kg, dissolved in 0.5% DMSO) was injected by endovenous route 30 min (n = 5) before administering sPLA2. The PKC inhibitor was able to significantly reduce edema induced by sPLA2, which was 0.123 ± 0.018 mL (n = 5).

About 20 μL of PLC inhibitor (U73122; Tocris; 30 mg/kg, dissolved in 0.5% DMSO) was injected intravenously 30 min prior to application of sPLA2, revealing that the peak of edema was 0.167 ± 0.021 mL (n = 5), which was significantly lower than the edema peak induced by sPLA2. In **Figure 2B**, we show the effect of the specific inhibitor against cPLA2 and COX2. To assess the effect of arachidonyl trifluoromethyl ketone (AACOCF3) (Sigma-Aldrich, 30 mg/kg, dissolved in 0.5% DMSO), each animal received 20 μL of the compound by endovenous route 30 min (n = 5) before injecting sPLA2; there was a significant decrease in the edema, revealing a maximum edema of 0.218 ± 0.018 mL (n = 5). About 20 μL of *N*-[2-(cyclohexyloxy)-4-nitrophenyl]methanesulfonamide (NS-398) (Cayman Chemical, 30 mg/kg, dissolved in 0.5% DMSO) was injected intravenously 30 min prior to application of sPLA2, and the peak of the resulting edema was 0.146 ± 0.021 mL (n = 5), which is also significantly lower than the edema peak induced by sPLA2.

The **Figures 1** and **2** show that sPLA2 triggers proinflammatory activity by a signaling pathway involving PKC and PLC. In the case of PLC, two products are generated, diacylglycerol (DAG) and inositol triphosphate (IP3), which can induce

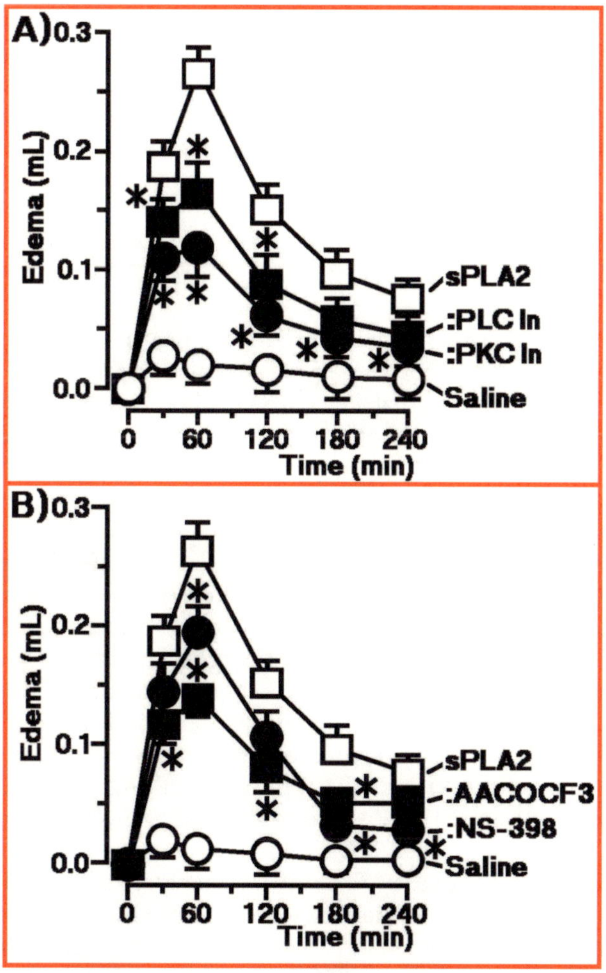

Figure 3.
Values of edema induced by sPLA2 of Cdt at the adjusted concentration of 10 μg/site (n = 5). (A) The effect of the inhibitor of PKC (PKC inhibitor 30′) and inhibitor of PLC (PLC inhibitor 30′). In (B), we evaluated the edema induced by sPLA2 in the presence of a specific inhibitor of cPLA2 (AACOCF3) and inhibitor of COX2 (NS-398).

the phosphorylation of several proteins [14, 39–43]. Thus, the sPLA2 of *Crotalus durissus terrificus* venom may induce an increase in AA metabolism through the interaction of Cdt sPLA2 with G-protein coupled cellular receptors, which activate PLC, generating PUFAs and AA. **Figures 2** and **3** present evidence of interconnections and pathways that generate AA, PLC, and PKC, with cPLA2 and COX2 revealing a possible route of signaling and mobilization of AA, and which could include PUFA release from membrane phospholipids. **Figure 2** also shows that the edema induced by sPLA2 involves the presence of ROS and lipid peroxidation, and that the AA produced can be oxidized to generate MDA as one of the byproducts [39, 44–46]. The results shown in **Figures 2** and **3** suggest that increased cellular oxidative stress and AA mobilization happen intensely and quickly. In this work, we have shown a possible mechanism of edema action induced by sPLA2 from *Crotalus durissus terrificus*, suggesting that the enzymatic activity of Cdt sPLA2 may participate in the inflammatory process, but this activity could also involve the presence of cellular receptors. sPLA2 induces two mechanisms. One mechanism increases oxidative stress, especially in the form of hydrogen peroxide, which leads to increased MDA concentrations; thus, increased oxidative stress has a relevant role in the course of edema. On the other hand, edema induced by sPLA2 also involves a PLC signaling pathway, which mobilizes IP3 (and intracellular calcium) and DAG. These two compounds potentiate the PKC signaling pathway and can lead to a significant increase of cPLA2 through cPLA2 phosphorylation, and this results in enhanced AA metabolism via COX2, an enzyme that could be a second important point in the control of induced inflammation by sPLA2 from *Crotalus durissus terrificus*.

5. "To be or not to be" enzymatically active important for Cdt sPLA2 inflammation

A great question that arises for characterizing the pharmacological and biological activity of Cdt sPLA2 is the importance of the enzymatic activity of sPLA2. For many years, several studies concluded that all biological, physiological, pharmacological, and pathological activity depended on the enzymatic activity of sPLA2, and this remained unanimous until the 1990s. In 1984, the structure and function of the basic sPLA2 of *Agkistrodon piscivorus* were elucidated, leading to the first structural characterization of basic Lys49 sPLA2 [47]. This enzyme also exhibits a moderate enzymatic activity on membrane phospholipids [47]. Subsequently, several works with purified Lys49 basic sPLA2 from snake (*Bothrops sp.*) were able to induce several pharmacological activities, such as pronounced edema, myonecrosis, oxidative stress, nephrotoxicity, insulin degranulation, and anticoagulant activity [17, 48–52]. In the case of the sPLA2 from Cdt, it was observed that its enzymatic activity can be practically abolished through treatment with certain compounds. Numerous natural compounds have the potential to downregulate or modulate the PLA2 activities, as well as other enzymes involved in AA metabolism, including cPLA2 or enzymes involved in prostaglandin metabolization [52–56]. One of the most abundant polyphenols in the human diet, 5-caffeoylquinic acid (5CQA), exerts potent anti-inflammatory, antibacterial, and antioxidant activities. The anti-inflammatory activity of 5CQA may involve multiple mechanisms of action, including the inhibition of the production and secretion of chemical mediators involved in the inflammatory process.

In **Figure 3A**, we show the effect of 5CQA on edema induced by purified sPLA2 from Cdt. When incubated with sPLA2, 5CQA forms a stable molecular complex and may interact with the catalytic site of the protein and strongly decrease its enzymatic activity, changing the secondary structure and leading to the virtual abolishment of sPLA2 enzymatic activity. The edematogenic assay performed with native sPLA2 and 5CQA incubated with sPLA2 clearly showed that edema induced by sPLA2:5CQA was not abolished, but significantly diminished (**Figure 4A**). Thus, in part, the anti-inflammatory effect of 5CQA probably involves the downregulation of pharmacological and enzymatic activity of sPLA2 [57, 58]. In **Figure 3B**, we show the effect of p-bromophenacyl bromide (p-BPB) and umbelliferone (7-HOC) on edema induced by sPLA2. These data reveal that previous treatment with sPLA2/7-HOC highly decreased the proinflammatory effect induced by sPLA2 purified from Cdt, whereas previous treatment with p-BPB abolished this effect.

Unlike flavonoids, both compounds 7-HOC and p-BPB chemically react with the structure of sPLA2 and form highly stable molecular complexes, both inducing large structural modifications that lead to the virtual abolishment of the enzymatic activity of sPLA2. However, the edematogenic experiments conducted with both compounds incubated with sPLA2 did not abolish the proinflammatory effect induced by the protein, as shown in **Figure 3B**. Thus, in this case, comparison between the results from pharmacological assays suggests that the abolishment of enzymatic activity did not suppress or inhibit the pharmacological effect of sPLA2. This paradox between enzymatic activity and pharmacological effect suggests that at least one more complex pharmacological mechanism is involved in the enzymatic activity, which is independent of the enzymatic activity only. These facts suggest the existence of a distinct pharmacological site, as already proposed by [10, 20].

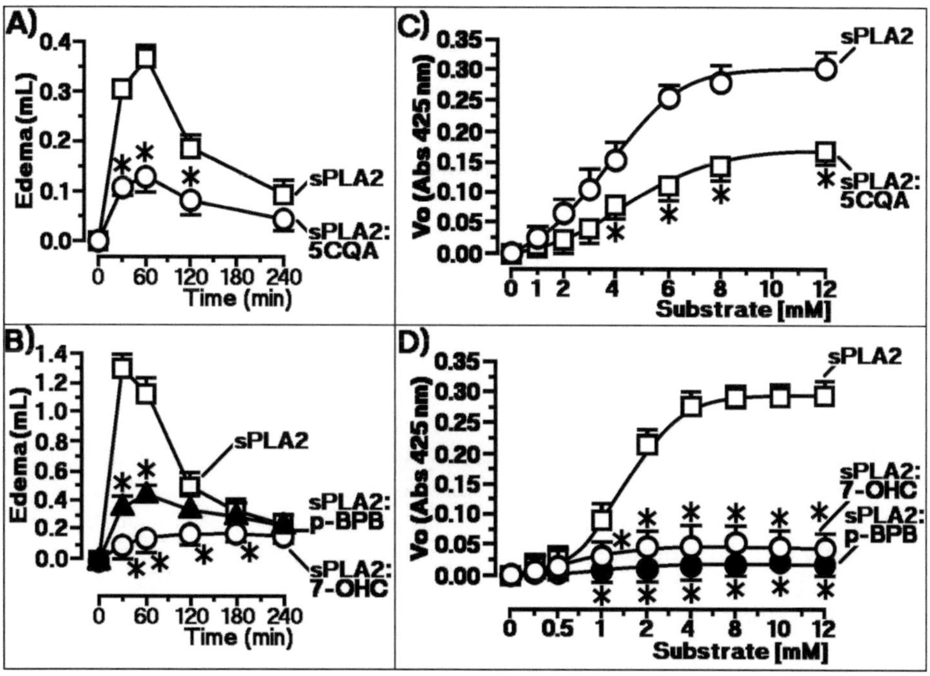

Figure 4.

*In (A), we show paw edema induced after the injection of sPLA2 and sPLA2:5CQA (10 μg/paw) into the right paw of Swiss mice. Measurements were performed after 30, 60, 120, 180, and 240 min, and statistical differences were observed with sPLA2 incubated with 5CQA. In (B), we show enzymatic activity analyzed using 4N3OBA as a substrate, then monitored at a wavelength of 425 nm. In this condition, we examined the effect of the substrate on the enzymatic activity of the native and 5CQA-pretreated sPLA2 (sPLA2:5CQA). Chemical treatment of sPLA2 with 5CQA shifts both the Km and Vmax of the native sPLA2. In (C), we show the mouse paw edema induced by untreated sPLA2 and sPLA2 treated with umbelliferone (sPLA2:7-HOC) or with p-bromophenacyl bromide (sPLA2:p-BPB). Doses of 10 μg/paw were used. Observations were conducted at intervals of 30, 60, 90, 120, and 180 min. (D) Results of enzymatic kinetic analysis of untreated (sPLA2) and 7-HOC- or p-BPB-treated sPLA2 (sPLAs:7-HOC) using 4N3OBA as substrate. sPLA2 Vmax; sPLA2:7-HOC Vmax. For the enzymatic assay results in (B) and (D), each point represents the mean ± SEM of n = 12 and *p < 0.05, and in (A) and (C), each point represents the mean ± SEM of five experiments and *p < 0.05.*

The authors performed several mutagenesis experiments besides those analyzing its catalytic site; there is another pharmacological site located in the calcium binding loop, and the presence of a second pharmacological site has also been considered by [8, 59, 60]. Thus, the enzymatic activity of sPLA2 from Cdt is not crucial for its pharmacological effect and involves other molecular regions, which are collectively designated as pharmacological sites [51, 61]. Some studies performed with sPLA2 from *Crotalus durissus ssp.* showed that the calcium binding loop is involved in the pharmacological activity [57], and others performed by [52] showed that regions close to the active site of sPLA2 could also be involved. According to [54], the C-terminal region could also participate in the interaction with pharmacological receptors. Even so, the crucial and commonly raised point is that the decreased enzymatic activity of Cdt sPLA2 is not accompanied by a proportional decrease in the proinflammatory activity of this enzymatic toxin, as shown by treatment of Cdt sPLA2 with p-BPB (**Figure 4**).

6. Analysis of peroxiredoxins during edema induced by sPLA2 from *Crotalus durissus terrificus*

Oxidative stress is implicated in numerous proinflammatory responses in mammalian cells. H_2O_2 is known to trigger the release and metabolism of AA in various cell types, but the mechanisms involved appear to diverge profoundly from one cell to another. Thus, mobilization of AA in response to oxidative stress appears to be a very complex process involving potentially multiple enzymes and pathways. Studies reveal that the pathological actions induced by sPLA2 from snake venom involve the induction of significant increases in proinflammatory mediators that may also induce a significant rise in reactive oxygen species levels, which can effectively lead to the establishment of numerous events. Thus, the decrease or control of the concentration of these reactive oxygen species may contribute to the decrease of several pathological actions induced by the A2 secretory phospholipase venom. This is evidenced in some studies, such as those that used plant extracts with antioxidant action. The increase in the cellular oxidative process resulting from the mobilization of AA is, in short, associated with the mobilization of H_2O_2 [62–64]; however, this event is not known to be the case for the sPLA2 found in several snake venoms. Some studies show that there is a direct cause and effect relationship between the increased expression of several calcium-dependent PLA2 isoforms and the increased concentration of hydrogen peroxide. Besides, this mechanism involves the presence of G-protein-bound cellular receptors and the consequent protein kinase activation. In addition, much data support the possible existence of cross talk between cPLA2 and sPLA2 while eliciting a full AA release response [63, 65, 66]. During the action of secretory and cytosolic A2 phospholipases, a large amount of AA is produced, which can be considered one of the major components that may be reduced via enzymatic peroxidation to prostaglandins, leukotrienes, thromboxanes, and other cyclooxygenase-, lipoxygenase-, or cytochrome P-450-derived products. Thus, during the process of oxidative stress, AA and other bioactive lipids can be converted into lipid hydroperoxide (LOOH). LOOHs are the primary products of lipid peroxidation, which are relatively stable and long lasting compared to other ROS. Among the many different aldehydes, which can be formed as secondary products during lipid peroxidation, MDA appears to be the most mutagenic [36, 56, 67].

The most accepted paradigm is that oxidative stress initiates a chain reaction of lipid peroxidation, which can be reduced by the presence of tocopherol (e.g., vitamin E) or some other chain-breaking antioxidant. However, several studies have shown that these antioxidants do not neutralize the oxidized phospholipids that were formed prior to the application of these compounds. Thus, lipid peroxidation is not spontaneously reversible, and enzymatic pathways that return lipids to their reduced states have been described. On the other hand, several authors showed that peroxiredoxins (Prxs), particularly Prx 6, play an essential role in the reduction of H_2O_2 and short hydroperoxides; besides, they can directly reduce phospholipid hydroperoxides. Prxs are thiol-dependent peroxidases that catalyze the reduction of a wide variety of hydroperoxides, and the catalytic activity is provided by the presence of a highly conserved catalytic cysteine residue, whose oxidation by hydroperoxide generates sulfenic acid (Cys-SOH). The Prx reduction mechanism involving Cys-SOH is a matter of debate, with glutaredoxin 2 (GRX2), thioredoxin 3 (Trx3), thioredoxin reductase 2 (Trr2), and ascorbate being proposed as possible reducers [68–70]. Several other studies revealed that, during oxidative stress, several Prxs are overexpressed, which can be used as a sensor of oxidative stress in several cells [71–73]. Thus, Prxs represent a group of antioxidant proteins able to decompose several types of hydroperoxides at rates of 10^{5-8} M/second. These enzymes utilize a cysteine residue, which, after the peroxide decomposition, oxidizes (CP-SOH), forming a disulfide bond with a second cysteine, which is reduced by the enzymes thioredoxin (Trx) and thioredoxin reductase (TrxR). In addition, several drugs have been characterized as peroxiredoxin inhibitors, and their use has been helpful in unraveling the physiological and biological roles of certain peroxiredoxins. Among these Prx inhibitors, the best known is adenanthin (Adn), which inhibits Prxs I, Prx II, and other thiol-dependent antioxidant enzymes [74, 75]. Another commercial drug is MJ33, which is described as a potent inhibitor of Prx 6, an extremely essential enzyme for regulating oxidative stress, inflammation, and NADPH oxidase (NOX)2 activation [76]. In addition, conoidin A (ConA) is characterized as a potent inhibitor of peroxiredoxin II, an antioxidant enzyme that acts in the intracellular signaling and defense against oxidative stress [77]. Enzyme inhibition is one of the ways in which enzyme activity is regulated experimentally and naturally.

In the case of the pharmacological tests, inoculation of 5 μg sPLA2 purified from the total venom of *Crotalus durissus terrificus* induced an inflammatory reaction, revealing a typical acute edema with a peak at 60 min (**Figure 5**). To assess the effects of inhibitors, MJ33, ConA, and Adn were injected intraperitoneally (2 μg/g mice) 30 min prior to administration of PLA2 isolated from Cdt venom. As shown in **Figure 5A**, MJ33 showed insignificant anti-inflammatory activity that was only observed along with the edema peak. **Figure 5B** shows the effect of ConA administrated before sPLA2, revealing insignificant inhibition of edema. Although both MJ33 and ConA are essential Prx inhibitors, they display some limitations, as found with MJ33, which is a specific inhibitor of Prx 6. Prx 6 is a complex Prx, exhibiting its maximal antioxidant activity only at acidic pH values [78].

Prx 6 shows calcium-independent phospholipase A2 enzyme activity that is also maximal at acidic pH [79]. The determination of its functional and enzymatic properties was recently elucidated. The low MJ33 inhibitory effect observed in our study could have been due to the presence of a calcium-independent PLA2 domain. Some studies showed that Prx 2 appear to be an essential negative regulator of LPS-induced inflammatory signaling through modulation of ROS synthesis via NADPH oxidase activities; therefore, Prx 2 is crucial for the prevention of excessive host responses to microbial products [80]. Although ConA shows the ability to covalently inhibit Prx 2 activity, the results presented in **Figure 5B** suggest that Prx 2 does not play a relevant role in reducing edema induced by Cdt sPLA2. On the other hand, LPS stimulates monocytes/macrophages through Toll-like receptor

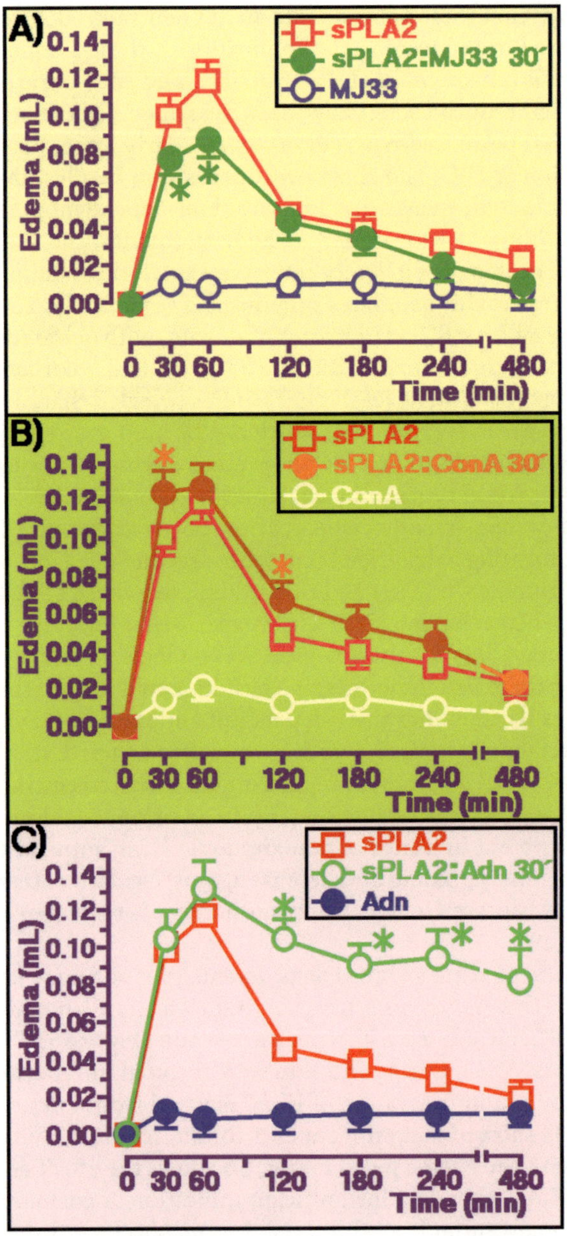

Figure 5.
*In (A), we show paw edema induced after the injection of sPLA2 and sPLA2:MJ33 (5 µg/paw) into the right paw of Swiss mice. Measurements were performed after 30, 60, 120, 180, 240 and 480 min, and statistical differences were observed with sPLA2 applied after MJ33 injection 30 minutes before sPLA2 injection. In (B), we show paw edema induced after the injection of sPLA2 and sPLA2:ConA (5 µg/paw) into the right paw of Swiss mice. Measurements were performed after 30, 60, 120, 180, 240 and 480 min, and statistical differences were observed with sPLA2 incubated with ConA (conoidin A) applied 30 minutes before sPLA2. In (C), we evaluate the effect of sPLA2 in comparison with adenanthin (Adn) previously applied 30 min before sPLA2. Each point represents the mean ± SEM of five experiments and *p < 0.05.*

4 (TLR4), resulting in a series of signaling activation events, which potentiate the production of inflammatory mediators, such as IL-6 and TNF-α [81, 82]. The results presented in **Figure 5C** clearly show that thiol-dependent antioxidant enzymes play an essential role in edema control and recovery induced by sPLA2 purified from

Cdt, and, similar to ConA and MJ33, these enzymes did not exhibit an inhibition or decrease of the edema peaks that occur at 60 min. **Figure 5C** also reveals that the edematogenic effect induced by sPLA2 diminished after 60–90 min, and the hind paw volume returned to its normal volume after 240 min. However, in animals treated with Adn 30 min before the sPLA2 injection, the edematogenic effect persisted for even 8 h after the experiment.

7. Conclusion

During inflammation (edema), induced by purified sPLA2, arachidonic acid generation and its metabolization by COX2 during the edema play crucial roles during this pharmacological event. Arachidonic acid can be mobilized by the catalytic activity of sPLA2 from *Crotalus durissus terrificus* (or other sources) or by activation of cytosolic PLA2. The enzymatic activity of secretory PLA2 (sPLA2) was not crucial for this initial mobilization, and the presence of sPLA2 receptors plays a crucial role in the mobilization of high amounts of arachidonic acid (AA). The classic AA production pathway, which basically involves cPLA2 modulation, also involves the interaction of a more complex pathway that includes the activation of PLC, producing IP3 and DAG. In turn, IP3 and DAG activate PKC, stimulating a strong increase of AA by cPLA2 [1, 83, 84]. However, AA is also mobilized by two other distinct pathways. One involves PLC activation, which has an essential role in AA production by DAG lipase and MAG lipase. In this pathway, catalysis leads to diacylglycerol hydrolysis, releasing a free fatty acid and monoacylglycerol as 2-acyl glycerol, which is converted to AA by MAG lipase action [85–87].

Another pathway that is initiated during AA mobilization involves the release of platelet aggregation factor (PAF)—another subproduct of the enzymatic hydrolysis of membrane phospholipids that cross through the cell membrane—and its specific receptor (PAF receptor or PAF-R) leads to the stimulation of PLC by G-protein [83, 88]. Thus, it is possible that sPLA2 from snake venom, such as venom from *Crotalus durissus terrificus*, mobilizes AA by three different pathways, and AA oxidative metabolism is a key factor that induces increased ROS and oxidative stress during edema. In addition, there are several studies that show AA production is an important way to increase the generation of hydrogen peroxide during inflammation. Thus, it is possible that the action of sPLA2 also increases cell oxidative stress and AA metabolism, culminating in the production of PGE2 and MDA [36]. All this occurs through the interaction of sPLA2 with its receptors to modulate the activity and function of cPLA2 and iPLA2, inducing a significant increase in AA metabolism and COX2 expression, a fact that contributes to the production of free radicals (**Figure 6**) [45, 89–95].

Several studies have shown that arachidonic acid produced by the action of sPLA2 and cPLA2 can activate NADPH oxidase (NOX) enzymes and induce a significant increase in hydrogen peroxide, which gains entry to the intracellular environment through aquaporins and has a predominant role in increasing cellular oxidative stress [91–96]. This would explain the importance of thiol-dependent antioxidant enzymes playing key roles in the control of edema induced by *Crotalus durissus terrificus* sPLA2. On other side, the inflammation (edema) induced by sPLA2 involves the mobilization of arachidonic acid and hydrogen peroxide, and both are the main elements involved in the inflammatory process. The data compiled in this work suggest that oxidative stress is integral in the progression and maintenance of inflammation (edema) induced by sPLA2 from

Crotalus durissus terrificus. Furthermore, our results show that *Crotalus durissus terrificus* sPLA2-induced edema is strongly regulated by thiol-dependent enzymes, and that adenanthin (Adn) was able to neutralize this control and the inflammatory process (edema).

On the other hand, several articles have reported that natural antioxidant compounds, such as flavonoids and related substances, when given prior to sPLA2 injection, have significant anti-inflammatory activities. This probably stems from the ability of many of these compounds to partially inhibit the enzymatic and pharmacological activities of sPLA2 from *Crotalus durissus terrificus*, as well as from their strong antioxidant activities [53–56, 97]. Thus, the search for new natural compounds with anti-inflammatory properties remains an important area of research.

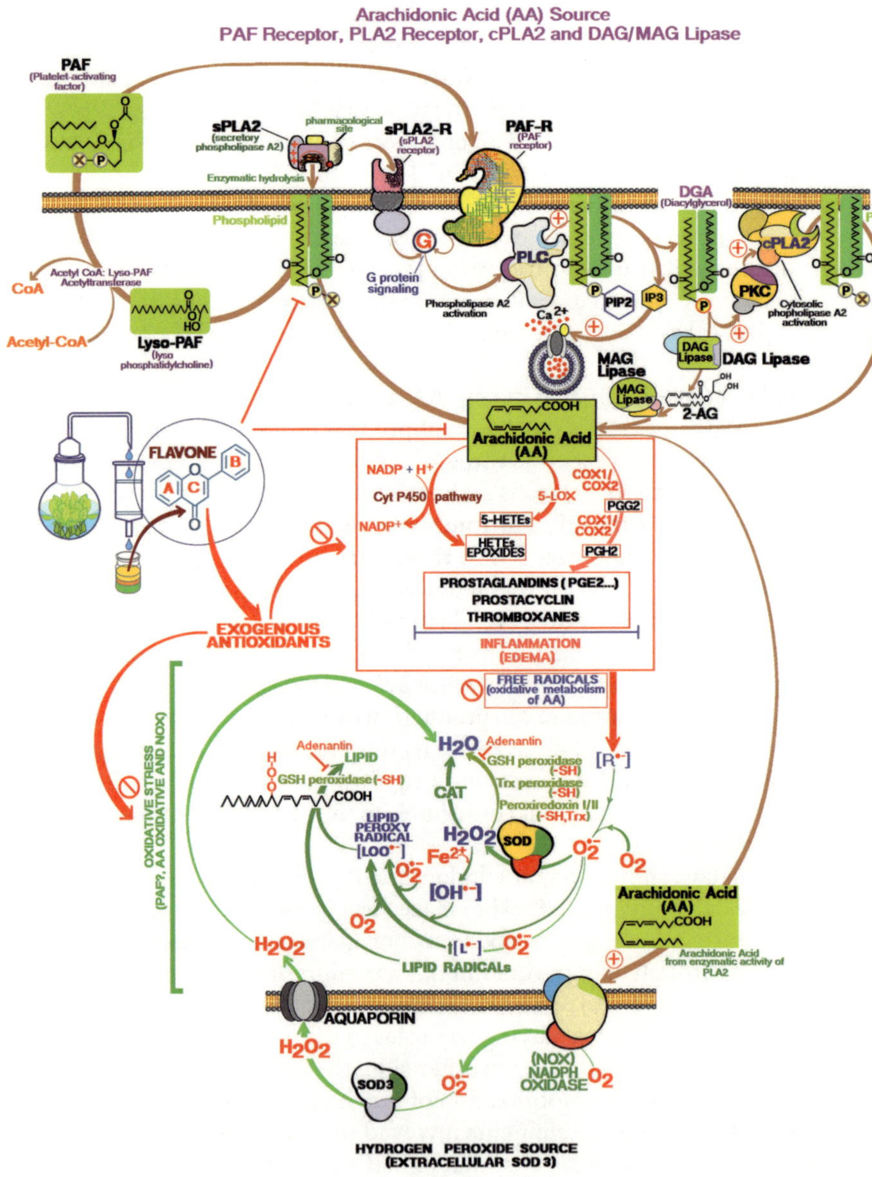

Figure 6.
Summary of possible inflammation mechanism of Cdt sPLA2 action during the inflammatory process.

Acknowledgements

The present project had the financial support of the FAPESP process no: 2017/20291-0 on the responsibility of Professor M.H. Toyama and the resources coming from the FAPESP process no: 2017/19942-7, to CNPq and UNESP.

Conflict of interest

The authors have no conflict of interests to declare.

Author details

Marcos H. Toyama[1*], Caroline R.C. Costa[1], Mariana N. Belchor[1], Danielle P. Novaes[1], Marcos A. de Oliveira[2], Rolando Ie[2], Henrique Hessel Gaeta[1] and Daniela de O. Toyama[1]

1 UNESP, Institute of Biosciences, Campus do Litoral Paulistac (CLP), BIOMOLPEP, São Vicente, São Paulo, Brasil

2 UNESP, Institute of Biosciences, Campus do Litoral Paulista (CLP), LABIMES, São Vicente, São Paulo, Brasil

*Address all correspondence to: marcoshikaritoyama@gmail.com

References

[1] Hanna VS, Hafez EAA. Synopsis of arachidonic acid metabolism: A review. Journal of Advanced Research. 2018;**11**:23-32

[2] Liu C et al. Arachidonic acid metabolism pathway is not only dominant in metabolic modulation but associated with phenotypic variation after acute hypoxia exposure. Frontiers in Physiology. 2018;**9**:236

[3] Hosford D, Braquet P. Platelet-activating factor (PAF), P. J. B. T.-E. of I. E. Delves, 2nd ed. Oxford: Elsevier, 1998, pp. 1971-1973.

[4] da Silva IA Jr, Chammas R, Lepique AP, Jancar S. Platelet-activating factor (PAF) receptor as a promising target for cancer cell repopulation after radiotherapy. Oncogene. 2017;**6**:e296

[5] Kasperska-Zajac A, Brzoza Z, Rogala B. Platelet-activating factor (PAF): A review of its role in asthma and clinical efficacy of PAF antagonists in the disease therapy. Recent Patents on Inflammation & Allergy Drug Discovery. 2008;**2**(1):72-76

[6] Xu B et al. Effects of platelet-activating factor and its differential regulation by androgens and steroid hormones in prostate cancers. British Journal of Cancer. 2013;**109**(5):1279-1286

[7] Murakami M, Taketomi Y, Miki Y, Sato H, Hirabayashi T, Yamamoto K. Recent progress in phospholipase A2 research: From cells to animals to humans. Progress in Lipid Research. 2011;**50**(2):152-192

[8] Murakami M, Sato H, Miki Y, Yamamoto K, Taketomi Y. A new era of secreted phospholipase A 2. Journal of Lipid Research. 2015;**56**(7):1248-1261

[9] Yarla NS, Bishayee A, Vadlakonda L, Chintala R, Duddukuri GR, Reddanna P, et al. Phospholipase A2 isoforms as novel targets for prevention and treatment of inflammatory and oncologic diseases. Current Drug Targets. 2016;**17**(16):1940-1962

[10] Murakami M, Lambeau G. Emerging roles of secreted phospholipase A2 enzymes: An update. Biochimie. 2013;**95**(1):43-50

[11] Pompeia C, Cury-Boaventura MF, Curi R. Arachidonic acid triggers an oxidative burst in leukocytes. Brazilian Journal of Medical and Biological Research. 2003;**36**(scielo):1549-1560

[12] Covey TM, Edes K, Fitzpatrick FA. Akt activation by arachidonic acid metabolism occurs via oxidation and inactivation of PTEN tumor suppressor. Oncogene. 2007;**26**:5784

[13] Chen J-K, Capdevila J, Harris RC. Cytochrome P450 Epoxygenase metabolism of arachidonic acid inhibits apoptosis. Molecular and Cellular Biology. 2001;**21**(18):6322-6331

[14] Balboa MA, Balsinde J. Oxidative stress and arachidonic acid mobilization. Biochimica et Biophysica Acta—Molecular and Cell Biology of Lipids. 2006;**1761**(4):385-391

[15] Yagami T et al., Human group IIA secretory phospholipase A2 induces neuronal cell death via apoptosis. Molecular Pharmacology. 2002;**61**(1):114-126

[16] Elena C, Seila F-F, Vincenza N, Angeles A, Pedro BJ, Gianfrancesco G. Group IIA secretory phospholipase A2 (GIIA) mediates apoptotic death during NMDA receptor activation in rat primary cortical neurons. Journal of Neurochemistry. 2010;**112**(6):1574-1583

[17] Fagundes FHR, Aparicio R, dos Santos ML, Filho EBSD, Oliveira SCB,

Toyama DO, et al. A catalytically inactive Lys49 PLA2 isoform from *Bothrops jararacussu* venom that stimulates insulin secretion in pancreatic beta cells. Protein & Peptide Letters. 2011;**18**(11):1133-1139

[18] Ximenes RM et al. Harpalycin 2 inhibits the enzymatic and platelet aggregation activities of PrTX-III, a D49 phospholipase A (2) from *Bothrops pirajai* venom. BMC Complementary and Alternative Medicine. 2012;**12**:139

[19] Murakami M, Taketomi Y. Secreted phospholipase A_2 and mast cells. Allergology International. 2015;**64**(1):4-10

[20] Lambeau G, Gelb MH. Biochemistry and physiology of mammalian secreted phospholipases A2. Annual Review of Biochemistry. 2008;**77**(1):495-520

[21] Farooqui AA, Horrocks LA. Phospholipase A_2-generated lipid mediators in the brain: The good, the bad, and the ugly. Neuroscience. 2006;**12**(3):245-260

[22] Halliwell B, Gutteridge JMC. Reactive species in disease: Friends or foes? In: Free Radicals in Biology and Medicine. 5th ed. Oxford: Oxford University Press; 2015

[23] Hoesel B, Schmid JA. The complexity of NF-κB signaling in inflammation and cancer. Molecular Cancer. 2013;**12**:86

[24] Kalisperati P et al. Inflammation, DNA damage, helicobacter pylori and gastric tumorigenesis. Frontiers in Genetics. 2017;**8**:20

[25] Szabó C. Hydrogen sulphide and its therapeutic potential. Nature Reviews. Drug Discovery. 2007;**6**:917

[26] Orient A, Donkó Á, Szabó A, Leto TL, Geiszt M. Novel sources of reactive oxygen species in the human body. Nephrology, Dialysis, Transplantation. 2007;**22**(5):1281-1288

[27] Lawrence T. The nuclear factor NF-κB pathway in inflammation. Cold Spring Harbor Perspectives in Biology. 2009;**1**(6):a001651

[28] Reuter S, Gupta SC, Chaturvedi MM, Aggarwal BB. Oxidative stress, inflammation, and cancer: How are they linked? Free Radical Biology & Medicine. 2010;**49**(11):1603-1616

[29] Ong ZY et al. Pro-inflammatory cytokines play a key role in the development of radiotherapy-induced gastrointestinal mucositis. Radiation Oncology. 2010;**5**(1):22

[30] Knoops B, Argyropoulou V, Becker S, Ferté L, Kuznetsova O. Multiple roles of peroxiredoxins in inflammation. Molecules and Cells. 2016;**39**(1):60-64

[31] Barros LO, Silva SV, Almeida FC, Silva ECB, Carneiro GF, Guerra MMP. Efeito da adição de glutationa peroxidase e cisteína ao diluidor de congelação do sêmen equino. Arquivo Brasileiro de Medicina Veterinária e Zootecnia. 2013;**65**(scielo):430-438

[32] Ribas V, García-Ruiz C, Fernández-Checa JC. Glutathione and mitochondria. Frontiers in Pharmacology. 2014;**5**:151

[33] Brown DI, Griendling KK. Regulation of signal transduction by reactive oxygen species in the cardiovascular system. Circulation Research. 2015;**116**(3):531-549

[34] Meléndez-Martínez D et al. Rattlesnake *Crotalus molossus nigrescens* venom induces oxidative stress on human erythrocytes. Journal of Venomous Animals and Toxins including Tropical Diseases. 2017;**23**:24

[35] Del Rio D, Stewart AJ, Pellegrini N. A review of recent studies on

malondialdehyde as toxic molecule and biological marker of oxidative stress. Nutrition, Metabolism, and Cardiovascular Diseases. 2005;**15**(4):316-328

[36] Ayala A, Muñoz MF, Argüelles S. Lipid peroxidation: Production, metabolism, and signaling mechanisms of malondialdehyde and 4-hydroxy-2-nonenal. Oxidative Medicine and Cellular Longevity. 2014;**2014**:360438

[37] Özyürek M, Bektaşoğlu B, Güçlü K, Güngör N, Apak R. A novel hydrogen peroxide scavenging assay of phenolics and flavonoids using cupric reducing antioxidant capacity (CUPRAC) methodology. Journal of Food Composition and Analysis. 2010;**23**(7):689-698

[38] Lee I-T, Lin C-C, Lin W-N, Wu W-L, Hsiao L-D, Yang C-M. Lung inflammation caused by adenosine-5′-triphosphate is mediated via Ca^{2+}/PKCs-dependent COX-2/PGE2 induction. The International Journal of Biochemistry & Cell Biology. 2013;**45**(8):1657-1668

[39] Fonteh AN, Atsumi G, LaPorte T, Chilton FH. Secretory phospholipase A2 receptor-mediated activation of cytosolic phospholipase A2 in murine bone marrow-derived mast cells. Journal of Immunology. 2000;**165**(5):2773-2782

[40] Reséndiz JC, Kroll MH, Lassila R. Protease-activated receptor-induced Akt activation—Regulation and possible function. Journal of Thrombosis and Haemostasis. 2007;**5**(12):2484-2493

[41] Holinstat M et al. Protease-activated receptor Signaling in platelets activates cytosolic phospholipase a(2) (α) differently for cyclooxygenase-1 and 12-lipoxygenase catalysis. Arteriosclerosis, Thrombosis, and Vascular Biology. 2011;**31**(2):435-442

[42] Carrim N et al. Thrombin-induced reactive oxygen species generation in platelets: A novel role for protease-activated receptor 4 and GPIbα. Redox Biology. 2015;**6**:640-647

[43] Duvernay MT, Matafonov A, Lindsley CW, Hamm HE. Platelet lipidomic profiling: Novel insight into cytosolic phospholipase A2α activity and its role in human platelet activation. Biochemistry. 2015;**54**(36):5578-5588

[44] Sun GY et al. Role of cytosolic phospholipase A(2) in oxidative and inflammatory signaling pathways in different cell types in the central nervous system. Molecular Neurobiology. 2014;**50**(1):6-14

[45] Quach ND, Arnold RD, Cummings BS. Secretory phospholipase A(2) enzymes as pharmacological targets for treatment of disease. Biochemical Pharmacology. 2014;**90**(4):338-348

[46] Soichiro T et al. C-type lectin-like domain and fibronectin-like type II domain of phospholipase A2 receptor 1 modulate binding and migratory responses to collagen. FEBS Letters. 2015;**589**(7):829-835

[47] Chen Y-C, Maraganore JM, Reardon I, Heinrikson RL. Characterization of the structure and function of three phospholipases A2 from the venom of Agkistrodon halys pallas. Toxicon. 1987;**25**(4):401-409

[48] Beghini DG, Toyama MH, Hyslop S, Sodek LC, Novello JC, Marangoni S. Enzymatic characterization of a novel phospholipase A2 from *Crotalus durissus cascavella* rattlesnake (maracambóia) venom. Protein Journal. 2000;**19**(8):679-684

[49] Lee W-H et al. Crystallization and preliminary X-ray diffraction studies of piratoxin II, a phospholipase A2 isolated from the venom of *Bothrops pirajai*. Acta Crystallographica. Section D, Biological Crystallography. 1998;**54** (6 II):1229-1230

[50] Hernandez-Oliveira S, Toyama MH, Toyama DO, Marangoni S, Hyslop S, Rodrigues-Simioni L. Biochemical, pharmacological and structural characterization of a new PLA2 from *Crotalus durissus terrificus* (South American Rattlesnake) venom. Protein Journal. 2005;**24**(4):233-242

[51] Dos Santos ML, Fagundes FHR, Teixeira BRF, Toyama MH, Aparicio R. Purification and preliminary crystallographic analysis of a new Lys49-PLA2 from *B. jararacussu*. International Journal of Molecular Sciences. 2008;**9**(5):736-750

[52] Ximenes RM et al. Inhibition of neurotoxic secretory phospholipases A2 enzymatic, edematogenic, and myotoxic activities by harpalycin 2, an isoflavone isolated from Harpalyce brasiliana Benth. Evidence-Based Complementary and Alternative Medicine. 2012;**12**:139

[53] Iglesias CV et al. Effects of morin on snake venom phospholipase A2 (PLA2). Toxicon. 2005;**46**(7):751-758

[54] Fonseca FV et al. Effect of the synthetic coumarin, ethyl 2-oxo-2H-chromene-3-carboxylate, on activity of *Crotalus durissus ruruima* sPLA2 as well as on edema and platelet aggregation induced by this factor. Toxicon. 2010;**55**(8):1527-1530

[55] Belchor MN et al. Evaluation of rhamnetin as an inhibitor of the pharmacological effect of secretory phospholipase A2. Molecules. 2017;**22**(9):1441

[56] Tamayose CI et al. Non-clinical studies for evaluation of 8-C-rhamnosyl apigenin purified from *Peperomia obtusifolia* against acute edema. International Journal of Molecular Sciences. 2017;**18**(9):1972

[57] Toyama DO, Ferreira MJP, Romoff P, Fávero OA, Gaeta HH, Toyama MH. Effect of chlorogenic acid (5-caffeoylquinic acid) isolated from *Baccharis oxyodonta* on the structure and pharmacological activities of secretory phospholipase A2 from *Crotalus durissus terrificus*. BioMed Research International. 2014;**2014**:1-10

[58] Toyama DDO et al. An evaluation of 3-rhamnosylquercetin, a glycosylated form of quercetin, against the myotoxic and edematogenic effects of sPLA2 from *Crotalus durissus terrificus*. BioMed Research International. 2014;**2014**(341270):11

[59] Chioato L, Ward RJ. Mapping structural determinants of biological activities in snake venom phospholipases A2 by sequence analysis and site directed mutagenesis. Toxicon. 2003;**42**(8):869-883

[60] Dennis EA, Cao J, Hsu Y-H, Magrioti V, Kokotos G. Phospholipase A2 enzymes: Physical structure, biological function, disease implication, chemical inhibition, and therapeutic intervention. Chemical Reviews. 2011;**111**(10):6130-6185

[61] Toyama DO, Marangoni S, Diz-Filho EBS, Oliveira SCB, Toyama MH. Effect of umbelliferone (7-hydroxycoumarin, 7-HOC) on the enzymatic, edematogenic and necrotic activities of secretory phospholipase A2 (sPLA2) isolated from *Crotalus durissus collilineatus* venom. Toxicon. 2009;**53**(4):417-426

[62] Balboa MA, Balsinde J. Involvement of calcium-independent phospholipase A2 in hydrogen peroxide-induced accumulation of free fatty acids in human U937 cells. The Journal of Biological Chemistry. 2002;**277**(43):40384-40389

[63] Han WK, Sapirstein A, Hung CC, Alessandrini A, Bonventre JV. Cross-talk between cytosolic phospholipase A2α (cPLA2α) and secretory phospholipase A2 (sPLA2) in

hydrogen peroxide-induced arachidonic acid release in murine mesangial cells: sPLA2 regulates cPLA2α activity that is responsible for arachidonic acid release. The Journal of Biological Chemistry. 2003;**278**(26):24153-24163

[64] Sun GY, Shelat PB, Jensen MB, He Y, Sun AY, Simonyi A. Phospholipases A2 and inflammatory responses in the central nervous system. Neuromolecular Medicine. 2010;**12**(2):133-148

[65] Martínez J, Moreno JJ. Role of Ca^{2+}-independent phospholipase A2 on arachidonic acid release induced by reactive oxygen species. Archives of Biochemistry and Biophysics. 2001;**392**(2):257-262

[66] Adibhatla RM, Hatcher JF. Phospholipase a(2), reactive oxygen species, and lipid peroxidation In CNS pathologies. BMB Reports. 2008;**41**(8):560-567

[67] Catalá A. Lipid peroxidation of membrane phospholipids generates hydroxy-alkenals and oxidized phospholipids active in physiological and/or pathological conditions. Chemistry and Physics of Lipids. 2009;**157**(1):1-11

[68] Wood ZA, Schröder E, Robin Harris J, Poole LB. Structure, mechanism and regulation of peroxiredoxins. Trends in Biochemical Sciences. 2003;**28**(1):32-40

[69] Cordray P, Doyle K, Edes K, Moos PJ, Fitzpatrick FA. Oxidation of 2-Cys-peroxiredoxins by arachidonic acid peroxide metabolites of lipoxygenases and Cyclooxygenase-2. The Journal of Biological Chemistry. 2007;**282**(45):32623-32629

[70] Rhee SG, Woo HA. Multiple functions of peroxiredoxins: Peroxidases, sensors and regulators of the intracellular messenger H_2O_2, and protein chaperones. Antioxidants & Redox Signaling. 2010;**15**(3):781-794

[71] Lee D, Moawad AR, Morielli T, Fernandez MC, O'Flaherty C. Peroxiredoxins prevent oxidative stress during human sperm capacitation. Molecular Human Reproduction. 2017;**23**(2):106-115

[72] Fisher AB. Peroxiredoxin 6 in the repair of peroxidized cell membranes and cell signaling. Archives of Biochemistry and Biophysics. 2017;**617**(Supplement C):68-83

[73] Fisher AB, Vasquez-Medina JP, Dodia C, Sorokina EM, Tao J-Q , Feinstein SI. Peroxiredoxin 6 phospholipid hydroperoxidase activity in the repair of peroxidized cell membranes. Redox Biology. 2018;**14**:41-46

[74] Soethoudt M, Peskin AV, Dickerhof N, Paton LN, Pace PE, Winterbourn CC. Interaction of adenanthin with glutathione and thiol enzymes: Selectivity for thioredoxin reductase and inhibition of peroxiredoxin recycling. Free Radical Biology & Medicine. 2014;**77**:331-339

[75] Siernicka M et al. Adenanthin, a new inhibitor of thiol-dependent antioxidant enzymes, impairs the effector functions of human natural killer cells. Immunology. 2015;**146**(1):173-183

[76] Lee I, Dodia C, Chatterjee S, Feinstein SI, Fisher AB. Therapeutic efficacy of MJ33, a novel inhibitor of phospholipase A2 (PLA2) of peroxiredoxin 6 (Prdx6), in LPS-induced acute lung injury (ALI). FASEB Journal. 2013;**27**(1_supplement):1107.11

[77] Haraldsen JD et al. Identification of conoidin A as a covalent inhibitor of peroxiredoxin II. Organic & Biomolecular Chemistry. 2009;**7**:3040-3048

[78] Chang C-H, Lo W-Y, Lee T-H. The antioxidant peroxiredoxin 6 (Prdx6)

exhibits different profiles in the livers of seawater- and fresh water-acclimated milkfish, Chanos chanos, upon hypothermal challenge. Frontiers in Physiology. 2016;**7**:580

[79] Manevich Y, Reddy KS, Shuvaeva T, Feinstein SI, Fisher AB. Structure and phospholipase function of peroxiredoxin 6: Identification of the catalytic triad and its role in phospholipid substrate binding. Journal of Lipid Research. 2007;**48**(10):2306-2318

[80] Yang C-S et al. Roles of peroxiredoxin II in the regulation of proinflammatory responses to LPS and protection against endotoxin-induced lethal shock. The Journal of Experimental Medicine. 2007;**204**(3):583-594

[81] Fang H et al. Lipopolysaccharide-induced macrophage inflammatory response is regulated by SHIP. Journal of Immunology. 2004;**173**(1):360-366

[82] Hoareau L et al. Signaling pathways involved in LPS induced TNFalpha production in human adipocytes. Journal of Inflammation (London). 2010;**7**:1

[83] Tang X, Edwards EM, Holmes BB, Falck JR, Campbell WB. Role of phospholipase C and diacylglyceride lipase pathway in arachidonic acid release and acetylcholine-induced vascular relaxation in rabbit aorta. American Journal of Physiology-Heart and Circulatory Physiology. 2006;**290**(1):H37-H45

[84] Reisenberg M, Singh PK, Williams G, Doherty P. The diacylglycerol lipases: Structure, regulation and roles in and beyond endocannabinoid signalling. Philosophical Tansactions of the Royal Society of London. Series B, Biological Sciences. 2012;**367**(1607):3264-3275

[85] Labar G, Wouters J, Lambert DM. A review on the monoacylglycerol lipase: At the Interface between fat and endocannabinoid signalling. Current Medicinal Chemistry. 2010;**17**(24):2588-2607

[86] Chang JW et al. Remarkably selective inhibitors of monoacylglycerol lipase bearing a reactive group that is bioisosteric with endocannabinoid substrates. Chemistry & Biology. 2012;**19**(5):579-588

[87] Grabner GF, Zimmermann R, Schicho R, Taschler U. Monoglyceride lipase as a drug target: At the crossroads of arachidonic acid metabolism and endocannabinoid signaling. Pharmacology & Therapeutics. 2017;**175**:35-46

[88] Soliman ML, Ohm JE, Rosenberger TA. Acetate reduces PGE(2) release and modulates phospholipase and cyclooxygenase levels in neuroglia stimulated with lipopolysaccharide. Lipids. 2013;**48**(7):651-662

[89] Rupprecht G, Scholz K, Beck K-F, Geiger H, Pfeilschifter J, Kaszkin M. Cross-talk between group IIA-phospholipase A(2) and inducible NO-synthase in rat renal mesangial cells. British Journal of Pharmacology. 1999;**127**(1):51-56

[90] Patel MI et al. Cytosolic phospholipase a(2)-α: A potential therapeutic target for prostate cancer. Clinical Cancer Research. 2008;**14**(24):8070-8079

[91] Drummond GR, Selemidis S, Griendling KK, Sobey CG. Combating oxidative stress in vascular disease: NADPH oxidases as therapeutic targets. Nature Reviews. Drug Discovery. 2011;**10**(6):453-471

[92] Nisimoto Y, Diebold BA, Constentino-Gomes D, Lambeth JD. Nox4: A hydrogen peroxide-generating oxygen sensor. Biochemistry. 2014;**53**(31):5111-5120

[93] Vieceli Dalla Sega F et al. Specific aquaporins facilitate Nox-produced hydrogen peroxide transport through plasma membrane in leukaemia cells. Biochimica et Biophysica Acta—Molecular and Cell Research. 2014;**1843**(4):806-814

[94] Montezano AC, Touyz RM. Reactive oxygen species, vascular Noxs, and hypertension: Focus on translational and clinical research. Antioxidants & Redox Signaling. 2014;**20**(1):164-182

[95] Lennicke C, Rahn J, Lichtenfels R, Wessjohann LA, Seliger B. Hydrogen peroxide—Production, fate and role in redox signaling of tumor cells. Cell Communication and Signaling: CCS. 2015;**13**:39

[96] Sies H. Hydrogen peroxide as a central redox signaling molecule in physiological oxidative stress: Oxidative eustress. Redox Biology. 2017;**11**:613-619

[97] Ximenes RM et al. Harpalycin 2 Inhibits the Enzymatic and Platelet Aggregation Activities of PrTX-III, a D49 Phospholipase A. BMC Complementary and Alternative Medicine. 2012;**12**:139

Chapter 5

Edema Management in Oral and Maxillofacial Surgery

Renato Yassutaka Faria Yaedu,
Marina de Almeida Barbosa Mello,
Juliana Specian Zabotini da Silveira and
Ana Carolina Bonetti Valente

Abstract

This chapter will discuss the expected edema and intercurrences in maxillofacial surgery, which involves important anatomical structures, such as the upper airways. It will also discuss important issues such as intrinsic and extrinsic enhancers of edema and the main consequences of a severe edema setting according to physiological, functional, and psychosocial points of view. Edema assessment and measurement is still performed subjectively in the clinical routine. However, for the accomplishment of studies, more objective forms are being tested, but still not very successful for clinical applicability. It is known that the best way to deal with edema is prevention; so in elective surgeries, much is discussed about the best management forms. This way, besides edema prevention, it is important not to cause unwanted reactions for the patient or in the performed procedure. Therefore, it will also be debated about preoperative medications and their consequences. Another point discussed involves main treatments for the underdeveloping edema and the one already installed, such as manual lymphatic drainage therapy, a treatment that is well known and used in other specialties, but is still very little widespread among maxillofacial surgeons.

Keywords: edema, oral surgery, maxillofacial surgery, postoperative period, postoperative care

1. Introduction

Every surgical procedure presents pain and edema in a variable degree, and many pharmacological and alternative methods have been used in an attempt to control and reduce them.

Maxillofacial surgery acts on the patient's face. The maxillofacial surgical procedures include outpatient surgeries using local anesthesia and also more extensive and invasive procedures under general anesthesia. The most used procedures are exodontia, biopsies, surgical cysts and tumors treatment, bone grafts, rehabilitations with osseous integrable implants, orthognathic surgery, face trauma treatment, and infections treatments.

An inflammatory response is expected after any injury or surgical procedure, in an attempt to defend and repair damage tissues. Inflammatory mediators (prostaglandins, leukotrienes, bradykinin, and others) are released, and consequently,

IntechOpen

there is an increase in vascular dilatation and permeability, resulting in an edema. However, when it comes to facial edema, the major concerns are related to airway permeability, making the care with this edema a fundamental step for the treatment. It is known that in outpatient surgeries, the extent and the consequence related to edema are smaller and more predictable than in hospital surgeries, but not less important, as we will discuss further on the topic of complications.

Many studies discuss the importance of edema for such surgeries, especially outpatient procedures, which not always presents significant amounts of edema. Besides that, the discussions about the treatment are not conclusive.

Edema is characterized by the excess of plasma proteins in the interstitial space. Its formation occurs when the lymphatic flow exceeds the transport capacity of the lymphatic system or when this system becomes inefficient in absorbing and transporting these proteins [1]. Although the primary edema is a condition usually developed by vascular and/or congenital diseases, the secondary edema occurs due to a lymphatic system injury, whether by infection, cancer, or surgery [2, 3].

2. Edema: risk factors

Despite the fact that the edema is part of the inflammatory process, and therefore, a consequence of the surgical process, the severity and localization of it can be related to some factors, intrinsic to the patient or related to the surgery.

The increase in the surgical procedure difficulty due to one or more of these factors directly influences on the severity and extension of the postoperative morbidities [4].

2.1 Preexisting conditions

Any condition that affects postsurgical inflammatory response directly interferes with the postoperative quality, recovery, and also with the edema formation. Therefore, all efforts are made to maintain airway permeability and prevent its obstruction.

An worrying condition is the angioedema, which results from changes in the immunoglobulins involved in the inflammatory response. Due to the fact that is a severe, acute, and rapidly evolving edema that mainly affects the larynx, pharynx, and face, there is a great risk of airways obstruction, and therefore, it is associated with reintubation and risk of death [5–8].

Unfortunately, the occurrence of angioedema is a difficult prediction factor, mainly if the patient never presented its manifestation. For this reason, a rapid and accurate diagnosis is essential, as well as the establishment of artificial airways and adequate drug treatment [6–8].

2.2 Body mass index (BMI)

The BMI consists in the division of ratio of body weight per height of the individual. Despite there is no consensus in the literature, some studies have related BMI with the severity of postoperative edema [4, 9–11].

Although is expected that individuals with higher BMI (overweight) develop greater edema, this correlation is not always found. Therefore, on those studies, other variables such as age and gender were considered more influential than BMI in the postoperative edema formation [4, 9].

The relation between BMI and the facial edema occurs because adipose tissue is responsible for most of the pro-inflammatory cytokines. So people with a higher BMI have more adipose tissue, more inflammatory biomarkers and, consequently, greater inflammation and greater edema [11, 12].

In the literature, a positive correlation between BMI values and developed edema is observed. Thus, individuals with higher BMI develop greater edema, but their rate of reduction is faster in the first postoperative days [10, 11]. However, individuals with lower BMI develop smaller edema, and although the rate of reduction in the first postoperative days is slower, the total resolution of edema occurs before than in people with a high BMI [10].

2.3 Operative time

The duration of surgery is appointed as one of the predictive factors for a greater or smaller postoperative edema. This is because a longer surgery requires a greater manipulation of the tissues, and consequently, a greater inflammatory process [4, 13–16].

The increasing of the surgical time can occur due to factors related to the surgery and intrinsic to the patient, such as age and anatomical variations. In addition of it, the surgeon's experience is related to the increasing or decreasing of the operative time [13, 15, 17].

The operative time is predictive not only for the amount of edema, but also to the intensity of pain and trismus. This is due to a bigger trauma or intraoperative complications, which is directly related to the increase in surgical time [4, 14, 16]. Thus, although studies indicate that there is a correlation between high surgical time and greater postoperative edema, factors that caused an increasing of the surgical time must be considered.

2.4 Type of surgery and surgical trauma

The type of surgery performed interferes directly in postoperative edema. Thus, large surgery (such as orthognathic surgery) is expected to cause a greater inflammatory process and, therefore, larger and more diffuse edema than minor surgery (third molar extraction, for example) [14, 18].

However, when it comes to the same type of surgery, variations can occur depending on the surgical difficulty level. It is expected that a major difficulty surgery occurs in a longer surgical time and causes a more intense and extensive surgical trauma. Therefore, the inflammatory process will be bigger, as well as the postoperative edema [4, 11, 14, 16, 19].

Some factors can contribute to the increasing of the surgery difficulty level, such as denser bones, teeth with roots formed and consolidated in the bone by masticatory stimuli, quantity of procedures, and unfavorable dental position [9, 11, 14].

The position of the third lower molar closer to the lingual wall appears to result in more severe postoperative edema, due to a more extensive surgical trauma in consequence of the bone amount removed [11]. In addition, the distal and horizontal position of the teeth is related to the greater postoperative edema, as the need to perform osteotomy and odontosection, which results in a greater surgical trauma [14].

In large surgeries such as orthognathic surgery, factors like the duration of the surgery, combined procedures (maxillary and mandibular osteotomy and mentoplasty) and bone density are related to the amount of postoperative edema. Thus, surgeries in only one of the jaws present less surgical trauma than the bimaxillaries, and therefore, develop smaller edema. When it comes to bone density, thicker and denser bones cause more difficulty in the osteotomies, increasing surgical trauma and inflammatory process [18, 20].

Surgeries involving maxilla, such as Le Fort I osteotomy, result in greater internal edema to the cavities, increasing the risk of airways obstruction [18].

2.5 Surgeon's experience

It is very difficult to evaluate the experience of one surgeon, since there are no preestablished protocols to separate experienced surgeons from inexperienced. Some papers use the classification based on the training phase in which the surgeon is, others how long the surgeon is graduated, or even the amount of surgeries already performed by the professional [14, 17, 21, 22].

Surgeon's experience indirectly interferes with postoperative edema. This is because it does not directly affect the factors that converge to the edema formation, but rather those that are related to the severity of the postoperative edema [14, 17, 21, 22].

The greater the experience of the surgeon, the lower is the occurrence of postoperative complications. In addition, the more experienced surgeon is capable to solve more quickly and efficiently intraoperative complications, as well as perform the surgical procedure accurately. And more, the surgeon's experience is closely related to possible planning errors (such as implant and orthognathic surgeries) and execution. Less experienced surgeons are more likely to make these mistakes, culminating in the prolongation in the surgery duration and even possible the need for surgical reintervention [17, 21, 22].

Therefore, the surgeon's experience interferes in the surgical time, trauma extension, and blood loss, which are decisive factors for the inflammatory process and, consequently, for postoperative edema [14, 21].

2.6 Blood loss

Although there are no studies relating the amount of transoperative bleeding to edema, it is known that there is a relation between blood loss and postoperative quality.

Lymphedema is characterized by the increasing volume of a body segment. However, this swelling is not always present only by edema, especially in the postoperative cases. Hematomas and clots also cause enlargement of the region volume. That way, trans- and postoperative bleeding contributes to swelling, as there is an increase in the body segment volume but, unfortunately, it is not possible to clearly distinguish whether it is edema, hematomas, or the combination of them [23].

Besides that, the amount of blood lost during surgery influences the inflammatory process. The greater the bleeding, the more intense and lasting is the inflammatory process, and the greater is the postoperative edema [18, 20].

Due the fact that these surgeries are performed in oral cavity, there is a possibility of swallowing blood during the surgical procedure. Besides the malaise caused by blood loss, postoperative vomiting increases the pressure in the newly operated region and causes an increasing of the edema. In addition, due to the bleeding caused by the pressure increasing, there may be formation and/or increasing of hematomas [24–26].

Therefore, strategies are necessary in order to reduce the amount of bleeding and, consequently, not only to improve postoperative quality, but also to help control facial edema and reduce the period of hospitalization after oral and maxillofacial surgeries.

2.7 Induced hypotension

The mean arterial pressure interferes directly in the bleeding and, thus in surgical time. Lower mean blood pressure reduces transoperative bleeding, reducing as well the amount of blood lost, improving the visualization of the surgical field, reducing surgical time, and the formation of hematomas and swelling [27–30].

The hypotension induced during surgery is a strategy to improve the surgical field through the reduction of bleeding and consequently reducing surgical time and postoperative inflammatory process [24, 27, 28, 31]. Induced hypotension, or controlled hypotension, is defined by the reduction of systolic blood pressure to 80–90 mmHg with a reduction in mean arterial pressure (MAP) to 50–65 mmHg or a 30% reduction in MAP [30, 32]. It is obtained through medicament during anesthesia. Despite being considered safe and presenting proven benefits, induced hypotension requires preparation and good skill of the anesthesiologist and should not be maintained for long time due to hypoperfusion risks of the organs such as the central nervous system (CNS), heart, liver, and kidneys [29, 32].

Although in the current literature have not yet been found studies that have investigated the correlation between hypotension induced in face surgeries and postoperative edema, hypotension is capable to improve several factors involved with the development and amount of edema.

2.8 Age

The age at which the patient is operated has been pointed out as one of the predictive factors for the development of bigger or smaller edema. Despite studies attempt to find this relation, there is still no consensus on the relation between age and severity of developed edema [4, 14, 15, 33, 34].

On the one hand, some authors argue that face surgery in younger individuals results in less difficulty in the procedure and consequently less surgical trauma and less edema [11]. On the other hand, there are authors who affirm that the reduction of the inflammatory response and diminution of the lymphatic system elasticity occur with the increase in the age. Thus, older individuals develop less edema and have less efficacy of the lymphatic system [4, 14–16, 33–35]. Besides that, older patients have a prolonged inflammatory process and, therefore, slower reduction of edema [15].

2.9 Gender

Another factor pointed as an influencer in the formation of edema and its quantity is gender. Although is expected that women develop greater swelling due to hormonal variations, use of oral contraceptives, and bigger risk for dry socket, the male gender is pointed out in studies as being more predisposed to a greater amount of postoperative edema [11, 13, 34].

Factors such as increased bone density and thickness and stronger muscles can do postoperative edema to be more severe in men than in women. This is because they are factors that directly interfere in the level of difficulty and quantity of surgical trauma, injuring more lymphatic structures and increasing the inflammatory response, generating more edema [11, 34].

However, the smaller thickness of the female mandible increases the chances of fracture of the mandibular ramus during third molar extraction, increasing surgical trauma [4, 13].

Anyway, this significant difference in the amount of developed edema is observed on the first postoperative day, but it is irrelevant on the seventh day [11, 34].

Thus, even in studies in which the amount of postoperative edema does not present a significant difference between the genders, the extent of surgical trauma and the occurrence of intraoperative complications are indicated as the main influential factors for the severity of postoperative edema [10, 19]. However, the occurrence and intensity of these factors are difficult to predict, so that is the reason to consider the gender and its risk factors and predict the level of the surgery difficulty.

2.10 Vomiting

The presence of nausea followed or not by vomiting is a factor that can be observed in clinical practice. Increased patient effort during vomiting increases facial edema and also stimulates postoperative bleeding. However, although the relation between nausea and vomiting with edema is not mentioned in the literature, it is a fact that can be verified in clinical practice, especially in the postoperative period of orthognathic surgery.

2.11 Postoperative rest

Another important factor related to the control or prevention of edema formation consists on the postoperative rest and positioning of the patient. It is known that the dorsal decubitus tilted by approximately 30° decreases the pressure in the face blood vessels and helps to control the bleeding and edema.

After surgery, the periosteum is detached in the operated region. Thus, the mobilization of this periosteum, by movement or compression of this region, stimulates the inflammatory response potentiating the edema.

Although these factors are not in specific scientific studies, clinical observation makes it possible to affirm the importance of both bedside and resting care in the postoperative period of face surgeries.

3. Forms of evaluation and edema measurement

In maxillofacial surgery, the observation, control, and reduction of edema are important postoperative factors, due to the possibility of airway compromise. In this way, surgeries with potential formation of exacerbated edema should present evaluation and control of this condition, in order to assist the decision related to the maintenance or replacement of the edema treatment protocol.

Between the techniques described for evaluating edema, the most used ones clinically are subjective, and are totally dependent on the professional's experience and on the patient's report. Although there are more objective methods of clinical evaluation with good reproducibility, these are limited to the upper and lower limbs, making it impossible to apply to regions such as head and neck [35, 36].

In the head and neck regions, most of the methods reported in the literature measure the edema by the distance between two points, based on anatomical points, such as mandibular angle, lateral, and medial epicanto of the eyes and middle of the chin.

Other measurement devices that provide more accurate data about the changes related to edema values include imaging exams. However, due to the fact that it involves high cost and exposes the patient to ionizing radiation, these techniques need specific indication [37]. Ultrasonography (US), magnetic resonance imaging, and computed tomography are examples of usable exams [38]. The US presents changes in the echogenicity of its images, which are not specific for volume changes caused by increasing of subcutaneous fluids [39]. In addition, to the face part, the echographic measurement does not always point the more swollen site due to the reproduction of the distances from the skin to the bone, which leads to imprecise and disproportionate results [40].

Bioelectrical impedance is another method described in the literature for the measurement of edema. This technique measures the amount of peripheral and total fluid in the body. However, low-cost and easily applicable devices for measuring body edemas as well as limbs are still scarce [36].

The evaluation methods developed for use in researches have evolved greatly. The first studies used subjective methods and difficult reproducibility, which made them less reliable in relation to the real magnitudes and behavior of edema. Van Gool et al. and Album et al. demonstrated the lack of correlation between subjective evaluations and objective measures of edema [41–43]

The measurement methods should be capable of being used in clinical and patient tolerable trials. Thus, portable devices were studied with the objective that they could be easily used with precision and transported to the place where the patient is, making possible to obtain early measures and follow-up of the edema [42, 44].

Therefore, objective measurement methods represent a more appropriate approach to the problem. However, these measurements should be evaluated and validated by doing repeated measurements on untreated individuals to verify its accuracy.

The methods already tested and used in studies were [45, 46]:

- facial bow method;
- ultrasound method;
- stereophotographic method;
- method of cuboid element;
- measurements with tape measure;
- sonographic evaluation;
- photo evaluation;
- face scanning; and
- evaluation with 3D mold.

4. Complications related to the postoperative edema

The early stage of inflammation presents accumulation of fibrin and polymorphonuclear neutrophils in the extracellular space of injured tissues. The processes that occur in this phase are vessel diameter change, increased vascular permeability, exudate formation and migration of neutrophil cellular exudates into the extravascular space. The chemical mediators of acute inflammation include histamine, prostaglandins, leukotrienes, serotonin, and various cytokines. It is known that prostaglandin associated to bradykinin has the most potent pain-activating effect [14, 47, 48].

The control of inflammation and, therefore, swelling aims to reduce pain and improve life quality in the postoperative period. The processes of the inflammatory mediator may last up to 96 hours.

Trismus occurs as a result of muscle spasm caused by the inflammatory process. In this process, there is compression of the nervous structures by the edema, leading to the limitation of movement accompanied by a painful sensation, which can be from discomfort to severe pain [14, 47, 49].

Although it is subjective and dependent on several factors, the evaluation of postoperative pain in maxillofacial surgeries is essential, since this is one of the main complaints of operated patients and is directly related to edema. Therefore, pain, edema and trismus are consequences of the formation and release of prostaglandins, bradykinins, and other mediators of inflammatory response [14, 47].

Patients with moderate and severe edema may be unable to discern pain from discomfort caused by stretching of the skin by increased facial volume. In addition, the pain is related to the patient's emotional state, being influenced directly by their mood, level of satisfaction, and well-being [18, 20, 50].

Therefore, edema can also cause psychological and emotional problems due to the esthetic alteration of the affected body segment [50]. The maxillofacial surgeries carry great esthetic and functional expectations. However, patients, although relieved to have undergone surgery, may present mood swings due to the difficulty of self-care, pain, and edema. Changes in body image are one of the major complaints related to edema [20].

Edema can also influence self-care. This is because it makes feeding and oral hygiene difficult because it prevents proper visualization of the oral cavity and limits the range of mandibular movement. In addition, patients submitted to orthognathic surgery have shown greater difficulty in removing and placing intermaxillary locking elastics according to the degree of edema they develop [20].

Internal edema to the cavities is a major concern in the postoperative period. This is because breathing may be affected by pressure and possible obstruction of upper airway structures, causing respiratory distress and discomfort, and even leading to the need for re-intubation or performing a tracheostomy in the most serious, life-threatening cases [6, 8].

Severe postoperative edema is an important complication that can affect upper airway permeability and may lead to obstruction in more severe cases. The procedure that presents the greatest risk of airway obstruction due to edema is the Le Fort I type osteotomy, performed in the maxilla and covering the floor of the nasal fossa [18]. Thus, severe edema can cause respiratory and functional problems, which increases hospitalization time and the need for ICU admission.

Peripheral nerve damage is the result of direct or indirect trauma to a nerve. The direct relationship between edema and paresthesia is known and can be explained by the spatial relationship of the nerve vessels with adjacent structures, such as muscles and bones.

Following the same mechanism of acute compressive neuropathies, facial edema caused by surgical trauma, infections, fractures, or injuries can compress the sensory and motor nerves of the face (trigeminal nerve and facial nerve). This compression, or even stretching of these nerve bundles, impairs the conduction of the nerve impulse, resulting in paresthesia and even temporary paralysis.

Studies on nerve conduction measured the magnitude of the conduction blockade of nerve action potentials and the focal slowing of conduction. Direct correlation between degree of changes and duration of compression was demonstrated. Another observation is related to local ischemia, which, in combination with direct pressure effects, contributes to the development of compressive neuropathies. In severe cases of acute compression, with direct relation to extensive and prolonged edema, remyelination of nerve fibers can take weeks or months after resolution of compression.

Another aspect in relation to the neurosensorial disorders is related to the inflammatory mediators that are released when a trauma to the tissue occurs. These are located in the edema region and act temporarily as chemical irritants to the nerves.

Thus, studies attempt to relate the use of corticosteroids with the improvement of neurosensory symptoms after tissue trauma with considerable edema. However, due to the lack of standardization of the applied tests and classification, only the presence or absence of the disorder was considered [51]. More controlled clinical trials need to be performed to obtain data on neurosensory disorders.

Some local factors (directly related to the wound) and systemic (linked to the individual) can interfere in the cicatricial process, facilitating complications and sequels and causing esthetic and functional damages to the tissue.

Local factors: dimension and depth of the lesion; level of contamination; presence of net collections (bruises, ecchymosis, edema); tissue necrosis and local infection; poor vascular supply; surgical technique used, material and technique of suture, types of bandages; and traction or mechanical pressure on the scar [52–54].

Systemic factors: age group, ethnic origin, nutritional status, presence of chronic diseases, and use of medicines.

Angiogenesis is essential to healing wounds as it provides restoration of blood flow and transport of nutrients to cells as well as transporting the components of the immune system. Edema makes this stage difficult, because the excessive distension of the tissues leads to compression of the newly formed vessels, altering the blood flow. In this way, the body's capability to carry defense cells and administered antibiotics is impaired, making healing more difficult.

Hypoxia in the area of the lesion stimulates angiogenesis responsively, aiming formation and remodeling of the extracellular matrix for tissue repair. However, this process is limited to the first 48 hours of the beginning of the repair process, being detrimental to vascular neoformation and regulation of healing factors.

Fibroblasts are involved in deposition of the extracellular matrix and also in approaching the edges of the wound. Thus, the tissue distension caused by edema compromises this narrowing and tissue reepithelialization, making it difficult to form the fibrin network and providing a disordered growth of collagen, which leads to the formation of hypertrophic scars [53].

With excessive edema, a lesion that could have first-intention healing with contact between the edges becomes second intention, due to tissue tension, causing dehiscences of suture and separation of the wound edges. In addition, local edema obstructs the lymphatic vessels, facilitating the accumulation of catabolites and producing a greater level of inflammation.

5. Medications used for edema control

5.1 Corticoids

Inflammation is the local physiological response to tissue injury. Although some amount of inflammation is needed for proper wound healing, the excess of inflammation leads to severe edema and pain that causes discomfort to the patient.

The use of corticosteroids during orthognathic surgery is a fairly common practice for faster resolution of facial edema [55]. However, there is no consensus on its uses, its benefits, and adverse effects. The comparison of drugs in published studies is difficult due to the variety of parameters and methods used. Corticosteroids help reduce facial edema by acting as immunosuppressants that block the early and late stages of inflammation, decreasing the dilation and permeability of blood vessels. From this, there is a reduction of the amounts of liquid, proteins, macrophages, and other inflammatory cells present in the areas of tissue injury. In this terms, corticoids have a beneficial effect on the inflammation control, and consequently, on edema [51].

The use of steroids in patients can be by mouth, intramuscular injection, or intravenous methods. A recent study compared the effects of different routes of methylprednisolone uses on edema and trismus after extraction of third molars [56]. It was concluded that the systemic application of a steroid is more effective for improving the range of motion. However, direct injection of the steroid into the musculature had the best effect in reducing postoperative swelling.

Another study by Ehsan et al. [57] analyzed the effect of preoperative submucosal uses of dexamethasone on swelling and trismus on third molar extraction. They found out that this injection was very effective in reducing these postoperative conditions. In another study, it was found that the uses of corticosteroids in the preoperative period through the parenteral route have a greater impact in the reduction of postoperative swelling and trismus [58]. In addition, patients with zygomatic bone fractures usually present swelling, pain, and trismus before surgery, requiring prolonged treatment than removal of the third molars. Therefore, in order to benefit from steroid medication, patients with facial fractures should receive higher doses than patients undergoing minor surgeries [45].

The use of intravenous systemic corticosteroids before orthognathic surgery helps to reduce facial edema, but adverse effects are not well described in literature [59]. The use of corticosteroids before, during, and after orthognathic surgery, independently of the dosages, promotes reduction in facial edema, mainly until the third postoperative day. The most commonly used corticosteroids are dexamethasone, methylprednisolone, and betamethasone [51, 60]. Betamethasone is considered a potent steroid because it has high anti-inflammatory activity and does not cause fluid retention [60]. Dexamethasone is a highly selective and long-acting synthetic corticosteroid that has potent anti-inflammatory action [61].

In oral surgery, of all pharmacological agents tested, steroids seem to be the most successful for inflammation control. Corticosteroids, such as dexamethasone, may inhibit the early stage of the inflammatory process and have been widely used in different regimens and pathways to decrease inflammatory process after third molar surgery [62].

Although steroids seem to be the most successful in relieving edema after extraction of the third molar, the immunosuppressive effects of cortisol and its synthetic analogues are well known [63]. Previous studies about dexamethasone in third molar surgeries have concluded the need of accurate clinical research for better evaluation protocols for corticosteroid use [64].

5.2 Analgesics

The use of analgesics and nonsteroidal anti-inflammatory drugs alone or in combination with corticosteroids or opioids is common after third molar surgeries to reduce facial edema and pain [65]. When nonsteroidal anti-inflammatory drugs are given prior to surgery, they significantly reduce postoperative edema [66]. One study compared the use of diclofenac potassium, etodolac, and naproxen sodium given in preoperative of third molar surgery and concluded that diclofenac potassium showed better edema reduction [67]. Another study compared the use of diclofenac potassium alone or in combination with dexamethasone and concluded that combined therapy was more effective in reducing pain, trismus, and edema after third molar surgery [68]. There is no consensus in literature about which analgesics to use, for how long, and what is the best dosage with the least adverse effects.

5.3 Hyaluronic acid (HA)

A new drug trend that has been used to control edema development is hyaluronic acid (HA). Nowadays, few studies are found in literature and their actual efficacy as well as their use is not well established yet. HA is a high molecular weight glycosaminoglycan, a major component of the extracellular matrix [69]. It can be found in several tissues, and one of its properties is formation induction of early granulation tissue, which helps the healing and improves inflammatory process [70]. HA turned out to be effective in reducing edema when used as spray after third molar extraction [70, 71]. The use of HA associated with platelet-rich fibrin was capable to decrease edema after third molar extraction surgery, compared to the isolated use of platelet fibrin [72]. Further studies using HA in larger groups and in other types of surgeries are necessary to establish a protocol use, consensus on its effects, and investigation of possible adverse effects.

5.4 Adverse effects of medications at the doses used

The adverse effects of corticosteroids are rare but important to evaluate. Complications are well known and include immune system suppression, hypertension, hyperglycemia, suppression of adrenal corticosteroid activity, allergic reactions, skin steroid acne, glaucoma, and psychiatric disorders. In addition, the use over 7 days may lead to development of Cushing's syndrome [54, 73].

Thus, it is noted that complications are related to prolonged use. In maxillofacial surgeries, it is generally used for a short time, at most 24–48 hours, so side effects are rare.

Also, it is known that anti-inflammatory drugs for edema control may increase bleeding by directly interfering in coagulation cascade. Thus, its benefit regarding edema control is compromised.

6. Most commonly used forms of edema control

6.1 Cryotherapy

Cryotherapy is the therapeutic use of cold applied for reducing skin and subcutaneous tissues temperature. It is indicated for inflammation control, pain, and edema after surgery or injury [65, 74]. Thus, physiological cooling exerts autonomic-mediated effect that induces vasoconstriction, favoring minimization and control of edema [75].

It is a treatment modality widely used because it is simple, inexpensive, and can be applied many times. Its therapeutic effects are due to alterations in blood flow, consequent vasoconstriction, and reduction of metabolism, also providing restriction of bacterial growth.

However, information concerning cryotherapy effects on edema is controversial [74]. Few studies report the effects of cryotherapy in maxillofacial surgeries, although its use is consecrated by the great majority of surgeons and in several types of surgeries.

Considering that during the first 10 minutes of ice application, most of the local temperature reduction occurs, most studies recommend the application for 10–20 minutes, having a rest period of the same time or twice as long [74]. The use of cryotherapy for 30 minutes every 1½ hours, for 48 hours after third molar extraction was quite effective in facial edema control [76].

Cryotherapy is contraindicated for patients with peripheral vascular disease, hypersensitivity or cold intolerance, as in Raynaud's phenomenon and in areas with impaired circulation. A disadvantage of cryotherapy is that its use normally starts at 0° and rapidly reaches room temperature [75].

The cryotherapy protocols use differ greatly from each other, especially regarding duration and application form [74]. Its efficacy has been questioned because despite its common and daily use in clinical practice after maxillofacial surgeries, there is no consensus or protocols on its use, so new studies are needed.

6.2 Hilotherapy

Hilotherapy began to be used recently in postoperative of maxillofacial surgeries for control and reduction of facial edema. It is a preformed polyurethane face mask, in which cold and sterile water stream passes through, promoting cryotherapy at regulated and maintained temperatures [77].

A recent systematic review showed that hilotherapy is used immediately after surgery, with temperatures of 14–15°C. However, in third molar extraction, single application was used for 45 minutes, and after orthognathic surgeries, the application was for continuous period from 48 to 72 hours. Both protocols had positive effect in reducing facial edema [78]. Therefore, it can be concluded that extensive surgeries require longer application.

Hilotherapy, when compared to facial cryotherapy performed using ice blocks, was more efficient in facial edema control and reduction after maxillofacial surgeries [77–80].

A recent study has shown that the use of facial hilotherapy performed at home after third molar extraction surgery is safe, easy to apply, brings benefits in reducing facial edema and also improves quality of life [75].

One of the difficulties in using hilotherapy is the cost of the device, which can reach high values. However, once this is resolved, its use will probably replace conventional cryotherapy in a few years as studies have shown beneficial effects in reducing edema and postoperative pain with greater patient comfort.

6.3 Laser

Low-power laser is a relatively recent method and has been used as an alternative to edema control because it is capable of promoting modulation of the inflammatory response, reducing pain, edema and trismus, in addition to accelerate tissue repair [71, 81]. It is considered easy to apply and does not cause adverse effects [65].

Laser acts in reduction of edema by controlling and decreasing inflammatory response. So, it promotes faster recovery of injured lymphatic vessels and potentiates the action of lymph nodes [82].

Despite this, there is still no consensus about which is the best protocol for use in maxillofacial surgeries, so that its effects can be better utilized. However, different protocols can be found in literature, especially regarding to which postoperative moment laser should be applied and how many sessions are necessary. In laboratory tests, low-power laser was able to improve pain by regulating inflammatory factors at doses around 7.5 J/cm^2. In addition, application in an area using more than one point promotes better results than the concentrated application in a single point.

The need to control inflammation in preoperative period is known. However, using laser before third molar extraction surgery seems to have only analgesic response [83].

The laser can be applied in minor surgeries, such as dental extractions and also larger, such as orthognathic surgery. Although the application of intraoral and extraoral laser at the end of the surgery does not show benefits in the immediate reduction of edema, when evaluated in the following days, the patients present a reduction in facial edema [82–84]. That occurs due to the latency period in which there is the biomodulation caused by the laser on the inflammatory response, with prolonged and residual effect [83], not requiring more than one application [84].

Therefore, the use of laser is questioned in small and controlled inflammatory processes, since benefits to patient do not justify treatment costs [85, 86]. Still, in some cases, laser seems to have analgesic effect only, not helping to reduce facial edema [87].

Thus, although low-power laser has potential to control inflammatory process and reduce complications, results depend on an indication that justifies its use and, mainly, the protocol used.

6.4 Manual lymphatic drainage (MDL)

Manual lymphatic drainage is a resource that, if applied correctly and by a trained professional, helps in the resolution of edema. By means of slow movements and gentle pressure (30–40 mmHg) following the lymph pathway, the MLD proposes to potentiate the function of the lymphatic system [88, 89]. Thus, it is a nondrug option in the treatment of edema.

The benefit of manual lymphatic drainage is undeniable; however, in maxillofacial surgeries, it is still little used and little known, due to the scarcity of studies that demonstrate its effectiveness in this type of surgery and also prove the safety of its application. In surgeries in other regions of the body, the use of MLD to decrease edema is quite consistent, with well-established protocols and benefits. In maxillofacial surgery, there are still no protocols for beginning and no consensus regarding their benefits due to the amount of work done so far.

The MLD had proven efficacy in the postoperative period of third molar extraction, alveolar bone graft, and orthognathic surgery [90–92]. In a clinical trial with a split mouth model, third molar extraction was performed by adding MLD on one side only in the postoperative period. Using reproducible facial measures and Visual Analogue Scale (VAS) for pain, it was concluded that MLD is able to significantly reduce postoperative swelling and pain in this surgery [93].

The same effect was observed in the postoperative period of alveolar bone graft with filling of the bone defect by spongy bone of the iliac crest. However, this study compared the MLD performed by a physiotherapist to an adapted drain that was taught and applied by the patient. Both groups showed improvement over the course of the day, but MLD applied by physiotherapist had better results on edema and pain compared to self-drainage [92]. Despite that, attention should be paid to the absence of a control group so that the study would effectively prove the benefits of MLD. However, it is possible to conclude the importance of the physical therapist in the postoperative period of this surgery, since this professional has skills that can contribute to the improvement of the discomfort caused by the edema and the referred pain.

In the orthognathic surgeries, MLD was very effective in reducing postoperative edema when compared to a placebo, both applied by a physiotherapist. In these cases, not only was drainage capable to accelerate the regression process of edema, but also to anticipate its peak. It was also observed that the maximum edema was lower in the patients who received the MLD. Thus, MLD is able to promote the control of edema when applied during its development period and also to accelerate the process of regression of swelling in the postoperative period [91, 94].

However, even in this study, MLD was not effective in relation to pain perception. The authors attribute this to two factors: the application of a placebo, which may have interfered in patients' perception of pain and the fact that the patients did not develop severe edema, and therefore, the pain or discomfort related to the edema may have been lower, as well as the perception of relief in the group that received the MLD [91].

Although the benefits of MLD in the postoperative period of oral and maxillofacial surgeries have been studied, there is still no agreement as to when the application of MLD should begin. However, it is known that the peak of edema in maxillofacial surgeries occurs between 48 and 72 hours after surgery, and therefore, the beginning of MLD before this period seems to anticipate the peak of edema and regression, causing the amount of edema at the peak being lower [91, 94].

It can be concluded that MLD represents a safe nondrug option in the treatment of postoperative edema, when well indicated and applied by a qualified professional. Despite all the proven benefits, it is necessary to observe the need for MLD in various oral and maxillofacial surgeries. It is known that it is able to accelerate the process of regression of edema and provide relief of pain, but the need should be questioned in cases of small surgeries with the formation of discrete and local edema. In those cases, typical of a small controlled inflammatory process, MLD can be an unnecessary treatment to the patient, increasing the costs of the treatment and not having all its benefits observed.

6.5 Kinesio taping (KT)

Elastic bandage, or Kinesio taping, was first used in athletes, to aid in the recovery of muscle injuries, provide more stability to the joints, and provide relief from pain. However, it was realized that due to its way of functioning, it could be beneficial in the treatment of lymphedema.

KT, through the formation of convolutions in the skin, increases the interstitial space. Thus, through this increased space, fluids tend to move from higher pressure areas (congesta) to areas of lower pressure, improving blood and lymphatic flow. This occurs following the placement of the KT, which is positioned according to the path of the lymphatic system. In that way, KT may be able to relieve swelling caused by bruising and edema [23, 45, 95, 96].

In maxillofacial surgeries, its efficacy has already been tested in several surgeries: surgical reduction of mandible fracture, surgery to reduce fractures of the zygomatic-orbital complex, third molar extraction, and orthognathic surgery [97].

In the surgical reduction of mandibular fracture and zygomatic-orbital complex, KT is effective in reducing edema, anticipating the day of peak edema, the amount of edema formed on this day, and accelerating its reduction. However, despite the more rapid resolution of edema, no effects on trismus or pain relief were found [95].

In third molar extraction surgeries, KT anticipates the day of maximum edema and the amount of edema formed on this day. However, the rate of edema reduction is lower when compared to patients who did not use KT. Despite that, patients who use KT postoperatively seem to have resolution of the edema earlier. Furthermore, KT was effective in relieving pain, but not in trismus [96].

Even so, in the exodontia, when compared to the placement of drains for the treatment of lymphedema, KT is not as effective. Drain placement at the surgical site is shown to be much more effective not only at the faster reduction of edema but also in relation to pain, although it is an invasive approach. Despite this, none of the treatments helped reduce trismus in this study. It should also be considered that drainage placement, despite being effective in reducing edema, may lead to other complications, in relation to the possibility of subcutaneous emphysema, infection, and external facial scar [98].

In orthognathic surgeries, the application of KT is beneficial in the treatment of postoperative edema, being capable to anticipate the day of maximum edema, reduce the maximum amount of edema formed, and accelerate the regression process of edema. However, it does not appear to have significant effects with regard to pain or trismus [97].

Thus, KT is a nonmedicated treatment option for the control and treatment of postoperative lymphedema of maxillofacial surgeries. However, its effects on pain and trismus need to be better elucidated. Although one of the goals of KT is to prevent the formation of bruises and/or to treat them, there is still no proof of it. Therefore, it is a function to be explored with great interest, since the increase in volume of a body segment is not only due to edema but also due to hematomas.

Therefore, KT is a relatively inexpensive treatment option, but it requires specific training and professional habilitation, as well as presurgery testing to check for allergy to the components of the bandage.

7. Conclusions

In this chapter, factors related to edema development in maxillofacial surgeries and alternatives for its control and treatment were presented. It is known that this condition is strictly related to the inflammatory process, and therefore, controlling edema also requires controlling postoperative inflammation.

Several factors contribute to edema severity, and knowing which factors cause these and their influence on inflammatory process, it is possible to predict the quality of the postoperative period. The inflammatory process control, and consequently edema restriction, is fundamental for the quality of healing process and postoperative. Thus, it is necessary to have attention and intervention of surgical team on controllable factors that lead to a most severe or mild formation of edema, such as surgical time and precise surgical planning.

In addition, knowing about the risks for each factor related to the edema development makes individual and personalized treatment possible, which brings great benefits to the patient. Aiming at reducing complications related to edema, better postoperative quality, increased satisfaction and reduction of hospitalization time and treatment costs, and several drug and nondrug methods may be employed. Currently, there is a tendency in reducing medicament use in order to reduce the occurrence and severity of adverse effects. In this way, nondrug methods are increasingly study targets and used in clinical practice.

Therefore, more studies are needed to prove the efficacy and safety of these methods. Also, the formation of a well-trained and integrated multiprofessional team is necessary, aiming for safety, comfort, and faster patient recovery in postoperative period of maxillofacial surgeries.

Conflict of interest

The authors declare that they have no conflict of interest.

Author details

Renato Yassutaka Faria Yaedu[1*], Marina de Almeida Barbosa Mello[2], Juliana Specian Zabotini da Silveira[2] and Ana Carolina Bonetti Valente[2]

1 Hospital for Rehabilitation of Craniofacial Anomalies, University of São Paulo and Bauru School of Dentistry, Bauru, São Paulo, Brazil

2 Hospital for Rehabilitation of Craniofacial Anomalies, University of São Paulo, Bauru, São Paulo, Brazil

*Address all correspondence to: yaedu@usp.br

References

[1] Ebert JR, Joss B, Jardine B, Wood DJ. Randomized trial investigating the efficacy of manual lymphatic drainage to improve early outcome after total knee arthroplasty. Archives of Physical Medicine and Rehabilitation. 2013;**94**(11):2103-2111

[2] Korpan MI, Crevenna R, Fialka-Moser V. Lymphedema: A therapeutic approach in the treatment and rehabilitation of cancer patients. American Journal of Physical Medicine & Rehabilitation. 2011;**90**(5 Suppl 1): S69-S75

[3] Smith BG, Lewin JS. Lymphedema management in head and neck cancer. Current Opinion in Otolaryngology & Head and Neck Surgery. 2010;**18**(3):153-158

[4] de Santana-Santos T, de Souza-Santos A-A-S, Martins-Filho P-R-S, da Silva L-C-F, De Oliveira E Silva E-D, Gomes A-C-A. Prediction of postoperative facial swelling, pain and trismus following third molar surgery based on preoperative variables. Medicina Oral, Patología Oral y Cirugía Bucal. 2013;**18**(1):e65-e70

[5] Bork K, Barnstedt S-E. Laryngeal edema and death from asphyxiation after tooth extraction in four patients with hereditary angioedema. Journal of the American Dental Association (1939). 2003;**134**(8):1088-1094

[6] Cifuentes J, Palisson F, Valladares S, Jerez D. Life-threatening complications following orthognathic surgery in a patient with undiagnosed hereditary angioedema. Journal of Oral and Maxillofacial Surgery. 2013;**71**(4):e185-e188

[7] Morcavallo PS, Leonida A, Rossi G, Mingardi M, Martini M, Monguzzi R, et al. Hereditary angioedema in oral surgery: Overview of the clinical picture and report of a case. Journal of Oral and Maxillofacial Surgery. 2010;**68**(9):2307-2311

[8] Puricelli E, Ponzoni D, Artuzi FE, Martins GL, Calcagnotto T. Clinical management of angioneurotic oedema patient post-orthognathic surgery. International Journal of Oral and Maxillofacial Surgery. 2011;**40**(1):106-109

[9] Carvalho RWF, do Egito Vasconcelos BC. Assessment of factors associated with surgical difficulty during removal of impacted lower third molars. Journal of Oral and Maxillofacial Surgery. 2011;**69**(11):2714-2721

[10] van der Vlis M, Dentino KM, Vervloet B, Padwa BL. Postoperative swelling after orthognathic surgery: A prospective volumetric analysis. Journal of Oral and Maxillofacial Surgery. 2014;**72**(11):2241-2247

[11] Pérez-González JM, Esparza-Villalpando V, Martínez-Rider R, Noyola-Frías MÁ, Pozos-Guillén A. Clinical and radiographic characteristics as predictive factors of swelling and trismus after mandibular third molar surgery: A longitudinal approach. Pain Research & Management. 2018;**2018**:7938492

[12] Kantor ED, Lampe JW, Kratz M, White E. Lifestyle factors and inflammation: Associations by body mass index. PLoS One. 2013;**8**(7):e67833

[13] Benediktsdóttir IS, Wenzel A, Petersen JK, Hintze H. Mandibular third molar removal: Risk indicators for extended operation time, postoperative pain, and complications. Oral Surgery, Oral Medicine, Oral Pathology, Oral Radiology, and Endodontics. 2004;**97**(4):438-446

[14] Bello SA, Adeyemo WL, Bamgbose BO, Obi EV, Adeyinka AA. Effect of age, impaction types and operative time on inflammatory tissue reactions following lower third molar surgery. Head & Face Medicine. 2011;**7**:8

[15] Pogrel MA. What is the effect of timing of removal on the incidence and severity of complications? Journal of Oral and Maxillofacial Surgery. 2012;**70**(9):S37-S40

[16] Mobilio N, Vecchiatini R, Vasquez M, Calura G, Catapano S. Effect of flap design and duration of surgery on acute postoperative symptoms and signs after extraction of lower third molars: A randomized prospective study. Journal of Dental Research, Dental Clinics, Dental Prospects. 2017;**11**(3):156-160

[17] Blondeau F, Daniel NG. Extraction of impacted mandibular third molars: Postoperative complications and their risk factors. Journal of the Canadian Dental Association. 2007;**73**(4):325

[18] Khattak ZG, Benington PCM, Khambay BS, Green L, Walker F, Ayoub AF. An assessment of the quality of care provided to orthognathic surgery patients through a multidisciplinary clinic. Journal of Cranio-Maxillo-Facial Surgery. 2012;**40**(3):243-247

[19] Osunde OD, Saheeb BD. Effect of age, sex and level of surgical difficulty on inflammatory complications after third molar surgery. Journal of Oral and Maxillofacial Surgery. 2015;**14**(1):7-12

[20] Robinson RC, Holm RL. Orthognathic surgery for patients with maxillofacial deformities. AORN Journal. 2010;**92**(1):28-49; quiz 50-2

[21] Jerjes W, El-Maaytah M, Swinson B, Banu B, Upile T, D'Sa S, et al. Experience versus complication rate in third molar surgery. Head & Face Medicine. 2006;**2**:14

[22] Cassetta M, Bellardini M. How much does experience in guided implant surgery play a role in accuracy? A randomized controlled pilot study. International Journal of Oral and Maxillofacial Surgery. 2017;**46**(7):922-930

[23] Ristow O, Pautke C, Kehl V, Koerdt S, Hahnefeld L, Hohlweg-Majert B. Kinesiologic taping reduces morbidity after oral and maxillofacial surgery: A pooled analysis. Physiotherapy Theory and Practice. 2014;**30**(6):390-398

[24] Lin S, Chen C, Yao C-F, Chen Y-A, Chen Y-R. Comparison of different hypotensive anaesthesia techniques in orthognathic surgery with regard to intraoperative blood loss, quality of the surgical field, and postoperative nausea and vomiting. International Journal of Oral and Maxillofacial Surgery. 2016;**45**(12):1526-1530

[25] Silva AC, O'Ryan F, Poor DB. Postoperative nausea and vomiting (PONV) after orthognathic surgery: A retrospective study and literature review. Journal of Oral and Maxillofacial Surgery. 2006;**64**(9):1385-1397

[26] Thomas JS, Maple IK, Norcross W, Muckler VC. Preoperative risk assessment to guide prophylaxis and reduce the incidence of postoperative nausea and vomiting. Journal of Perianesthesia Nursing. 23 Jun 2018. DOI: 10.1016/j.jopan.2018.02.007

[27] Yu CN, Chow TK, Kwan AS, Wong SL, Fung SC. Intra-operative blood loss and operating time in orthognathic surgery using induced hypotensive general anaesthesia: Prospective study. Hong Kong Medical Journal. 2000;**6**(3):307-311

[28] Praveen K, Narayanan V, Muthusekhar MR, Baig MF. Hypotensive anaesthesia and

blood loss in orthognathic surgery: A clinical study. The British Journal of Oral & Maxillofacial Surgery. 2001;**39**(2):138-140

[29] Choi WS, Samman N. Risks and benefits of deliberate hypotension in anaesthesia: A systematic review. International Journal of Oral and Maxillofacial Surgery. 2008;**37**(8):687-703

[30] Prasant MC, Kar S, Rastogi S, Hada P, Ali FM, Mudhol A. Comparative study of blood loss, quality of surgical field and duration of surgery in maxillofacial cases with and without hypotensive anesthesia. Journal of International Oral Health. 2014;**6**(6):18-21

[31] Phillips C, Brookes CD, Rich J, Arbon J, Turvey TA. Postoperative nausea and vomiting following orthognathic surgery. International Journal of Oral and Maxillofacial Surgery. 2015;**44**(6):745-751

[32] Degoute C-S. Controlled hypotension. Drugs. 2007;**67**(7): 1053-1076

[33] Olmedo-Gaya MV, Vallecillo-Capilla M, Galvez-Mateos R. Relation of patient and surgical variables to postoperative pain and inflammation in the extraction of third molars. Medicina Oral. 2002;**7**(5):360-369

[34] Yuasa H, Sugiura M. Clinical postoperative findings after removal of impacted mandibular third molars: Prediction of postoperative facial swelling and pain based on preoperative variables. The British Journal of Oral & Maxillofacial Surgery. 2004;**42**(3):209-214

[35] Stanton AWB, Northfield JW, Holroyd B, Mortimer PS, Levick JR. Validation of an optoelectronic limb volumeter (Perometer®). Lymphology. 1997;**30**(2):77-97

[36] Nuutinen J, Ikäheimo R, Lahtinen T. Validation of a new dielectric device to assess changes of tissue water in skin and subcutaneous fat. Physiological Measurement. 2004;**25**(2):447-454

[37] Haaverstad R, Nilsen G, Rinck PA, Myhre HO. The use of MRI in the diagnosis of chronic lymphedema of the lower extremity. International Angiology. 1994;**13**(2):115-118

[38] Lahtinen T, Nuutinen J. A new device for clinical and radiobiological research to measure local development of edema induced by radiotherapy, drugs or surgery. Radiotherapy and Oncology. 2005;**76**:S47

[39] Gniadecka M, Quistorff B. Assessment of dermal water by high-frequency ultrasound: Comparative studies with nuclear magnetic resonance. The British Journal of Dermatology. 1996;**135**(2):218-224. Available from: https://onlinelibrary.wiley.com/doi/abs/10.1111/j.1365-2133.1996.tb01150.x

[40] Piso DU, Eckardt A, Liebermann A, Gutenbrunner C, Schäfer P, Gehrke A. Early rehabilitation of head-neck edema after curative surgery for orofacial tumors. American Journal of Physical Medicine & Rehabilitation. 2001;**80**(4):261-269

[41] Van Gool AV, Ten Bosch JJ, Boering G. A photographic method of assessing swelling following third molar removal. International Journal of Oral Surgery. 1975;**4**(3):121-129

[42] Album B, Olsen I, Løkken P. Bilateral surgical removal of impacted mandibular third molar teeth as a model for drug evaluation: A test with oxyphenbutazone (Tanderil®). International Journal of Oral and Maxillofacial Surgery. 1977;**6**(3):177-189

[43] Holland CS. The development of a method of assessing swelling following

third molar surgery. The British Journal of Oral Surgery. 1979;**17**(2):104-114

[44] Ågren E. High-speed or conventional dental engines for the removal of bone in oral surgery: I. A study of the reactions following removal of bilateral impacted lower third molars. Acta Odontologica Scandinavica. 1963;**21**(6):585-625

[45] Ristow O, Pautke C, Kehl V, Koerdt S, Schwärzler K, Hahnefeld L, et al. Influence of kinesiologic tape on postoperative swelling, pain and trismus after zygomatico-orbital fractures. Journal of Cranio-Maxillo-Facial Surgery. 2014;**42**(5):469-476

[46] Yamamoto S, Miyachi H, Fujii H, Ochiai S, Watanabe S, Shimozato K. Intuitive facial imaging method for evaluation of postoperative swelling: A combination of 3-dimensional computed tomography and laser surface scanning in orthognathic surgery. Journal of Oral and Maxillofacial Surgery. 2016;**74**(12):2506.e1-2506.e10

[47] Garcia AG, Sampedro FG, Rey JG. Trismus and pain after removal of impacted lower third molars. Journal of Oral and Maxillofacial Surgery. 1997;**55**(11):1223-1226. Available from: https://www.joms.org/article/S0278-2391(97)90172-5/abstract

[48] Gunes N. A comparison of the effects of methylprednisolone and tenoxicam on pain, edema, and trismus after impacted lower third molar extraction. Medical Science Monitor. 2014;**20**:147-152

[49] Laureano Filho JR, Maurette PE, Allais M, Cotinho M, Fernandes C. Clinical comparative study of the effectiveness of two dosages of Dexamethasone to control postoperative swelling, trismus and pain after the surgical extraction of mandibular impacted third molars. Medicina Oral, Patología Oral y Cirugía Bucal. 2008;**13**(2):E129-E132

[50] Ridner SH. The psycho-social impact of lymphedema. Lymphatic Research and Biology. 2009;**7**(2):109-112

[51] de Lima VN, Lemos CAA, Faverani LP, Santiago Júnior JF, Pellizzer EP. Effectiveness of corticoid administration in orthognathic surgery for edema and neurosensorial disturbance: A systematic literature review. Journal of Oral and Maxillofacial Surgery. 2017;**75**(7):1528.e1-1528.e8

[52] Deodhar AK, Rana RE. Surgical physiology of wound healing: A review. Journal of Postgraduate Medicine. 1997;**43**(2):52-56

[53] Steinbrech DS, Longaker MT, Mehrara BJ, Saadeh PB, Chin GS, Gerrets RP, et al. Fibroblast response to hypoxia: The relationship between angiogenesis and matrix regulation. The Journal of Surgical Research. 1999;**84**(2):127-133

[54] Lawrence WT, Diegelmann RF. Growth factors in wound healing. Clinics in Dermatology. 1994;**12**(1):157-169

[55] Chegini S, Dhariwal DK. Review of evidence for the use of steroids in orthognathic surgery. The British Journal of Oral & Maxillofacial Surgery. 2012;**50**(2):97-101

[56] Koçer G, Yuce E, Tuzuner Oncul A, Dereci O, Koskan O. Effect of the route of administration of methylprednisolone on oedema and trismus in impacted lower third molar surgery. International Journal of Oral and Maxillofacial Surgery. 2014;**43**(5):639-643

[57] Ehsan A, Ali Bukhari SG, Ashar AM, Manzoor A, Junaid M. Effects of pre-operative submucosal

dexamethasone injection on the postoperative swelling and trismus following surgical extraction of mandibular third molar. Journal of the College of Physicians and Surgeons–Pakistan. Jul 2014;**24**(7):489-492

[58] Herrera-Briones FJ, Prados Sánchez E, Reyes Botella C, Vallecillo CM. Update on the use of corticosteroids in third molar surgery: Systematic review of the literature. Oral Surgery, Oral Medicine, Oral Pathology, Oral Radiology. 2013;**116**(5):e342-e351

[59] Jean S, Dionne P-L, Bouchard C, Giasson L, Turgeon AF. Perioperative systemic corticosteroids in orthognathic surgery: A systematic review and meta-analysis. Journal of Oral and Maxillofacial Surgery. 2017;**75**(12):2638-2649

[60] Widar F, Kashani H, Alsén B, Dahlin C, Rasmusson L. The effects of steroids in preventing facial oedema, pain, and neurosensory disturbances after bilateral sagittal split osteotomy: A randomized controlled trial. International Journal of Oral and Maxillofacial Surgery. 2015;**44**(2):252-258

[61] Tripathi KD. Essentials of Medical Pharmacology. New Delhi, India: JP Medical Ltd; 2013. p. 1002

[62] ElHag M, Coghlan K, Christmas P, Harvey W, Harris M. The anti-inflammatory effects of dexamethasone and therapeutic ultrasound in oral surgery. The British Journal of Oral & Maxillofacial Surgery. 1985;**23**(1):17-23

[63] Asimakopoulos G, Thompson R, Nourshargh S, Lidington EA, Mason JC, Ratnatunga CP, et al. An anti-inflammatory property of aprotinin detected at the level of leukocyte extravasation. The Journal of Thoracic and Cardiovascular Surgery. 2000;**120**(2):361-369

[64] Alexander RE, Throndson RR. A review of perioperative corticosteroid use in dentoalveolar surgery. Oral Surgery, Oral Medicine, Oral Pathology, Oral Radiology, and Endodontics. 2000;**90**(4):406-415

[65] Osunde OD, Adebola RA, Omeje UK. Management of inflammatory complications in third molar surgery: A review of the literature. African Health Sciences. 2011;**11**(3):530-537

[66] Zor ZF, Isik B, Cetiner S. Efficacy of preemptive lornoxicam on postoperative analgesia after surgical removal of mandibular third molars. Oral Surgery, Oral Medicine, Oral Pathology, Oral Radiology. 2014;**117**(1):27-31

[67] Akbulut N, Üstüner E, Atakan C, Çölok G. Comparison of the effect of naproxen, etodolac and diclofenac on postoperative sequels following third molar surgery: A randomised, double-blind, crossover study. Medicina Oral, Patología Oral y Cirugía Bucal. 2014;**19**(2):e149-e156

[68] Bamgbose BO, Akinwande JA, Adeyemo WL, Ladeinde AL, Arotiba GT, Ogunlewe MO. Effects of co-administered dexamethasone and diclofenac potassium on pain, swelling and trismus following third molar surgery. Head & Face Medicine. 2005;**1**:11

[69] Gocmen G, Gonul O, Oktay NS, Yarat A, Goker K. The antioxidant and anti-inflammatory efficiency of hyaluronic acid after third molar extraction. Journal of Cranio-Maxillo-Facial Surgery. 2015;**43**(7):1033-1037

[70] Koray M, Ofluoglu D, Onal EA, Ozgul M, Ersev H. Efficacy of hyaluronic acid spray on swelling, pain, and trismus after surgical extraction of impacted mandibular third molars. International Journal of Oral and Maxillofacial Surgery. 2014;**43**(11):1399-1403. Available from:

https://www.sciencedirect.com/science/article/pii/S0901502714001799

[71] Drew SJ. Best practices for management of pain, swelling, nausea, and vomiting in dentoalveolar surgery. Oral and Maxillofacial Surgery Clinics of North America. 2015;**27**(3):393-404

[72] Afat İM, Akdoğan ET, Gönül O. Effects of leukocyte- and platelet-rich fibrin alone and combined with hyaluronic acid on pain, edema, and trismus after surgical extraction of impacted mandibular third molars. Journal of Oral and Maxillofacial Surgery. 2018;**76**(5):926-932

[73] Semper-Hogg W, Fuessinger MA, Dirlewanger TW, Cornelius CP, Metzger MC. The influence of dexamethasone on postoperative swelling and neurosensory disturbances after orthognathic surgery: A randomized controlled clinical trial. Head & Face Medicine. 2017;**13**(1):19

[74] Greenstein G. Therapeutic efficacy of cold therapy after intraoral surgical procedures: A literature review. Journal of Periodontology. 2007;**78**(5):790-800

[75] Beech AN, Haworth S, Knepil GJ. Effect of a domiciliary facial cooling system on generic quality of life after removal of mandibular third molars. The British Journal of Oral & Maxillofacial Surgery. 2018;**56**(4):315-321

[76] Laureano Filho JR, de Oliveira e Silva ED, Batista CI, FMV G. The influence of cryotherapy on reduction of swelling, pain and trismus after third-molar extraction: A preliminary study. Journal of the American Dental Association (1939). 2005;**136**(6):774-778 quiz 807

[77] Moro A, Gasparini G, Marianetti TM, Boniello R, Cervelli D, Di Nardo F, et al. Hilotherm efficacy in controlling postoperative facial edema in patients treated for maxillomandibular malformations. The Journal of Craniofacial Surgery. 2011;**22**(6):2114-2117

[78] Glass GE, Waterhouse N, Shakib K. Hilotherapy for the management of perioperative pain and swelling in facial surgery: A systematic review and meta-analysis. The British Journal of Oral & Maxillofacial Surgery. 2016;**54**(8):851-856

[79] Rana M, Gellrich NC, Joos U, Piffkó J, Kater W. 3D evaluation of postoperative swelling using two different cooling methods following orthognathic surgery: A randomised observer blind prospective pilot study. International Journal of Oral and Maxillofacial Surgery. 2011;**40**(7):690-696

[80] Veitz-Keenan A. Continuous cooling mask devices reduce patient discomfort and postoperative pain and swelling in patients undergoing orofacial surgery. Evidence-Based Dentistry. 2016;**17**(4):121-122

[81] Oliveira Sierra S, Melo Deana A, Agnelli Mesquita Ferrari R, Maia Albarello P, Kalil Bussadori S, Porta Santos Fernandes K. Effect of low-level laser therapy on the post-surgical inflammatory process after third molar removal: Study protocol for a double-blind randomized controlled trial. Trials. 2013;**14**(1):373

[82] He WL, Yu FY, Li CJ, Pan J, Zhuang R, Duan PJ. A systematic review and meta-analysis on the efficacy of low-level laser therapy in the management of complication after mandibular third molar surgery. Lasers in Medical Science. 2015;**30**(6):1779-1788

[83] Petrini M, Ferrante M, Trentini P, Perfetti G, Spoto G. Effect of pre-operatory low-level laser therapy on pain, swelling, and trismus associated

with third-molar surgery. Medicina Oral, Patología Oral y Cirugía Bucal. 2017;**22**(4):e467-e472

[84] Koparal M, Ozcan KA. Effects of low-level laser therapy following surgical extraction of the lower third molar with objective measurement of swelling using a three-dimensional system. Experimental and Therapeutic Medicine. 2018;**15**(4):3820-3826. Available from: https://www.spandidos-publications.com/etm/15/4/3820

[85] Brignardello-Petersen R, Carrasco-Labra A, Araya I, Yanine N, Beyene J, Shah PS. Is adjuvant laser therapy effective for preventing pain, swelling, and trismus after surgical removal of impacted mandibular third molars? A systematic review and meta-analysis. Journal of Oral and Maxillofacial Surgery. 2012;**70**(8):1789-1801

[86] Farhadi F, Eslami H, Majidi A, Fakhrzadeh V, Ghanizadeh M, KhademNeghad S. Evaluation of adjunctive effect of low-level laser therapy on pain, swelling and trismus after surgical removal of impacted lower third molar: A double blind randomized clinical trial. Laser Therapy. 2017;**26**(3):181-187

[87] Raiesian S, Khani M, Khiabani K, Hemmati E, Pouretezad M. Assessment of low-level laser therapy effects after extraction of impacted lower third molar surgery. Journal of Lasers in Medical Sciences. 2017;**8**(1):42-45

[88] Kasseroller RG. The Vodder school: The Vodder method. Cancer. 1998;**83**(12 Suppl American):2840-2842

[89] Rockson SG, Miller LT, Senie R, Brennan MJ, Casley-Smith JR, Földi E, et al. American Cancer Society Lymphedema Workshop. Workgroup III: Diagnosis and management of lymphedema. Cancer. 1998;**83**(S12B):2882-2885

[90] Szolnoky G, Mohos G, Dobozy A, Kemény L. Manual lymph drainage reduces trapdoor effect in subcutaneous island pedicle flaps. International Journal of Dermatology. 2006;**45**(12):1468-1470

[91] Yaedú RYF, Mello MAB, Tucunduva RA, JSZ d S, Takahashi MPMS, ACB V. Postoperative orthognathic surgery edema assessment with and without manual lymphatic drainage. The Journal of Craniofacial Surgery. 2017;**28**(7):1816-1820

[92] Ferreira T, Sabatella MZ, Silva T. Facial edema reduction after alveolar bone grafting surgery in cleft lip and palate patients: A new lymphatic drainage protocol. RGO - Rev Gaúcha Odontol. 2013. Available from: http://www.revistargo.com.br/viewarticle.php?id=2893&

[93] Szolnoky G, Szendi-Horváth K, Seres L, Boda K, Kemény L. Manual lymph drainage efficiently reduces postoperative facial swelling and discomfort after removal of impacted third molars. Lymphology. 2007;**40**(3):138-142

[94] Modabber A, Rana M, Ghassemi A, Gerressen M, Gellrich N-C, Hölzle F, et al. Three-dimensional evaluation of postoperative swelling in treatment of zygomatic bone fractures using two different cooling therapy methods: A randomized, observer-blind, prospective study. Trials. 2013;**14**:238

[95] Ristow O, Hohlweg-Majert B, Kehl V, Koerdt S, Hahnefeld L, Pautke C. Does elastic therapeutic tape reduce postoperative swelling, pain, and trismus after open reduction and internal fixation of mandibular fractures? Journal of Oral and Maxillofacial Surgery. 2013;**71**(8):1387-1396

[96] Ristow O, Hohlweg-Majert B, Stürzenbaum SR, Kehl V, Koerdt S,

Hahnefeld L, et al. Therapeutic elastic tape reduces morbidity after wisdom teeth removal—A clinical trial. Clinical Oral Investigations. 2014;**18**(4):1205-1212

[97] Tozzi U, Santagata M, Sellitto A, Tartaro GP. influence of kinesiologic tape on post-operative swelling after orthognathic surgery. Journal of Oral and Maxillofacial Surgery. 2016;**15**(1):52-58

[98] Genc A, Cakarer S, Yalcin BK, Kilic BB, Isler SC, Keskin C. A comparative study of surgical drain placement and the use of kinesiologic tape to reduce postoperative morbidity after third molar surgery. Clinical Oral Investigations. 19 Apr 2018. DOI: 10.1007/s00784-018-2442-x

Section 3

Neutrophils in Immunity and Inflammation

Chapter 6

Neutrophil Counts and Rates in Otorhinolaryngology

Erkan Yildiz

Abstract

Complete blood count is a fairly inexpensive test that is widely used in the clinic. Neutrophils are also one of the most important parameters in complete blood count. They play a critical role in upper respiratory tract infection, as well as in many chronic otolaryngology diseases. It also has widespread uses in otorhinolaryngology practice. There are many publications on neutrophil counts and neutrophil lymphocyte ratios in patients. Neutrophil counts and rates play an important role in the follow-up and prognosis of many important otolaryngology diseases such as bell palsy, sudden hearing loss, allergic rhinitis, chronic otitis media, nasal polyposis, and chronic rhinosinusitis. In this chapter, the importance of neutrophils in these diseases will be discussed with the literature.

Keywords: neutrophil, neutrophil lymphocyte ratios, otolaryngology

1. Introduction

Neutrophils are known as basic defense cells in humans. However, recent research has shown that they do much more than defense. Neutrophil migration and its roles in inflammation gradually attracted the attention of researchers. The use of advanced technology has been effective in demonstrating the behavior of neutrophils in tissues. Neutrophils follow multiple ways to advance to the site of injury and infection [1].

Neutrophils are the most abundant leukocytes in the blood. They trigger the first damage in the host during the infection phase. They provide these roles thanks to phagocytosis, degranulation and reactive oxygen types. Overactivation of neutrophils sometimes leads to excessive tissue damage. Neutrophils causing chronic inflammation can cause loss of function in organs. When the number of neutrophils decreases, the response to inflammation decreases and this turns into immune deficiency. Neutrophils are produced in the bone marrow; this number may increase up to 1000 times in case of need.

Recently, neutrophil counts, and neutrophil lymphocyte ratios have been used in the diagnosis and follow-up of clinical errors. Numerous researches have been done on this subject and its widespread use has started in otolaryngology [2, 3].

2. Neutrophils in rhinology

In many nose-related diseases, nasal congestion is the main symptom. The most important of these diseases are allergic rhinitis, septum deviation, rhinosinusitis,

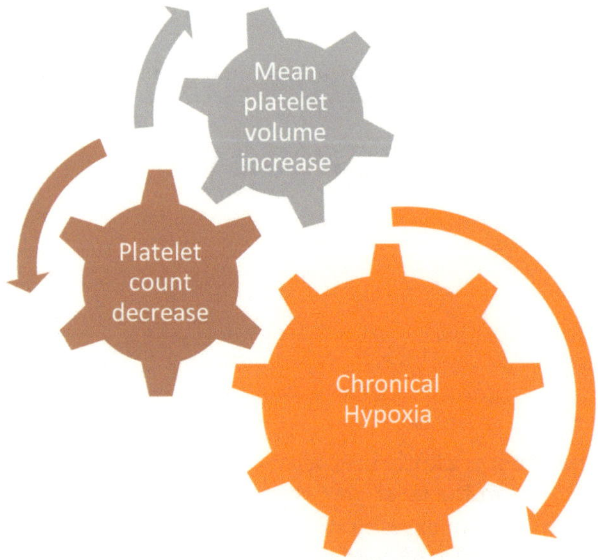

Figure 1.
Change of hematological parameters in hypoxia caused by nasal congestion [1].

nasal polyp, and antrochoanal polyp. These diseases have chronic hypoxia and are caused by airway resistances. Hypoxia increases the mean platelet volume (**Figure 1**). Erythropoiesis develops again due to hypoxia. Therefore, change begins in hematological markers. In the study of patients with nasal septum deviation, the number of platelets decreased while the mean platelet volume increased [1]. Similarly, similar results were obtained in sleep apnea syndrome. No relation was found between laboratory values and apnea in pediatric sleep apnea children [2]. No significant difference was observed in pre- and postoperative studies in children with adenoid hypertrophy [3]. NLR has also been shown to be prognostic in patients with allergic rhinitis. Neutrophils, eosinophils, and basophils can be monitored in nasal cytology.

3. Neutrophils in otology

Neutrophils, which are effective in many areas of otolaryngology, are also important in otology. In autology, inflammatory cells increase and inflammatory changes are observed in diseases such as acute otitis media, serous otitis media, chronic suppurative otitis media, cholesteatoma, facial paralysis, sudden idiopathic sensorineural hearing loss, tinnitus, and vertigo. There are many studies on hematological markers in sudden idiopathic sensorineural hearing loss. NLR, PLR, neutrophil and lymphocyte count are known to be prognostic [4]. No relationship was found between the degree of hearing loss in the audiogram and hematological parameters [5]. Another study showed that there were laboratory parameters such as lymphocyte, lymphocyte%, platelet, mean platelet volume, platelet distribution width (MPV), neutrophil-lymphocyte ratio, platelet-lymphocyte ratio, mean corpuscular hemoglobin, and mean corpuscular hemoglobin concentration [6] NLR Adult Bell While it can be used prognostically in paralysis, PLR has been reported to be meaningless [7]. In pediatric Bell palsy, it was observed that both NLR and PLR were significant [8]. In otitis media with effusion, hematological parameters were important markers determining viscosity [9]. In a study conducted with inactive patients with active chronic otitis media, no difference was observed in both patient groups [10]. In chronic otitis media, both NLR and PLR and MPV values are found to be high, as well as normal studies [11]. In the cholesteatoma, there is an invasive transition of the outer ear epithelium to the middle ear. During this transition, inflammatory cytokines are produced. No difference in NLR levels from control groups was found in cholesteatoma [12]. In a study of tinnitus patients, a connection was found between tinnitus and MPV values [13].

4. Neutrophils in infections in the oral region

In recurrent aphthous stomatitis, no relation was found between hematological parameters and infection. There was no difference between these patients and the control group in terms of WBC, Hb, neutrophil, lymphocyte, platelet, MPV, NLR, PLR, ESR, and CRP levels [14]. Although tonsillectomy and adenoidectomy are common surgical procedures, the effects of these operations on the immune system have not been fully established. Studies in patients with chronic tonsillitis and adenoid hypertrophy show that chronic tonsillitis and adenoid hypertrophy disrupt neutrophil chemotaxis functions and these values become normal after adenotonsillectomy. In addition, oxidant values appear to improve after this procedure [15]. It has been shown that it can be used in chronic tonsillitis patients as an effective assistant method in determining neutrophil-lymphocyte ratio, tonsillectomy, and postoperative follow-up [16]. It was stated that the mean platelet volume and neutrophil lymphocyte ratio can be used as markers in peritonsillar abscess [17].

5. Neutrophils in head and neck infections

NLR values can be used as a prognostic indicator in deep neck infections occurring after acute bacterial tonsillitis [18]. It can also be used seriously in the evaluation of chronic tonsillitis [19]. NLR values were not found statistically significant in children with obstructive sleep apnea undergoing adenoidectomy [2].

6. Neutrophils in head and neck cancers

Neutrophils play an important role in cancer formation and progression [20]. In head and neck cancers with high degree of systemic inflammation, an increase in the number of neutrophils is detected. Many studies have also been done on the prognosis of head and neck cancers. The study showed that increased neutrophil lymphocyte ratios (NLR) worsened head and neck cancer prognosis. Similar results have emerged in another study [21, 22]. In another study, a significant correlation was found between high cut-off value before treatment and poor prognosis [23]. In another study, it was determined that the rate of NLR in the nasopharyngeal carcinoma was a poor prognosis factor [24]. In patients who received pre-treatment adjuvant or primary chemotherapy in squamous cell head and neck cancers, the NLR ratio has been indicated as an important marker in demonstrating treatment success [25]. In another study related to the rates of laryngeal cancer, it was shown that the NLR rate did not change in benign lesions, premalignant or malignant laryngeal lesions of the larynx, but was prognostic in lymph node metastases. In Ref. [26], it was shown that it can help early confirmation of treatment failure in patients with metastatic HNSCC [27]. In patients with head and neck cancer of unknown P16-negative primer, NLR-6.0 was significantly associated with poor prognosis [28]. In a study in patients with oral squamous

Neutrophil/lymphocyte ratio in head and neck carcinoma.		
Study	**Region**	**Ratio**
Takenaka et al. [21]	Head and neck (all)	Elevated
Takenaka et al. [24]	Nasopharynx	Elevated
Bojaxhiu et al. [25]	Head and neck (chemotherapy before/after)	Elevated
Eskiizmir et al. [26]	Laryngeal neoplasm	Elevated only in lymph node metastasis
Mascarella et al. [22]	Head and neck (all)	Elevated
Zhang et al. [29]	Oral squamous cell carcinoma	Elevated
Xu et al. [28]	Unknown primary head and neck carcinoma(p16-)	Elevated (worse prognosis)

Table 1.
Neutrophil/lymphocyte ratio in head and neck carcinoma.

cell cancers, increased NLR values have been shown to be a sign of poor prognosis [29]. It has higher NLR, MLR, PLR, and RDW values in children with histopathologically diagnosed lymphoma than in children with reactive LAP. Anywhere NLR, MLR, PLR, and RDW tests can be used to determine which LAP patients should be selected for biopsy (**Table 1**) [30].

Author details

Erkan Yildiz
Department of Otorhinolaryngology, Afyonkarahisar Şuhut State Hospital, Şuhut/Afyonkarahisar, Turkey

*Address all correspondence to: dr.erkanyildiz@hotmail.com

References

[1] Unlu I, Kesici GG, Oneç B, Yaman H, Guclu E. The effect of duration of nasal obstruction on mean platelet volume in patients with marked nasal septal deviation. European Archives of Oto-Rhino-Laryngology. 2016;**273**:401-405. DOI: 10.1007/s00405-015-3580-2

[2] Derin S, Erdogan S, Sahan M, Topal H, Sozen H. Neutrophil-lymphocyte ratio in patients with adenoidectomy. Journal of Clinical and Diagnostic Research. 2016;**10**(3):MC03-MC05. DOI: 10.7860/JCDR/2016/16549.7360

[3] Onder S, Caypinar B, Sahin-Yilmaz A, Toros SZ, Oysu C. Relation of mean platelet volume with obstructive adenoid hypertrophy in children. International Journal of Pediatric Otorhinolaryngology. 2014;**78**:1449-1451. DOI: 10.1016/j.ijporl.2014.06.001

[4] Cao Z, Li Z, Xiang H, Huang S, Gao J, Zhan X, et al. Prognostic role of haematological indices in sudden sensorineural hearing loss: Review and meta-analysis. Clinica Chimica Acta. 2018;**483**:104-111. DOI: 10.1016/j.cca.2018.04.025

[5] Salvago P, Rizzo S, Bianco A, Martines F. Sudden sensorineural hearing loss: Is there a relationship between routine haematological parameters and audiogram shapes? International Journal of Audiology. 2017;**56**:148-153. DOI: 10.1080/14992027.2016.1236418

[6] Durmus K, Terzi H, Karatas TD, Dogan M, Uysal IO, Sencan M, et al. Assessment of hematological factors involved in development and prognosis of idiopathic sudden sensorineural hearing loss. The Journal of Craniofacial Surgery. 2016;**27**:e85-e91. DOI: 10.1097/SCS.0000000000002241

[7] Oya R, Takenaka Y, Imai T, Sato T, Oshima K, Ohta Y, et al. Neutrophil-to-lymphocyte ratio and platelet-to-lymphocyte ratio as prognostic hematologic markers of Bell's palsy: A meta-analysis. Otology & Neurotology. 2019;**40**:681-687. DOI: 10.1097/MAO.0000000000002166

[8] Kim DH, Oh JH, Kim J, Cho CH, Lee JH. Predictive values of neutrophil-to-lymphocyte ratio, platelet-to-lymphocyte ratio, and other prognostic factors in pediatric patients with Bell's palsy. Ear, Nose, & Throat Journal. 2020. DOI: 10.1177/0145561320922097

[9] Elbistanli MS, Koçak HE, Acipayam H, Yiğider AP, Keskin M, Kayhan FT. The predictive value of neutrophil-lymphocyte and platelet-lymphocyte ratio for the effusion viscosity in otitis media with chronic effusion. The Journal of Craniofacial Surgery. 2017;**28**:e244-e247. DOI: 10.1097/SCS.0000000000003452

[10] Tansuker HD, Eroğlu S, Yenigün A, Taşkin Ü, Oktay MF. Can serum neutrophil-to-lymphocyte ratio Be a predictive biomarker to help differentiate active chronic otitis media from inactive chronic otitis media? The Journal of Craniofacial Surgery. 2017;**28**:e260-e263. DOI: 10.1097/SCS.0000000000003484

[11] Yigit E, Onerci Celebi O, Araz Server E, Longur ES. Neutrophil-to-lymphocyte ratio and mean platelet volume in chronic otitis media with or without cholesteatoma. Istanbul Medical Journal. 2018;**19**:162-166. DOI: 10.5152/imj.2018.77854

[12] Klllçkaya MM, Aynali G, Tuz M, Bagcl Ö. Is There A Systemic inflammatory effect of cholesteatoma? International Archives of Otorhinolaryngology 2017;**21**:42-45. doi:10.1055/s-0036-1584363

[13] Ulusoy B, Bozdemir K, Akyol M, Mişe HI, Kutluhan A, Korkmaz MH. Investigationofneutrophil-to-lymphocyte ratio, platelet-to-lymphocyte ratio and mean platelet volume in patients with tinnitus. The Journal of Laryngology & Otology. 2018;**132**(2):129-132. DOI: 10.1017/S0022215117002481

[14] Karaer IC. Mean platelet volume, neutrophil-to-lymphocyte ratio, and platelet-to-lymphocyte ratio as İnflammatory markers in patients with recurrent aphthous stomatitis. Eurasian Journal of Medicine. 2020;**52**:38-40. DOI: 10.5152/eurasianjmed.2019.18486

[15] Sennaroglu L, Onerci M, Hascelik G. The effect of tonsillectomy and adenoidectomy on neutrophil chemotaxis. Laryngoscope. 1993;**103**(12):1349-1351. DOI: 10.1288/00005537-199312000-00005

[16] Yenigun A. The efficacy of tonsillectomy in chronic tonsillitis patients as demonstrated by the neutrophil-to-lymphocyte ratio. The Journal of Laryngology and Otology. 2015;**129**:386-391. DOI: 10.1017/S0022215115000559

[17] Şentürk M, Azgın İ, Övet G, Alataş N, Ağırgöl B, Yılmaz E. O papel do volume plaquetário médio e a relação neutrófilos/linfócitos em abscesso periamigdaliano. Brazilian Journal of Otorhinolaryngology. 2016;**82**:662-667. DOI: 10.1016/j.bjorl.2015.11.018

[18] Bakshi SS. Letter to the editor regarding "predictive value of the neutrophil-to-lymphocyte ratio in patients with deep neck space infection secondary to acute bacterial tonsillitis". International Journal of Pediatric Otorhinolaryngology. 2017;**92**:193. DOI: 10.1016/j.ijporl.2015.10.028

[19] Yenigun A, Sezen S, Calim OF, Ozturan O. Evaluation of the eosinophil-to-lymphocyte ratio in pediatric patients with allergic rhinitis. American Journal of Rhinology & Allergy. n.d.;**30**:e21-e25. DOI: 10.2500/ajra.2016.30.4296

[20] Available from: https://neurosurgery.directory/2019/07/07/neutrophil-to-lymphocyte-ratio-for-glioma/

[21] Takenaka Y, Oya R, Kitamiura T, Ashida N, Shimizu K, Takemura K, et al. Prognostic role of neutrophil-to-lymphocyte ratio in head and neck cancer: A meta-analysis. Head & Neck. 2018;**40**:647-655. DOI: 10.1002/hed.24986

[22] Mascarella MA, Mannard E, Silva SD, Zeitouni A. Neutrophil-to-lymphocyte ratio in head and neck cancer prognosis: A systematic review and meta-analysis. Head & Neck. 2018;**40**:1091-1100. DOI: 10.1002/hed.25075

[23] Cho JK, Kim MW, Choi IS, Moon UY, Kim MJ, Sohn I, et al. Optimal cutoff of pretreatment neutrophil-to-lymphocyte ratio in head and neck cancer patients: A meta-analysis and validation study. BMC Cancer. 2018;**18**. DOI: 10.1186/s12885-018-4876-6

[24] Takenaka Y, Kitamura T, Oya R, Ashida N, Shimizu K, Takemura K, et al. Prognostic role of neutrophil–lymphocyte ratio in nasopharyngeal carcinoma: A meta-analysis. PLOS One. 2017;**12**. DOI: 10.1371/journal.pone.0181478

[25] Bojaxhiu B, Templeton AJ, Elicin O, Shelan M, Zaugg K, Walser M, et al. Relation of baseline neutrophil-to-lymphocyte ratio to survival and toxicity in head and neck cancer patients treated with (chemo-) radiation. Radiation Oncology. 2018;**13**. DOI: 10.1186/s13014-018-1159-y

[26] Eskiizmir G, Uz U, Onur E, Ozyurt B, Karaca Cikrikci G, Sahin N,

et al. The evaluation of pretreatment neutrophil–lymphocyte ratio and derived neutrophil–lymphocyte ratio in patients with laryngeal neoplasms. Brazilian Journal of Otorhinolaryngology. 2019;**85**:578-587. DOI: 10.1016/j.bjorl.2018.04.013

[27] Ueda T, Chikuie N, Takumida M, Furuie H, Kono T, Taruya T, et al. Baseline neutrophil-to-lymphocyte ratio (NLR) is associated with clinical outcome in recurrent or metastatic head and neck cancer patients treated with nivolumab. Acta Oto-Laryngologica. 2020;**140**:181-187. DOI: 10.1080/00016489.2019.1699250

[28] Xu C, Yuan J, Du W, Wu J, Fang Q, Zhang X, et al. Significance of the neutrophil-to-lymphocyte ratio in p16-negative squamous cell carcinoma of unknown primary in head and neck. Frontiers in Oncology. 2020;**10**. DOI: 10.3389/fonc.2020.00039

[29] Zhang B, Du W, Gan K, Fang Q, Zhang X. Significance of the neutrophil-to-lymphocyte ratio in young patients with oral squamous cell carcinoma. Cancer Management and Research. 2019;**11**:7597-7603. DOI: 10.2147/CMAR.S211847

[30] Tezol O, Bozlu G, Sagcan F, Tuncel Daloglu F, Citak C. Value of neutrophil-to-lymphocyte ratio, monocyte-to-lymphocyte ratio, platelet-to-lymphocyte ratio and red blood cell distribution width in distinguishing between reactive lymphadenopathy and lymphoma in children. Bratislava Medical Journal. 2020;**121**:287-292. DOI: 10.4149/bll_2020_045

Chapter 7

Neutrophil Gelatinase-Associated Lipocalin as a Promising Biomarker in Acute Kidney Injury

Camila Lima, Maria de Fatima Vattimo and Etienne Macedo

Abstract

Acute kidney injury (AKI) is a common complication in several settings inside and outside hospitals. It affects millions of people around the world, and despite high levels of research funding, there is no specific treatment that changes the disease course. The basis for unfavorable outcomes related to this disease is the failure to provide early diagnosis. Currently, the diagnosis of AKI is based on serum creatinine and urine output, and both measures have several limitations, making early diagnosis difficult. In recent decades, several biomarkers of kidney injury have been proposed, with neutrophil gelatinase-associated lipocalin (NGAL) being one of most studied and promising for use in early diagnosis. Despite there being several studies on NGAL, it has not yet been applied in clinical practice; thus, furthering the understanding of the development, interpretation, and limitations of NGAL in the diagnosis of AKI is the objective of this chapter.

Keywords: acute kidney injury, biomarkers, neutrophil gelatinase-associated lipocalin

1. Introduction

Acute kidney injury (AKI) is a frequent complication in several clinical settings, including large surgeries [1], emergency departments [2, 3], and intensive care units (ICUs) [4]. The incidence of AKI has been increasing over the years, with about 2 million people being affected in 2010 [5], despite the efforts of researchers and organizations [6–8]. AKI is commonly followed by worse outcomes: prolonged length of ICU and hospital stay, need for dialysis, decreases in the glomerular filtration rate (GRF), development of chronic kidney disease (CKD), and increases in mortality [9–11].

In recent decades, therapeutic interventions aimed at reversing kidney dysfunction have had disappointing results in multiple settings; thus, the research focus has shifted from treatment to prevention and early detection by focusing on two main issues: diagnostic criteria and early diagnosis. In 2004, the Acute Dialysis Quality Initiative (ADQI) sought a more uniform definition of AKI, and the most recent consensus definition was published in 2012 by Kidney Disease: Improving Global Outcomes (KDIGO) [8]. The diagnosis of AKI is based on changes in serum creatinine (Scr) and urine output (UO), but neither marker is kidney specific. Efforts have been made to identify novel biomarkers that have high sensitivity and specificity.

The standardization of the diagnosis of AKI allowed us to compare the diagnoses made in different settings. However, the issue of early diagnosis is still a challenge. First, there are limitations regarding the use of Scr and UO. Second, determining the need for renal replacement therapy is difficult due to a lack of information about whether the AKI is transient or persistent. Last, the research advances identifying early biomarkers have thus far been inaccessible in clinical practice [12].

Neutrophil gelatinase-associated lipocalin (NGAL) [13] has been far and away the most promising biomarker to help fill this gap, and its diagnostic capabilities as a biomarker have been confirmed in a large number of clinical trials. This chapter aims to present information on the role of NGAL in the renal injury process, its expression in the kidney, confounding factors, the type of assay used, whether plasma or urine NGAL has better accuracy, the cutoff values in normal individuals, the accuracy of NGAL for diagnosing AKI, and the evaluation of other outcomes.

2. The role of NGAL

In 1993, Kjeldsen et al. [13] isolated lipocalin as a protease-resistant polypeptide covalently bound to neutrophil gelatinase, named neutrophil gelatinase associated lipocalin (NGAL), also known as siderocalin, lipocalin 2 or oncogene 24p [14].

NGAL is a 25 kilodalton (kDa) protein covalently bound to gelatinase in neutrophil-specific granules. NGAL is expressed at very low levels in various human tissues, including the kidneys, uterus, prostate, salivary gland, trachea, lungs, stomach, and adult and fetal colon [15, 16]. The anti-inflammatory function of NGAL is demonstrated by increased NGAL expression in proliferative epithelia, inflammatory areas, and intestinal malignancies [17].

In normal kidneys, the expression of NGAL is mainly released by the thick ascending limb and the intercalated cells of the thick collecting duct. Some NGAL expression is also present in the proximal tubular epithelium, once NGAL is filtered by the glomerulus and reabsorbed by the proximal tubule in a megalin-dependent manner [17, 18]. The physiological function of NGAL in the kidneys is unknown; however, the role of NGAL in renal morphogenesis is under consideration [19]. NGAL also has a predominant role in the regulation of cell proliferation, repair processes, and tubular reepithelization. NGAL expression corresponds to an additional iron transport pathway, which increases the transcription of hemeoxygenase, an enzyme with proliferative and antiapoptotic effects that protects and preserves proximal tubular cells [20, 21].

Several biological functions for NGAL have been suggested; in the kidney, NGAL release is associated with ischemic or nephrotoxic insults. Additionally, a decrease in tubular reabsorption after AKI may lead to a further increase in urinary NGAL concentration, resulting acquiring a status of the "troponin" of the kidneys [22–24].

KEY POINT: The role of NGAL remains unclear, but its release mainly from the distal tubule has been associated with an increase in kidney injury.

3. Confounding factors affecting NGAL

The conditions that can interfere with the performance, sensitivity, and specificity of NGAL, already identified as a biomarker, are sepsis, chronic obstructive pulmonary disease, and cardiac dysfunction, and the presence of these conditions may act as confounding factors for NGAL measurements. The predictive performance of NGAL seems to also be influenced by age (higher predictive value in children than in older patients), sex (higher predictive value in female patients than in male patients), urinary tract infection, and impaired renal function (higher predictive value in patients with chronic kidney disease) [25–27].

Sepsis will be more thoroughly addressed in the next chapter.

KEY POINT. Controlling for confounding factors in clinical trials is vital to maintain the internal validity of a study.

4. Types of NGAL assays

The commercialization of NGAL as the gold standard for the diagnosis of AKI is somewhat controversial [28]. There are many types of NGAL assays available on the market that use different nonautomated ELISA platforms, which makes it difficult for comparisons to be made among studies from around the world.

The first kit for the quantitative and automated determination of NGAL by the ELISA method was developed by Abbott Laboratories (Abbott Park, IL, USA) for the urinary evaluation of NGAL, with a cutoff value of 141 μg/L (95% CI 125–158 μg/L). An EDTA plasma blood test was created by the Triage Meter platform (Biosite-Inverness Medical, Waltham, USA) with a cutoff value of 163 μ/L (CI 109–221 μ/L) [29].

Bioporto (Bioporto Diagnostics A/S, Gentfte, Denmark) developed a new particle-enhanced turbidimetric immunoassay (PETIA) that has the advantages of flexibility (adaptation for clinical use in different analyzers), automation (closer to clinical practice), and applicability in different biological matrices (urine and plasma) [30].

The chemiluminescence test is an alternative to assess NGAL, and it is commonly used to analyze studies with small animals since it is possible to do the analysis with few substrates [31].

Because there are three known molecular forms of NGAL, the assay of interest should differentiate the 25 kDa NGAL monomer produced by the monocyte tubular epithelial cells from other forms of NGAL: 45 kDa NGAL, from the homodimer predominantly secreted by neutrophils, and the 145 kDa NGAL/matrix metalloproteinase-9 (MMP9) covalently complexed heterodimer [32, 33].

According to Mårtensson et al. [34] and Cai et al. [33], the combination of two ELISAs, may improve the diagnostic accuracy of NGAL, one to determine the monomeric form and the other to determine the homodimeric form.

The confounding factor of sepsis is described herein and is dependent on the assay method, as well as whether the chosen kit is less sensitive to 25 kDa NGAL expressed by tubular epithelial cells. The test can also measure the 45 kDa homodimer predominantly secreted by neutrophils, which are common in sepsis, and the increase in neutrophils increases homodimeric NGAL expression and results in false positives.

KEY POINT: Choose a method closer to those used in clinical practice and a test more accurate for measuring the monomeric form of NGAL expressed by tubular epithelial cells after injury.

5. Plasma or urine NGAL measurement and normalization of urine values

The consensus is clear that NGAL measured in urine has better performance [35], because the release and increase in NGAL will occur first in urine. However, the collection of urine depends on the urine output, which is sometimes not available. Some benefits of plasma NGAL are that it is available at any time and is more accurate in anuric or oliguric patients.

The issue about the normalization of urinary NGAL by correction for the urinary creatinine level is debatable, but it has been used to correct for urine output in cases of oliguria or pollakiuria, avoiding inaccurate concentration or dilution measurements of the biomarkers. The fact is that the creatinine release time is different from the biomarker release time, and the normalized level will be affected by this difference and will not represent a real physiological value [36].

KEY POINT: Urinary NGAL is released earlier than plasma NGAL, and the accuracy of the normalization of urinary NGAL by creatinine is debatable.

6. Cutoff values of NGAL in normal individuals

The determination of normal NGAL levels in healthy adults has been inadequately described in the literature. However, some studies have been performed, such as that of Cullen et al. [26], which analyzed urine by the Abbot-Architec assay in 174 healthy people (100 men and 74 women aged between 19 and 88 years). The value of the immunoassay result was normalized by urinary creatinine, and the cut-off value was 107 μ/mmol (13 μ/mmol). There was a higher concentration of creatinine-normalized urinary NGAL in women, in the elderly and in patients with leukocyturia.

The study reported by Stejkal et al. [37] analyzed BioVendor's NGAL assay using the serum of 136 healthy, nonobese individuals (53 men and 83 women). The authors reported median NGAL values (78.8 μg/L for men and 80 μg/L for women). Pernnemans et al. [27] analyzed the NGAL ELISA (RD System Europe, Abingdon, UK) and other urinary biomarkers in 338 healthy individuals (199 women and 139 men, aged 0 to 95 years). They reported that the NGAL reference range of the 21–95 years age group was 73.88–211.16 μg/L in women and 149.26–182.58 μg/L in men, and there was higher expression in elderly individuals.

An NGAL PETIA (Bioporto Diagnostics A/S, Gentfte, Denmark) [36] was evaluated for 200 healthy nonobese individuals (137 men and 63 women, with a mean age of 39 years (SD 11.2)). They proposed reference plasma concentrations from 38.7–157.6 ng/ml for women and 24.4–142.5 ng/ml for men and proposed reference urine concentrations of <9–54.5 ng/ml for both sexes. The authors reported that the mean values in men were higher than in women, 78.9 ng/ml vs. 73.8 ng/ml, respectively; there was a significant difference in NGAL in relation to age.

In addition to the variability of the chosen immunoassay, the unit of measurement in the interpretation of the NGAL studies should be considered—the most commonly found are ng/ml, μg/L, ng/dl, mg/ml and μg/mmol.

KEY POINT: The median cutoff value for urinary NGAL in healthy men was between 78.8 and 182.58 μg/L, and the median plasma value was between 24.4 and 142.5 ng/ml in men. The broad variability of the results difficult to interpret.

7. NGAL to predict AKI

NGAL is the most widely investigated AKI biomarker. Its performance for predicting AKI has been evaluated in various settings, such as in pediatric and adult cardiac surgery patients, in critically ill patients, and in patients in the emergency room, as well in kidney transplant and other settings [38, 39].

Numerous studies have demonstrated the ability of NGAL to diagnose AKI. For example, the study reported by Constantin et al. [40], that evaluated the plasma NGAL of 88 patients at ICU admission, found a sensitivity of 82%, specificity of 97% and AUC of 0.92 to cut-off value of 155 mmol/L to predictor of AKI.

A multicenter study, reported by Di Somma et al. [41], with 665 patients admitted to the emergency department, assessed plasma NGAL in several points after admission. Serial evaluation of NGAL at times zero and six hours provided a high negative predictive value (NPV) (98%) to rule out the diagnosis of AKI within six hours of the arrival of patients to the emergency department. The NGAL value at admission could demonstrated a strong predictive value for in-hospital mortality of the patient, with a cut-off value of 400 ng/ml.

In the meta-analysis by Haase et al. [42]—with 19 studies, totaling 2538 patients, of whom 487 (19.2%) developed AKI—NGAL was demonstrated to have diagnostic and prognostic value for AKI, with an OR of 18.6 (95% CI 9–38.1) and AUC of 0.81 (95% CI 0.73–0.89). The cut-off value ranged from 100 to 270 ng/ml, but a value of 150 ng/dl was suggested for the diagnosis of AKI.

In another recent meta-analysis by Zhou et al. [39]—with 24 studies, a total of 4066 patients from 9 countries, including studies with serum and urinary NGAL—the sensitivity for the diagnosis of AKI was 0.68 (95% CI, 65–0.70), and the specificity was 0.79 (95% CI 0.77–0.80).

In the study by Singer et al. [38], urinary NGAL was useful for classifying and stratifying patients with established AKI: the level of NGAL>104 μg/L indicated intrinsic AKI (odds ratio of 5.97), while the level of NGAL <47 μg/L indicated unlikely intrinsic AKI (odds ratio of 0.2). In the logistic regression analysis, NGAL was able to predict the worsening of the RIFLE class, the need for RRT and in-hospital mortality. The performance of NGAL to evaluate other outcomes will be discussed in the next chapter.

KEY POINT: Despite the good results of NGAL for predicting AKI, the variability of the cutoff value is still a challenge for applying NGAL in clinical practice.

8. The early timing diagnosis by NGAL versus standard serum creatinine

The study by Bennett et al. [43] clearly indicated that urinary NGAL is a powerful early biomarker of AKI after cardiopulmonary bypass that preceded the increase in serum creatinine by 2–3 days. Studies have shown that elevation of NGAL is detectable after 3 hours and peaks approximately 6–12 hours after injury. The elevation can persist up to 5 days according to the severity of injury [44–46]. In addition to Benett's study, other studies in general have failed to reach conclusions about the early timing diagnosis of NGAL, which is the main finding required to reach a therapeutic window and better evaluate future medication targets in AKI.

KEY POINT: If you perform a study or analyze a biomarker, remember to compare the pattern of biomarker early timing diagnosis with serum creatinine.

9. Evaluation of other outcomes by NGAL

Several studies have assessed the diagnostic value of NGAL to predict AKI, but only a few have analyzed the early diagnosis in hours/days and compared it with serum creatinine, as seen in the last chapter. Still fewer studies have evaluated the predictive performance of NGAL in other outcomes, such as the need for RRT, recovery of renal function, progression to end stage renal disease (ESRD) and mortality, which will be discussed in this chapter.

In the meta-analysis by Hall et al. [47], for 91 kidney transplant patients, the incidence of need for RRT was 4.3%, and NGAL, in this scenario, had an OR of 12.9 and AUC of 0.78. In the same study, NGAL and urinary IL18 were predictors of the need for RRT up to 1 week after transplantation. NGAL presented a good AUC of

0.81 (95% CI 0.70–0.92) 6 hours after transplantation and was also a predictor of graft recovery for up to 3 months.

In the study conducted by Constantin et al. [40], the cutoff value of NGAL to assess the need for RRT was 330 mmol/L. The value of urinary NGAL (Architect, Abbot Park, IL) was correlated with the need for dialysis (r: 0.48 P: 0.01), presenting an AUC of 0.86 2 hours after cardiopulmonary bypass in children [43].

A recent meta-analysis by Klein et al. analyzed 12 studies to predict the need for RRT and found an AUC of 0.70 (95% CI 0.63–0.80) for NGAL [48].

Bhavsar et al. [49] concluded that higher levels of NGAL (measured by the Luminex assay) were associated with stage 3 CKD incidence. Some researchers have discussed whether the association of NGAL level is not exclusively related to the increase in neutrophils already described by Tian et al. [50] and maintain that further studies would be needed to elucidate this issue.

In the meta-analysis by Haase et al. [42], the incidence of mortality was 5.4%, and NGAL, in this scenario, showed an OR of 8.8 and AUC of 0.70.

In the Ariza study [51], PNGAL and UNGAL were demonstrated to be strong predictors of prognosis, and UNGAL was significantly predictive of the MELD score using the 28-day mortality score AUC of 0.88 (0.83–0.92).

In the study by Bennett et al. [43], the value of urinary NGAL (Architect, Abbot Park, IL) was also correlated with mortality (r: 0.53 p 0.01), with an AUC of 0.91, 2 hours after cardiopulmonary bypass in children.

The study by Dent et al. [52], using PNGAL (Biosite Inc., San Diego, USA) in 120 children undergoing cardiopulmonary bypass (CBP) and a cut-off value of 150 ng/ml and AKI prediction, found an AUC of 0.96 2 hours after CBP. PNGAL was also strongly correlated with the duration of AKI ($r = 0.57$, $p < 0.001$) and hospital stay time ($r = 0.44$, $p < 0.001$), and PNGAL at 12 hours was correlated with mortality ($r = 0.48$, p: 0.004).

In the study by Daniels et al. [53], PNGAL (Alere Inc., Waltham, USA) was measured in 1393 adult patients with cardiovascular disease (CVD) who were followed for 11 years. Of these, 436 did not survive, and 169 died from CVD. PNGAL was a predictor of CVD mortality, with a risk ratio of 1.33% and a risk ratio of 1.19% for all causes of mortality.

KEY POINT: Evaluating outcomes by NGAL beyond the limitation of only the diagnosis of AKI is important to know how more than one parameter evaluates the outcome and prognosis, and it could help physicians by indicating an early need for RRT, for example.

10. Conclusion

This brief review, based on accumulated evidence, discussed the role and value of NGAL in the diagnosis and prognosis of AKI. Studies' findings suggest that induction of NGAL plays an important role in kidney function preservation, reducing apoptosis, and enhancing proliferative responses. In kidney injury, rapid and massive upregulated synthesis of NGAL occurs in the distal tubule, which quickly increases the concentration of NGAL in urine [54]. In addition, other important considerations have been provided as "key point" to help researchers move the NGAL analysis to clinical practice as soon possible.

Conflict of interest

The authors declare that there are no conflicts of interest regarding the publication of this chapter.

Author details

Camila Lima[1*†], Maria de Fatima Vattimo[2‡] and Etienne Macedo[1,3§]

1 Internal Medicine Department, Nephrology Division, University of Sao Paulo, Sao Paulo, Brazil

2 Medical Surgical Department, School of Nursing, University of Sao Paulo, Sao Paulo, Brazil

3 Department of Medicine, Nephrology Division, University of California, San Diego, USA

*Address all correspondence to: camilaxlima@gmail.com

† Current Address: 455 Av. Arnaldo Dr, 01246-903, Cerqueira Cesar, Sao Paulo, Brazil.

‡ Current Address: 419 Av Dr Eneas de Carvalho Aguiar, Cerqueira Cesar, Sao Paulo, Brazil.

§ Current Address: 9500 Gilman Dr, MC 0892, La Jolla, California, United States of America.

References

[1] Zhou F, Luo Q, Wang L, Han L. Diagnostic value of neutrophil gelatinase-associated lipocalin for early diagnosis of cardiac surgery-associated acute kidney injury: A meta-analysis. European Journal of Cardio-Thoracic Surgery. 2016;**49**(3):746-755. DOI: 10.1093/ejcts/ezv199

[2] Nickolas TL, O'Rourke MJ, Yang J, Sise ME, Canetta PA, Barasch N, et al. Sensitivity and specificity of a single emergency department measurement of urinary neutrophil gelatinase-associated lipocalin for diagnosing acute kidney injury. Annals of Internal Medicine. 2008;**148**:810-819

[3] Di Somma S, Magrini L, Berardinis B, Marino R, Ferri E, Moscatelli P, et al. Additive value of blood neutrophil gelatinase associated lipocalin to clinical judgement in acute kidney injury diagnosis and mortality prediction in patients hospitalized from the emergency department. Critical Care. 2013;**17**(29):1-13. DOI: 10.1186/cc12510

[4] Constantin JM, Futier E, Perbet S, Roszyk L, Lautrette A, Gillart T, et al. Plasma neutrophil gelatinase-associated lipocalin is an early marker of acute kidney injury in adult critically ill patients: A prospective study. Journal of Critical Care. 2010;**25**(1):176.e1-176.e6. DOI: 10.1016/j.jcrc.2009.05.010

[5] Ali T, Roderick P. Epidemiology of Acute Kidney Injury. Berlin Heidelberg: Springer; 2010

[6] Chawla LS, Bellomo R, Bihorac A, et al. Acute kidney disease and renal recovery: Consensus report of the acute disease quality initiative (ADQI) 16 workgroup. Nature Reviews. Nephrology. 2017;**13**(4):241-257

[7] Mehta RL, Kellum JA, Shah SV, Molitoris BA, Ronco C, et al. Acute kidney injury network: Report of an initiative to improve outcomes in acute kidney injury. Critical Care. 2007;**11**(2):1-8

[8] Kidney. Disease improving global outcomes (KDIGO) acute kidney injury work group. KDIGO clinical practice guideline for acute kidney injury. Kidney International. Supplement. 2012;**2**:1-138

[9] Afonso RC, Hidalgo R, Zurstrassen MP, Fonseca LE, Pandullo FL, Rezende MB, et al. Impact of renal failure on liver transplantation survival. Transplantation Proceedings. 2008;**40**:808-810

[10] Chertow GM, Burdick E, Honour M, Bonventre JV, Bates DW. Acute kidney injury, mortality, length of stay, and costs in hospitalized patients. Journal of the American Society of Nephrology. 2005;**16**:3365-3370

[11] Fabrizi F, Dixit V, Martin P, Messa P. Chronic kidney disease after liver transplantation: Recent evidence. The International Journal of Artificial Organs. 2010;**33**(11):803-811

[12] Lima C, Macedo E. Urinary biochemistry in the diagnosis of acute kidney injury. Disease Markers. 2018;**2018**:4907024. DOI: 10.1155/2018/4907024

[13] Kjeldsen L, Johnsen AH, Sengelov H, Borregaard N. Isolation and primary structure of NGAL, a novel protein associated with human neutrophil gelatinase. The Journal of Biological Chemistry. 1993;**268**:10425-10432

[14] Kashani K, Cheungpasitporn W, Ronco C. Biomarkers of acute kidney injury: The pathway from discovery to clinical adoption. Clinical Chemistry and Laboratory Medicine. 2017;**55**(8):1074-1089. DOI: 10.1515/cclm-2016-0973

[15] Cowland JB, Borregaard N. Molecular characterization and pattern of tissue expression of the gene for neutrophil gelatinaseassociated lipocalin from humans. Genomics. 1997;**45**:17-23

[16] Zappitelli M, Washburn KK, Arikan AA, Loftis L, Ma Q, Devarajan P, et al. Urine neutrophil gelatinase-associated lipocalin is an early marker of acute kidney injury in critically ill children: A prospective cohort study. Critical Care (London, England). 2007;**11**:R84

[17] Nielsen B, Borregaard N, Bundgaard J, Timshel S, Sehested M, Kjeldsen L. Induction of NGAL synthesis in epithelial cells of human colorectal neoplasia and inflammatory bowel diseases. Gut. 1996;**38**:414-420

[18] Hvidberg V, Jacobsen C, Strong RK, et al. The endocytic receptor megalin binds the iron transporting neutrophil-gelatinase-associated lipocalin with high affinity and mediates its cellular uptake. FEBS Letters. 2005;**579**:773-777

[19] Schmidt-Ott KM, Chen X, Paragas N, Levinson RS, Mendelsohn CL, Barasch J. C-kit delineates a distinct domain of progenitors in the developing kidney. Developmental Biology. 2006;**299**(1):238-249

[20] Kiyoshi M, Thomas HL, Dana R, Ian RD, Kirk F, Jun Y, et al. Endocytic delivery of lipocalin-siderophore-iron complex rescues the kidney from ischemia-reperfusion injury. Journal of Clinical Investigation. 2005;**115**:610-621

[21] Yang J, Goetz D, Li JY, Wang W, Mori K, Setlik D, et al. An iron delivery pathway mediated by a lipocalin. Molecular Cell. 2002;**10**:1045-1056

[22] Schrezenmeier EV, Barasch J, Budde K, Westhoff T, Schmidt-Ott KM. Biomarkers in acute kidney injury – Pathophysiological basis and clinical performance. Acta Physiologica. 2017;**219**:556-574

[23] Mishra J, Ma Q, Prada A, et al. Identification of neutrophil gelatinase-associated lipocalin as a novel early urinary biomarker for ischemic renal injury. Journal of the American Society of Nephrology. 2003;**14**:2534-2543

[24] Mishra J, Mori K, Ma Q, Kelly C, Barasch J, Devarajan P. Neutrophil gelatinase-associated lipocalin: A novel early urinary biomarker for cisplatin nephrotoxicity. American Journal of Nephrology. 2004;**24**:307-315

[25] Legrand M, Darmon M, Joannidis M. NGAL and AKI: The end of a myth? Intensive Care Medicine. 2013;**39**:1861-1863. DOI: 10.1007/s00134-013-3061-2

[26] Cullen MR, Murray PT, Fitzgibbon MC. Establishment of a reference interval for urinary neutrophil gelatinase-associated lipocalin. Annals of Clinical Biochemistry. 2012;**49**(2):190-193

[27] Pennemans V, Rigo JM, Faes C, Reynders C, Penders J, Swennen Q. Establishment of reference values for novel urinary biomarkers for renal damage in the healthy population: Are age and gender an issue? Clinical Chemistry and Laboratory Medicine. 2013;**51**(9):1795-1802

[28] Cervellin G, Di Somma S. Neutrophil gelatinase-associated lipocalin (NGAL): The clinician's perspective. Clinical Chemistry and Laboratory Medicine. 2012;**50**(9):1489-1493. DOI: 10.1515/cclm-2012-0433

[29] Cavalier E, Bekaert AC, Carlisi A, Legrand D, Krzesinski JM, Delanaye P. Neutrophil gelatinase-associated lipocalin (NGAL) determined in urine with the Abbott architect or in plasma with the biosite triage? The laboratory's point of view. Clinical Chemistry and Laboratory Medicine. 2011;**49**:339-341

[30] Bargnoux AS, Piéroni L, Cristol JP. Analytical study of a new turbidimetric assay for urinary neutrophil gelatinase-associated lipocalin (NGAL) determination. Clinical Chemistry and Laboratory Medicine. 2013;**51**(12):293-296

[31] Krzeminska E, Wyczalkowska-Tomasik A, Korytowska N, Paczek L. Comparison of two methods for determination of NGAL levels in urine: ELISA and CMIA. Journal of Clinical Laboratory Analysis. 2016;**30**(6): 956-960. DOI: 10.1002/jcla.21962

[32] ILippi G, Plebani M. Neutrophil gelatinase-associated lipocalin (NGAL): The laboratory perspective. Clinical Chemistry and Laboratory Medicine. 2012;**50**:1483-1487

[33] Cai L, Rubin J, Han W, Venge P, Xu S. The origin of multiple molecular forms in urine of HNL/NGAL. Clinical Journal of the American Society of Nephrology. 2010;**5**(12):2229-2235

[34] Mårtensson J, Xu S, Bell M, Martling CR, Venge P. Immunoassays distinguishing between HNL/NGAL released in urine from kidney epithelial cells and neutrophils. Clinica Chimica Acta. 2012;**413**(19-20):1661-1667

[35] Lima C, de Paiva Haddad LB, de Melo PDV, Malbouisson LM, do Carmo LPF, D'Albuquerque LAC, et al. Early detection of acute kidney injury in the perioperative period of liver transplant with neutrophil gelatinase-associated lipocalin. BMC Nephrology. 2019;**20**(1):367. DOI: 10.1186/s12882-019-1566-9

[36] Makris K, Stefani D, Makri E, Panagou I, Lagiou M, Sarli A, et al. Evaluation of a particle enhanced turbidimetric assay for the measurement of neutrophil gelatinase-associated lipocalin in plasma and urine on Architect-8000: Analytical performance and establishment of reference values. Clinical Biochemistry. 2015;**48**(18):1291-1297. DOI: 10.1016/j.clinbiochem.2015.08.003

[37] Stejskal D, Karpísek M, Humenanska V, Hanulova Z, Stejskal P, Kusnierova P, et al. Lipocalin-2: Development, analytical characterization, and clinical testing of a new ELISA. Hormone and Metabolic Research. 2008;**40**(6):381-385

[38] Singer E, Elger A, Elitok S, Kettritz R, Nickolas T, Barasch J, et al. Urinary neutrophil gelatinase-associated lipocalin distinguishes pre-renal from intrinsic renal failure and predicts outcomes. Kidney International. 2011;**80**:405-411. DOI: 10.1038/ki.2011.41

[39] Zhou F, Luo Q, Wang L, Han L. Diagnostic value of neutrophil gelatinase-associated lipocalin for early diagnosis of cardiac surgery-associated acute kidney injury: A meta-analysis. European Journal of Cardio-Thoracic Surgery. 2016;**49**(3):746-755

[40] Constantin JM, Futier E, Perbet S, Roszyk L, Lautrette A, Gillart T, et al. Plasma neutrophil gelatinase-associated lipocalin is an early marker of acute kidney injury in adult critically ill patients: A prospective study. Journal of Critical Care. 2010;**25**:176

[41] Di Somma S, Magrini L, Berardinis B, Marino R, Ferri E, Moscatelli P, et al. Additive value of blood neutrophil gelatinase associated lipocalin to clinical judgement in acute kidney injury diagnosis and mortality prediction in patients hospitalized from the emergency department. Critical Care. 2013;**17**(29):1-13

[42] Haase M, Bellomo R, Devarajan P, Schlattmann P, Haase-Fielitz A. NGAL meta-analysis Investigator Group. Accuracy of neutrophil gelatinase-associated lipocalin (NGAL) in diagnosis and prognosis in acute

kidney injury: A systematic review and metaanalysis. American Journal of Kidney Diseases. 2009;**54**(6): 1012-1024. DOI: 10.1053/j.ajkd.2009.07.020

[43] Bennett M, Dent CL, Ma Q, Dastrala S, Grenier F, Workman R, et al. Urine NGAL predicts severity of acute kidney injury after cardiac surgery: A prospective study. Clinical Journal of the American Society of Nephrology. 2008;**3**:665-673. DOI: 10.2215/CJN.04010907

[44] Devarajan P. Review: Neutrophil gelatinase-associated lipocalin - A troponin-like biomarker for human acute kidney injury. Nephrology (Carlton, Vic.). 2010;**15**:419-428

[45] Mishra J, Dent C, Tarabishi R, Mitsnefes MM, Ma Q, Kelly C, et al. Neutrophil gelatinase-associated lipocalin (NGAL) as a biomarker for acute renal injury after cardiac surgery. The Lancet. 2005;**365**:1231-1238

[46] Parikh CR, Coca SG, Thiessen-Philbrook H, Shlipak MG, Koyner JL, Wang Z, et al. Postoperative biomarkers predict acute kidney injury and poor outcomes after adult cardiac surgery. Journal of the American Society of Nephrology. 2011;**22**:1748-1757

[47] Hall IE, Yarlagadda SG, Coca SG, Wang Z, Doshi M, Devarajan P, et al. IL-18 and urinary NGAL predict dialysis andgraft recovery after kidney transplantation. Journal of the American Society of Nephrology. 2010;**21**:189-197

[48] Klein SJ, Brandtner AK, Lehner GF, Ulmer H, Bagshaw SM, Wiedermann CJ, et al. Biomarkers for prediction of renal replacement therapy in acute kidney injury: A systematic review and meta-analysis. Intensive Care Medicine. 2018;**44**:323-336. DOI: 10.1007/s00134-018-5126-8

[49] Bhavsar NA, Köttgen A, Coresh J, Astor BC. Neutrophil gelatinase-associated lipocalin (NGAL) and kidney injury molecule 1 (KIM-1) as predictors of incident CKD stage 3: The atherosclerosis risk in communities (ARIC) study. American Journal of Kidney Diseases. 2012;**60**(2):865-867

[50] Tian N, Penman AD, Manning RD Jr, Flessner MF, Mawson AR. Association between circulating specific leukocyte types and incident chronic kidney disease: The atherosclerosis risk in communities (ARIC) study. Journal of the American Society of Hypertension. 2012;**6**(2):100-108

[51] Ariza X, Graupera I, Coll M, Solà E, Barreto R, García E, et al. Neutrophil gelatinase-associated lipocalin is a biomarker of acute-on-chronic liver failure and prognosis in cirrhosis. Journal of Hepatology. 2016;**65**(1):57-65. DOI: 10.1016/j.jhep.2016.03.002

[52] Dent CL, Ma Q, Dastrala S, Bennett M, Mitsnefes MM, Barasch J, et al. Plasma neutrophil gelatinase-associated lipocalin predicts acute kidney injury, morbidity and mortality after pediatric cardiac surgery: A prospective uncontrolled cohort study. Critical Care. 2007;**11**(6):1-8. DOI: 10.1186/cc6192

[53] Daniels LB, Barrett-Connor E, Clopton P, Laughlin GA, Ix JH, Maisel AS. Plasma neutrophil gelatinase-associated lipocalin is independently associated with cardiovascular disease and mortality in community-dwelling older adults. The rancho Bernardo study. Journal of the American College of Cardiology. 2012;**59**:1101-1109

[54] Misha J, Mori K, Ma Q. Amelioration of ischemic acute renal injury by neutrophil gelatinase-associated lipocalim. Journal of the American Society of Nephrology. 2004;**15**:3073-3082

Chapter 8

The Role of Neutrophil Extracellular Traps (NETs) in the Pathogenesis and Complications of Malignant Diseases

Sheniz Yuzeir and Liana Gercheva

Abstract

It was recently proved that neutrophils and platelets are active participants in some inflammatory processes as well as a number of pathological conditions, including neoplastic diseases and thrombosis. It has been found that circulating neutrophils actively affect the mechanisms of tumour genesis, and along with platelets, act as independent regulators of different complications in infectious and malignant diseases. A few years ago, it was found that neutrophils have the ability to release extracellular traps (called neutrophil extracellular traps or NETs). Thus, neutrophils use both intracellular and extracellular mechanisms to limit inflammatory complications. Several recent studies confirmed that NETs increase considerably in malignant diseases, demonstrating that tumour-induced NETosis is a clinically significant process. It is recognised as an element of tumour biology, as it participates in tumour progression and angiogenesis. Neutrophils and the NETs released from them are stimulators of thrombotic processes in physiological and pathological conditions. Several reports demonstrate the connection between NETs and thrombosis. The presence of NETosis serves as a potential risk factor for thrombotic complications in malignant diseases. This chapter summarises the current knowledge of NETosis and the mechanisms that lead to the formation of NETs, including the role of circulating platelet–neutrophil complexes as regulators of tumour-induced NETosis in malignant diseases.

Keywords: NETosis, neutrophils, platelets, malignant diseases, infections

1. Introduction

One of the important causes of increased mortality in patients suffering from different inflammatory and neoplastic diseases is thrombosis of a large artery or vein. Recently, the attention of study groups has been drawn to the newly discovered functions of neutrophils, which confirm their significant role in not only inflammatory processes but also a number of pathological conditions, including neoplastic diseases and thrombosis [1, 2].

Neutrophils, as inherent mediators of immune defence, play an important role in various inflammatory processes [1]. Studies of the content of neutrophil granules reveal that an abundance of enzymes and macromolecules have roles in the different cellular interactions of granulocytes [3]. Enzyme-rich content reflects the active participation of neutrophils in the protective inflammatory response to bacteria, fungi and, to a lesser extent, other infections. These enzyme-mediated reactions are activated after membrane signalisation from the granulocyte plasmalemma, which possesses adhesive proteins, receptor molecules and ionic channels with pump mechanisms [4, 5]. Some receptor molecules have enzyme activity that inactivates cytokines and interleukins or activates intracellular processes for chemotactic movement of neutrophils through circulation from endothelial pores to tissues [6, 7]. Their ability to absorb pathogens and activate apoptosis through intracellular phagolysosomes is well known. After apoptosis was first described in 1972, several other mechanisms of cellular death were revealed, and decoding the paths leading to cellular death has remained a subject of discussion. In 2004, a group of scientists led by Brinkman [8] proved that stimulation of neutrophils with interleukin 8 (IL-8) or lipopolysaccharides (LPSs) causes liberation of chromatin in the extracellular space. Thus, these specific inflammatory cells release neutrophilic extracellular traps (NETs), which are formed mainly by decondensed nucleosomes and chromatin extracted from intracellular granules, such as neutrophil elastase and myeloperoxidase. So, it has been proven that neutrophils use both intracellular and extracellular mechanisms to confine infections.

2. Neutrophil Extracellular Traps (NETs)

The process of NET formation is called NETosis. This is characterised as a new process of cellular death that leads to chromatin decondensation, followed by cellular protein disintegration, lysis of the cytoplasm membrane and release of NETs [9]. The process of NETosis is dependent on enzyme peptidylarginine deaminase 4 (PAD4), which catalyses the transformation of histone-associated arginine residues into citrulline. It is mediated through the transformation of the α-amino group of arginine into a ketone group with subsequent chromatin decondensation [10–12].

The molecular mechanisms leading to NET formation remain unclear. According to recent data, the release of NETs in the extracellular space depends on two important processes: generation of reactive oxygen species (ROS) and decondensation of chromatin. The production of ROS is realised by activating nicotinamide adenine dinucleotide phosphate, (NADPH) oxydase as well as by including additional signal paths that mediate different forms of NETosis. The activation of protein kinase C leads to the assembly of a NOX 2 complex in the phagosome membrane and subsequent electronic transport and formation of hydrogen peroxide (H_2O_2), which is a powerful inductor for the generation of NETs [9, 13].

The second process leading to the formation of NETs is decondensation of chromatin. Interestingly, the additional release of lipopolysaccharides demonstrates that neutrophil elastase from azurophilic granules is the etiologic agent of this phenomenon. After neutrophil activation, the enzyme moves to the cellular nucleus and decomposes histones, particularly histone 4, while the nuclear changes and decondensation of chromatin are both proportional to the level of histone 4 decomposition [14]. This implies that the other enzyme included in the process of NET formation is myeloperoxidase [15]. An important step in NET formation is epigenetic modification of the histones, so-called histone citrullination through activation of the enzyme peptidyl-arginine deaminase (PAD4). Histone citrullination prevents histone methylation and further transcription, eventually resulting in chromatin decondensation [12, 16]. Releasing NET into the extracellular space involves a series of interconnected processes. The first process occurs when the nuclear and granular membrane disintegrates and elastase enters the nucleus; the second process involves the hypercytrulinisation of histones; the third process includes decondensation in the cytoplasm; and the fourth process transpires when the plasma membrane ruptures and nuclear material is extruded from the cell in the outer space. Certain enzymes, such as peptidyl arginine deminase type IV (PAD4), neutrophil elastase (NE) and myeloperoxidase (MPO), play key roles in the chromatin decondensation process [17, 18]. Extracellular DNA, histones and granular enzymes form a network of NETs that capture endogenous (e.g. platelets) and external (e.g. bacteria) particles. In addition, molecules are involved in the formation of HETs. Negatively charged DNA has been determined to act as the basis for NET and to interact with other NET components through a positive electrostatic charge. Although a number of studies have used PMA as an inducer of NET, the exact intracellular pathway that leads to the release of NET has yet to be determined [19, 20].

Most studies have concluded that an important autophagy process is activated in the formation of NETs. Autophagy is an anti-apoptotic mechanism that activates in response to cell stress. It occurs in order to regulate protein and organelle turnover, ensuring cell survival [21]. The protein kinase mammalian target of rapamycin (mTOR) negatively regulates autophagy, which is also involved in the formation of NET [22, 23]. Most studies have indicated that an important autophagy process is activated during the formation of NETs. Some intracellular signalling pathways, such as the PICK3 blocking autophagy, inhibit the release of NETS. It has been presumed that autophagy is critical to the release of NET in both infectious and non-infectious diseases, such as sepsis, familiar Mediterranean fever (FMF), gout and inflammatory-driven fibrosis [24, 25].

The main components of NETs are DNA, histones and proteases, which have pro-coagulation properties. Histones have a marked cytotoxic effect on the vascular endothelium and can induce thrombosis [26]. Sulphurous proteases, such as neutrophil elastase, inactivate the tissue factor pathway inhibitor and lead to hypercoagulation and fibrin deposition [27].

The critical role of neutrophils in the processes of tumour genesis has been emphasised in a number of publications. As inflammatory cells, they release different types of cytokines and chemokines that, through activation of intercellular interactions and modulation of the immune response, influence the tumour microenvironment [28]. In addition, the proteases secreted by neutrophils have a specific role in regulation of the proliferation of tumour cells, tumour angiogenesis and the metastasis process. Different activating cytokines [IL-8, granulocyte colony-stimulating factor (G-CSF) and tumour necrosis factor alpha], myeloperoxidase, neutrophil elastase and histone citrullination are included in the NET release process [21].

Some studies emphasise the critical role of G-CSF in tumour-induced NETosis. It is known that a major proportion of tumour cells produce G-CSF, which induces neutrophilia, a common finding in malignant diseases, which is usually related to poor prognosis. By releasing NETs, neutrophils provide a scaffold and stimulate the processes of platelet adhesion and aggregation. They are closely linked to tumour cells in vivo and in the tumour vasculature, but their role in tumour biology is still a subject of discussion.

Tumour-induced neutrophils have both pro- and anti-tumour potential. On the one hand, they secrete cytokines, generate thrombin and initiate positive feedback for stimulation of tumour growth, tumour invasion and maintenance of tumour angiogenesis. On the other hand, the anti-tumour potential of neutrophils is explained by their direct cytotoxic interaction with cancer cells, which stimulates the apoptotic decomposition of tumour cells due to their antibody-dependent cell-mediated cytotoxicity and favours their migration [29]. A number of studies have confirmed that tumours expressing high levels of G-CSF are powerful inductors of NETosis [30]. Also, cytokine IL-8, which is frequently expressed by different tumour cells, is described as a NET-inducing factor and has recently been proven to be essential for tumour-induced NETosis [31].

NETosis occurs in some infectious diseases as well as a number of non-infectious diseases. Some years ago, Hakkim and colleagues demonstrated that its incidence has increased in autoimmune diseases, such as lupus erythematodes [32]. Also, NETosis has recently been described to have a role in diabetes. It has been proven that hyperglycaemia is the cause of more frequent neutrophil activation and NET formation [33]. Additionally, it is assumed that NETs are included in the pathogenesis of some conditions, such as atherosclerosis [34].

The neutrophils and NETs released from them are important stimulators of thrombus formation processes in individuals with physiological and pathological conditions. Malignant diseases are risk factors for different types of thrombosis, and most often this is associated with the process of hypercoagulation as well as with increases in the capacity of activated neutrophils to form NETs. In the nineteenth century, Armand Trousseau reported the first data confirming the association of cancer with thrombosis, later called Trousseau's syndrome. The connection between NETs and thrombosis was demonstrated later, when Fuchs and colleagues showed that neutrophil extracellular traps provide a scaffold for activation of circulating platelets [35]. Since then, NETs have been considered to be involved in thrombosis processes related to cancer, and NETosis has been suggested to be a potential target for preventing thrombotic complications in malignant diseases [36]. Higher levels of NETs in blood stimulate the development of both arterial and venous thrombi.

Tumour-induced platelets have a critical role in the process of NETs' release. Their immunomodulating effects are partially connected to their interactions with the inherent mediators of the immune system. The hyperactive condition of platelets in individuals with malignant diseases is due to the fact that many tumours express a tissue factor that leads to fibrin formation and platelet activation [37]. Their increased activation leads to the development of thrombosis and influences tumour genesis [38]. Therefore, it is generally accepted that neutrophils and platelets are important regulators of tumour-induced NETosis.

It is established that the number of activated neutrophils and platelets increases in the presence of inflammatory and neoplastic diseases. The formation of complexes between these cells is the main mechanism that connects haemostasis with inflammatory processes [39, 40]. About 50 years ago, the phenomenon of platelets adhering to neutrophils was described and termed 'platelet satellitism' [41]. These complexes are observed in a number of pathological conditions, such as bronchial asthma, chronic ulcerative colitis, sepsis, rheumatoid arthritis and acute coronary syndrome [42–45]. The first time these interactions were observed specifically in patients with cancer of the prostate gland was in 1975 [46]. The platelet–neutrophil complexes that were formed led to the mutual activation of platelets and neutrophils as well as the release of cytokines, exposition of adhesion molecules and receptors on the cell surface [39, 40]. This process of complex interaction is realised between the adhesion molecule P-selectin (CD62 P), which is located on the platelet surface, and the ligand P-selectin glycoprotein ligand-1 (PSGL-1), which is situated on neutrophils [47]. The important role of the interactions between integrated receptor molecules, such as glycoprotein 1b-IX-V and glycoprotein IIB/IIa on the platelets and alpha-M-beta-2 on neutrophils, which initiate intracellular signal transduction [48–51], is emphasised. A number of studies demonstrated that activated neutrophils cause activation of platelets, similar to the way that activated platelets stimulate greater synthesis of NETs. Some interesting facts show that these circulating platelet–neutrophil complexes form the so-called 'metastatic niche' and accelerate the process of metastasis formation [52]. Tumour-induced NETosis is a promoter of subsequent pathological processes connected to the development and progression of cancer [53].

Some prospective studies cite data confirming increased levels of circulating platelet–neutrophil complexes in patients with myeloproliferative diseases. The correlation of these complexes with the stage of the disease, the clinical course and treatment is of great interest. It has been found that patients with advanced stages of disease have higher levels of circulating complexes in their blood. In addition, the process of neutrophil activation, which is characterised by increased membrane expression of CD11b, release of proteolytic enzymes and platelet–neutrophil aggregates, contributes to the development of thrombosis [54].

Chemotherapy is related to an increased risk of developing thrombosis, but the pathogenetic mechanisms and the cytostatic agents that modulate haemostasis have not been fully clarified [55]. It is known that some of the cytostatics (e.g. doxorubicin, epirubicin) used in therapy for malignant haemopathies and solid tumours induce tissue factor (TF) expression on the cancer cells, monocytes and the vascular smooth muscle fibres [56, 57]. Global coagulation assays are used to examine the effects of chemotherapeutic agents on the haemostatic balance, providing a good assessment of the pro- and anti-coagulant activity of these cells. Interestingly, treating patients with doxorubicin and epirubicin stimulates the expression of tissue factor and increases thrombin generation in defibrinated plasma. The procoagulant effect of anthracyclines on endothelial cells can cause an increase in the exposure of phosphatidylserine by caspase activation. Their effects on the activation of protein C have also been studied [58, 59]. To summarise, studies performed in vitro suggest that doxorubicin and epirubicin have the greatest prothrombotic potential to induce a procoagulant phenotype, as they provoke both apoptosis and NETosis.

In most publications, the preferred method to evaluate and assess the levels of circulating platelet–neutrophil complexes is flow cytometric analysis of venous blood after stimulation of the complexes with adenosine diphosphate and phorbol 12-myristate 13-acetate. The conjugated antibody CD62 P (P-selectin) is used to assess the expression of CD11b and platelet–neutrophil complexes (CD41, CD45). Using this method, it has been established that the higher the percentage of circulating complexes in blood, the higher the risk of thrombotic complications [60].

In conclusion, it should be emphasised that neutrophils and platelets are key regulators of tumour-induced NETosis. The neutrophils and formed NETs are important stimulators of the thrombotic processes. The identification of NETs and the characterisation of their role in disease have revived the overlooked role of neutrophils in disease pathogenesis. The analysis and evaluation of the levels of the circulating platelet–neutrophil complexes in blood in neoplastic diseases can be used as potential predictors of the occurrence of thrombosis. The flow cytometric method used for evaluation of the interaction between neutrophils and platelets achieves accurate and reproducible results.

Author details

Sheniz Yuzeir* and Liana Gercheva
Clinic of Hematology, St. Marina University Hospital, Medical University of Varna, Varna, Bulgaria

*Address all correspondence to: shenizyuzeir@abv.bg

References

[1] Amulic B, Cazalet C, Hayes GL, et al. Neutrrophil function: From mechanisms to disease. Annual Review of Immunology. 2012;**30**:459-489

[2] Mocsai A. Diverse novel functions of neutrophils in immunity, inflammation, and beyond. The Journal of Experimental Medicine. 2013;**210**(7):1283-1299

[3] Stone R. The difficult problem of acute myeloid leukemia in the older adult. Cancer Journal for Clinicians. 2002;**52**:363

[4] Armitage J. Emerging applications of recombinant human granulocyte-macrophage colony-stimulating factor. Blood. 1998;**12**:4491-4508

[5] Awanson G et al. Growth factor usage and outcomes in the community setting: Collection through a practice-based computerized clinical information system. Journal of Clinical Oncology. 2000;**18**(8):1764

[6] Kuter D, Begley C. Recombinant human thrombopoetin: Basic biology and evaluation of clinical studies. Blood. 2002;**100**:3457-3469

[7] Pamphilon D. Transfusion policy. In: Apperly JK, Glickman E, Gratwohl A, editors. Blood and Marrow Transplantation. European Group for Blood and Marrow Transplantation; 2000. pp. 120-132

[8] Brinkmann V, Reichard U, Goosmann C, et al. Neutrophil extracellular traps kill bacteria. Science. 2004;**303**(5663):1532-1535

[9] Fuchs TA, Abed U, Goosmann C, et al. Novel cell death program leads to neutrophil extracellular traps. The Journal of Cell Biology. 2007;**176**(2):231-241

[10] Li P, Li M, Lindberg MR, et al. PAD4 is essential for antibacterial innate immunity mediated by neutrophil extracellular traps. The Journal of Experimental Medicine. 2010;**207**(9):1853-1862

[11] Martinod K, Demers M, Fuchs TA, et al. Neutrophil histone modification by peptidylarginine deiminase 4 is critical for deep vein thrombosis in mice. Proceedings of the National Academy of Sciences of the United States of America. 2013;**110**(21):8674-8679

[12] Wang Y, Li M, Stadler S, et al. Histone hypercitrullination mediates chromatin decondensation and neutrophil extracellular trap formation. The Journal of Cell Biology. 2009;**184**(2):205-213

[13] Brinkmann V, Zychlinsky A. Beneficial suicide: Why neutrophils die to make NETs. Nature Reviews. Microbiology. 2007;**5**(8):577-582

[14] Papayannopoulos V, Metzler KD, Hakkim A, et al. Neutrophil elastase and myeloperoxidase regulate the formation of neutrophil extracellular traps. The Journal of Cell Biology. 2010;**191**(3):677-691

[15] Metzler KD, Fuchs TA, Nauseef WM, et al. Myeloperoxidase is required for neutrophil extracellular trap formation: Implications for innate immunity. Blood. 2011;**117**(3):953-959

[16] Remijsen Q, Kuijpers TW, Wirawan E, et al. Dying for a cause: NETosis, mechanisms behind an antimicrobial cell death modality. Cell Death and Differentiation. 2011;**18**(4): 581-588

[17] Wang Y, Li M, Stadler S, Correll S, Li P, Wang D, et al. Histone hyper-citrullination mediates chromatin decondensation and neutrophil extracellular trap formation. The Journal of Cell Biology. 2009;**184**(2):205-213. DOI: 10.1083/jcb.200806072

[18] Kolaczkowska E, Jenne CN, Surewaard BGJ, Thanabalasuriar A, Lee W-Y, Sanz M-J, et al. Molecular mechanisms of NET formation and degradation revealed by intravital imaging in the liver vasculature. Nature Communications. 2015;**6**:6673. DOI: 10.1038/ncomms7673

[19] Kusunoki Y, Nakazawa D, Shida H, Hattanda F, Miyoshi A, Masuda S, et al. Peptidylarginine deiminase inhibitor suppresses neutrophil extracellular trap formation and MPO-ANCA production. Frontiers in Immunology. 2016;**7**:227. DOI: 10.3389/fimmu.2016.00227

[20] Li P, Li M, Lindberg MR, Kennett MJ, Xiong N, Wang Y. PAD4 is essential for antibacterial innate immunity mediated by neutrophil extracellular traps. The Journal of Experimental Medicine. 2010;**207**(9):1853-1862. DOI: 10.1084/jem.20100239

[21] Remijsen Q, Kuijpers TW, Wirawan E, Lippens S, Vandenabeele P, Vanden BT. Dying for a cause: NETosis, mechanisms behind an antimicrobial cell death modality. Cell Death and Differentiation. 2011;**18**(4):581-588. DOI: 10.1038/cdd.2011.1

[22] Eisenberg-Lerner A, Bialik S, Simon H-U, Kimchi A. Life and death partners: Apoptosis, autophagy and the cross-talk between them. Cell Death and Differentiation. 2009;**16**(7):966-975. DOI: 10.1038/cdd.2009.33

[23] Cuervo AM. Autophagy: Many paths to the same end. Molecular and Cellular Biochemistry. 2004;**263**(1-2):55-72. DOI: 10.1023/B:MCBI.0000041848.57020.57

[24] Remijsen Q, Vanden Berghe T, Wirawan E, Asselbergh B, Parthoens E, De Rycke R, et al. Cell Research. 2011;**21**(2):290-304. DOI: 10.1038/cr.2010.150

[25] Papayannopoulos V, Zychlinsky A, et al. Trends in Immunology. 2009;**30**(11):513-521. DOI: 10.1016/j.it.2009.07.011

[26] Xu J, Zhang X, Pelayo R, et al. Extracellular histones are major mediators of death in sepsis. Nature Medicine. 2009;**15**(11):1318-1321

[27] Massberg S, Grahl L, von Bruehl ML, et al. Reciprocal coupling of coagulation and innate immunity via neutrophil serine proteases. Nature Medicine. 2010;**16**(8):887-896

[28] Nathan C. Neutrophils and immunity: Challenges and opportunities. Nature Reviews. Immunology. 2006;**6**:173-182

[29] Gregory AD, Houghton AM. Tumor-associated neutrophils: New targets for cancer therapy. Cancer Research. 2011;**71**:2411-2416. DOI: 10.1158/0008-5472.CAN-10-2583

[30] Cedervall J, Zhang Y, Huang H, et al. Neutrrophil extracellular traps accumulate in peripheral blood vessels and compromise organ function in tumor-bearing animals. Cancer Research. 2015;**75**:2653-2662. DOI: 10.1158/0008-5472. CAN-14-3299

[31] Alfaro C, Teijeira A, Onate C, et al. Tumor-produced interleukin-8 attracts human myeloid- derived suppressor cells and elicits extrusion of neutrop extracellular traps(NETs). Clinical Cancer Research. 2016;**22**(15):3924, 10.1158/1078-00432.CCR-15-2463-3936

[32] Hakkim A, Furnrohr BG, Amann K, et al. Impairment of neutrophil extracellular trap degradation is associated with lupus nephritis. Proceedings of the National Academy of Sciences of the United States of America. 2010;**107**:9813-9818

[33] Wong SL, Demers M, Martinod K, et al. Diabetes primes neutrophils to undergo NETosis, which impairs wound healing. Nature Medicine. 2015;**21**:815-817

[34] Warnatsch A, Ioannou M, Wang Q, et al. Inflammation. Neutrophil extracellular traps license macrophages for cytokine production in atherosclerosis. Science. 2015;**349**: 316-320

[35] Fuchs TA, Brill A, Duerschmied D, et al. Extracellular DNA traps promote thrombosis. Proceedings of the National Academy of Sciences of the United States of America. 2010;**107**:15880-15885

[36] Demers M, Krause DS, Schatzberg D, et al. Cancer spread is pose neutrophils to release extracellular DNA traps that contribute to cancer. 7 August 2012;**109**(32):13076-13081. Epub: [23 July 2012]. [Pub Med] DOI: 10.1073/pnas.1200419109

[37] Van den Berg YW, Osanto S, Reitsma PH, et al. The relationship between tissue factor and cancer progression: Insights from bench and bedside. Blood. 2012;**119**:924-932. DOI: 10.1182/blood-2011-06-317685

[38] Cedervall J, Olsson AK. Platelet Regulation of Angiogenesis, Tumor Growth and Metastasis. Tumour Angiogenesis. InTech: Rijeka; 2012

[39] Peters MJ, Dixon, et al. Circulating platelet-neutrophil complexes represent a subpopulation of activated neutrophils primed for adhesion, phagocytosis and intracellular killing. British Journal of Haematology. 1999;**106**:391-399.2

[40] Huo Y, Schober A, Forlow SB, et al. Circulating activated platelets exacerbate atherosclerosis in mice deficient in apolipoprotein E. Nature Medicine. 2003;**9**:61-67

[41] Kjeldsberg CR, Swanson J. Platelet satellitism. Blood. 1974;**43**:831-836

[42] Bunescu A, Seideman P, Lenkei R, et al. Enhanced Fcgamma receptor I, alphaMbeta2 integrin receptor expression by monocytes and neutrophils in rheumatoid arthritis: Interaction with platelets. The Journal of Rheumatology. 2004;**31**:2347-2355

[43] Ferroni P, Basili S, Martini F, et al. Soluble P-selectin as a marker of platelet hyperactivity in patients with chronic obstructive pulmonary disease. Journal of Investigative Medicine. 2000;**48**:21-27

[44] Irving PM, Macey MG, Feakins RM, et al. European Journal of Gastroenterology & Hepatology. 2008;**20**: 283-289. DOI: 10.1097/MEG.0b013e3282f246c2

[45] Setianto BY, Hartopo AB, Gharini PP, et al. Circulating soluble CD40 ligand mediates the interaction between neutrophils and platelets in acute coronary syndrome. Heart and Vessels. 2010;**25**:282-287. DOI: 10.1007/s00380-009-1199-1

[46] Bauer HM. In-vitro platelet-neutrophil adherence. American Journal of Clinical Pathology. 1975;**63**:824-827. DOI: 10.1093/ajcp/63.6.824

[47] Théorêt JF, Bienvenu JG, Kumar A, et al. P-Selectin antagonism with recombinant P-selectin glycoprotein ligand-1 (rPSGLIg) inhibits circulating activated platelet binding to neutrophils induced by damaged arterial surfaces. The Journal of Pharmacology and Experimental Therapeutics. 2001;**298**:658-664

[48] Ruggeri ZM, Mendolicchio GL. Adhesion mechanisms in platelet function. Circulation Research. 2007;**100**:1673-1685. DOI: 10.1161/01.RES.0000267878.97021.ab

[49] van Gils JM, Zwaginga JJ, Hordijk PL. Molecular and functional interactions among monocytes, platelets, and endothelial cells and their relevance for cardiovascular diseases. Journal of Leukocyte Biology. 2009;**85**:195-204. DOI: 10.1189/jlb.0708400

[50] Diacovo TG, defougerolles AR, Bainton DF, et al. A functional integrin ligand on the surface of platelets: Intercellular adhesion molecule-2. The Journal of Clinical Investigation. 1994;**94**:1243-1251. DOI: 10.1172/JCI117442

[51] Kuijper PH, Gallardo Tores HI, Lammers JW, et al. Platelet associated fibrinogen and ICAM-2 induce firm adhesion of neutrophils under flow conditions. Thrombosis and Haemostasis. 1998;**80**:443-448

[52] Labelle M, Begum S, Hynes RO. Platelets guide the formation of early metastatic niches. Proceedings of the National Academy of Sciences of the United States of America. 2014;**111**:E3053-E3061. DOI: 10.1073/pnas.1411082111

[53] Cools-Lartigue J, Spicer J, McDonald B, et al. The Journal of Clinical Investigation. 2013;**123**:3446-3458. DOI: 10.1172/JCI67484

[54] Marin Oyarzún CP, Carestia A, et al. Neutrophil extracellular trap formation and circulating nucleosomes in patients with chronic myeloproliferative neopla. Scientific Reports. 2016;**6**:38738

[55] McMahon BJ, Kwaan HC. Thrombotic and bleeding complications associated with chemotherapy. Seminars in Thrombosis and Hemostasis. 2012;**38**(8):808-817

[56] Boles JC, Williams JC, Hollingsworth RM, et al. Antracycline treatment of the human monocytic leukemia cell line THP-I increase phosphatidylserine exposure and tissue factor activity. Thrombosis Research. 2011;**129**(2012):197-203. DOI: 10.1016/j.thrombres.2011.06.022

[57] Robert J, Vrignaud P, Nguyen-Ngoc T, et al. Comparative pharmacokinetics and metabolism of doxorubicin and epirubicin in patients with metastatic breast cancer. Cancer Treatment Reports. 1985;**69**:633-640

[58] Muller I, Niethammer D, Bruchelt G. Anthracycline-derived chemotherapeutics in apoptosis and free radical cytotoxicity (review). International Journal of Molecular Medicine. 1998;**1**:491-494

[59] Santucci L, Mencarelli A, Renga B, et al. Nitric oxide modulates proapoptotic and antiapoptotic properties of chemotherapy agents: The case of NO-pegylated epirubicin. The FASEB Journal. 2006;**20**:765

[60] Mauler M et al. Platelet-neutrophil complex formation—A detailed in vitro analysis of murine and human blood samples. November 2015;**98**(5):683-874. DOI: 10.1189/jlb.3TA0315-082R

Section 4

Introns in Inflammation

Chapter 9

The Role of Introns for the Development of Inflammation-Mediated Cancer Cell

Begum Rokeya, Mohammad Asrafuzzaman, Maliha Tabassum Rashid and Shaeri Nawar

Abstract

Cancer and inflammation are connected by intrinsic pathways and extrinsic pathway where the intrinsic pathway is activated by genetic events including mutation, chromosomal rearrangement or amplification, and the inactivation of tumor-suppressor genes, as well as the extrinsic pathway, is the inflammatory or infectious conditions that increase the cancer risk. On the other hand, introns are non-coding elements of the genome and play a functional role to generate more gene products through splicing out, transcription, polyadenylation, mRNA export, and translation. Moreover, introns also may act as a primary element of some of the most highly expressed genes in the genome. Intron may contain their regulatory function as CRISPR system which is activated after the demand of specific gene for specific protein formation where those are required for gene expression, they go for transcription and rest of them form splicing. This chapter will focus on the plausible role of introns to influence the genetic events of inflammation-mediated cancer cell development.

Keywords: inflammation, cancer, intron retention, CRISPR, transcription, PcGs

1. Introduction

The functioning links between cancer and inflammation was approached by a great scientist and physician Rudolf Ludwing Carl Virchow in 1863 [1–3]. Thereafter, for long Virchow's idea had almost been unevaluated and discussed insufficiently [1]. Balkwill and colleagues (2001) supported Virchow's idea and stated that if molecular deregulation is the "match that lights the fire" of cancer, then some types of inflammation may act as the fuel that stimulates the flame. For instance, the inflammatory process act as a cofactor in malignancy in the bladder, cervical, ovarian, gastric, MALT (mucosa-associated lymphoid tissue) lymphoma, esophageal, colorectal, hepatocellular, bronchial, mesothelioma, and Kaposi sarcoma [3].

Currently, it is scientifically proven that inflammation promotes all stages of tumor formation as well as the development of cancer where chronic inflammation or non-resolving inflammation is playing a principal role in the initiation, promotion, malignant transformation, invasion and metastasis of cancer [4–9]. Interestingly, cancer-related inflammation is representing its 7th position as a cancer hallmark and catching the current research attention in human cancer biology [5]. Basically, Inflammation act on cancer development by linking extrinsic and intrinsic pathway [9]. The extrinsic pathway develops inflammatory condition or microenvironment by inflammatory leukocytes particularly macrophages and soluble mediators (vasoactive amines such as histamine and serotonin, peptide such as bradykinin, and eicosanoids such as thromboxanes, leukotrienes, and prostaglandins) that raises cancer risk [9–11]. Intrinsic pathway is driven by genetic events (e.g. oncogenes, genetic aberrations) causing neoplastic transformation, initiate the expression of inflammation-related programs which guide the construction of an inflammatory microenvironment [11]. Inflammatory system involves the dynamic regulations of hundreds of genes and complex transcriptional program [12]. Moreover, the gene regulations by intron are often expressed in most of the cell through the effects of splicing or specific features [13–15]. Recently, several scientific reports claim that retained intron deregulates splicing machine in tumor transcriptoms [16–18]. Intron retention is considered as mis-splicing in which rather than being spliced out intron stays back and retained in mature mRNA [17]. However, the broad gap exists in monitoring of introns role in understanding of gene expression which could be a powerful tool in biotechnological and therapeutic applications. This chapter will cover intron's role in the development of inflammation, intron retaining genes causing inflammation to cancer and finally unfolding of a hypothesis about CRISPR like machine to monitor introns function.

2. Inflammation to cancer

2.1 Extrinsic pathway

Inflammation is activated by leukocytes which make inflammatory mediators in the extrinsic pathway and this pathway is also triggered by various infections and toxic agents such as gastric acid reflux, autoimmune disease etc. [9]. Patients with inflammatory bowel diseases have an increased chance of getting colorectal cancer. As an example, about 43% of patients with ulcerative colitis develop colorectal cancer [19]. Moreover, *in vivo* and *in vitro* experiments have shown that DNA can be damaged by reactive oxygen species (ROS) and nitrogen intermediates which are known as inflammation generated mediators [20, 21]. For example, the enzymes of nitrogen production (iNOS) are overly expressed in many cancer cells [22]. It has been shown scientifically that over expressed iNOS involves in free radical-mediated DNA damage as well as creates an inflammatory microenvironment [23–27]. In a hypoxic atmosphere, a heterodimeric transcription factor known as HIF-1 (HIF-1α & HIF-1β) binds to hypoxia regulated genes and triggers the activation of iNOS and vascular endothelium growth factor (VEGF) [28, 29]. Thus hypoxia-responsive molecules such as HIF-1α & HIF-1β play an integral role in tumor and cancer development [30]. Matsumoto et al., 2007 have shown that *Helicobacter pylori* produce cytidinedeaminase (AID) in gastric epithelium which induce chronic inflammation mediated cholangiocarcinoma [31, 32].

2.2 Intrinsic pathway

Intrinsic pathway is activated by genetic variation such as proto-oncogene activation, inactivated tumor suppressor genes, and chromosomal multiplication as well as mutation which develops neoplasia [22]. A gene coding protein namely tyrosine kinase RET shows rapid and ample genetic variation in human papillary thyroid carcinoma (PTC) and initiates the transcriptional program that links to the development of inflammation [33]. Transcriptome profile is activated by tyrosine kinase RET in human papillary carcinoma and comprises with colony-stimulating factors (CSFs), interleukin 1β (IL-1β), cyclo-oxygenase 2 (COX2), chemokines attacking monocytes and dendritic cells (CCL2 & CCL20), angiogenicchemokines (CXCL8), matrix-degrading enzymes and inhibitors, chemokine receptor (CXCR4) [34]. For example, patients with lymph nodes metastasis have shown an elevated level of tyrosine kinase RET activated inflammatory molecules in their biopsy results which demonstrate that genetic events have taken place in the pathogenesis of tumor and constructed an inflammatory environment [33–35]. Moreover, *Ras* oncogenes were known to be the most dominant genes that tend to get mutated rapidly and play a significant role in tumorigenesis. *Ras* oncogenes family includes KRAS, HRAS, and NRAS and their mutation has been observed in 25–30% of tumor specimens which has an impact on the KRAS locus [22]. For instance cervical cancer has shown that shifting of *RAS* oncogenes makes a chemokine named CXCL8 which participates in tumor development [36, 37]. Furthermore, polycomb complex target genes (PcGs) play a salient role in the growth of the embryo and aging through epigenetic rearranging. These groups of genes also involve in abnormal DNA methylation and histone modification in cancer cells [38]. As an example, Yu H and colleagues (2007) reported that a mouse model with intestinal inflammation and cancer shows abnormal DNA methylation where over 70% of abnormal methylated genes were observed in PcGs [38].

3. Functional role of intron for development of cancer

Intron is defined as any intervening nucleotide sequence that formed splicing at the RNA level [39]. Intron was first discovered in 1970s with a traditional views that the coding region of eukaryotic genes are interrupted by introns which are spliced out from pre mature mRNA transcripts before the formation of mature mRNA [39–41]. After the elucidation of intron splicing mechanism, scientist became excited about its function on gene expression and speculated that may be introns carry out some function like regulation of splicing function, regulation of transcription, evolutionary function or coding capacity but there was no clear examples of their active functions on gene expression [41]. From the starting 21st century, many researches have claimed about the intron function on gene expression or intron mediated enhancement of gene expression [13, 42–47]. However, a question remains unclear that within the genome, who is responsible to remember or decide which intron or parts of nucleotide sequences are necessary to stay within the mature mRNA stand for inflammatory gene expression rather than form splicing that result in cancer? Current chapter sheds light on the above question and hypothesize CRISPR like machine in perspective of inflammation mediated cancer development.

After the discovery of alternative splicing (AS), the transcriptomic and proteomic complexity has increases significantly [47, 48]. Recent breakthrough studies in high-throughput sequencing have explored a pivotal role of AS in normal biology that more than 95% of human multi exonic genes are subject to AS and produce at least two alternative isoforms [49, 50]. Moreover, Braunschweig and colleague compared 11 vertebrate species and observed that about 50–75% of multi-exonic genes are affected by intron retention (IR) which is one kind of AS [47, 48, 51]. While another study showed that IR affects near about 80% of protein coding genes in humans [52]. Some scientific reports also considered IR as a harmful process for the body by slowing down splicing kinetics and delaying the onset of gene expression, by raising pre-mRNA degradation in the nucleus through nuclear exosomes and finally by enhancing cytoplasmic pre-mRNA degradation through nonsense-mediated decay [51, 53, 54].

This statement is also supported by the Green and colleague's research as the genes that encoded the regulators of macrophage transcription, signaling inflammation, and phagocytosis has increased their expression when the IR events decreased [55]. As it is known, that intron retention (IR) is the process where instead of typically being spliced out, the introns remain intact in the mature mRNAs and thus whole process of IR supposedly has numerous physiological drawbacks resulting in different diseases [47, 48]. Currently, many researchers strongly claim that IR is a key mechanism to control gene expression during the development, differentiation and activation of several types of mammalian cell [56–63]. A recent study by Green and colleague claimed that intron retention affected the expression of key genes *(ID2, IRF7, ENG,* and *LAT*) involved in the development and function of macrophages those are the key inflammatory regulator [55]. So IR gene might be acting as one of the major causes of inflammation mediated cancer development (**Table 1**).

3.1 *TGIF2* gene

PCR technique revealed two alternate splice forms of *TGIF2* gene that were found in mice. The coding sequence of *TGIF2* gene both in human and mice consists with intron that is retained [78]. The splicing phenomenon depends on the *TGIF2* coding sequence where both splice forms encoded for an active transcriptional repressor protein that is used to repress independent TGFβ and dependent TGFβ transcription [79]. Moreover, Melhuish and colleague have shown that the transcriptional core-repressor mSin3 interacts with human and mice*TGIF2* and also revealed that the *TGIF2* gene retains intron at a negligible amount which is not spliced out from human mRNA but a bigger amount is spliced out from the mice and thus correlated with variant cancers [79]. These findings are also supported by the study of Imoto et al., 2020 where the authors claimed that amplification and over-expression of *TGIF2* gene lead to ovarian cancer [80]. The *TGIF2* gene is located in chromosome 20q11.2–12 [80]. Often in solid human tumors, it has been observed that the long arm of chromosome 20 is highly amplificated [64]. Rapid amplification of *TGIF2* in chromosome 20 leads to ovarian cancer which is observed in the cell lines of ovaries [80]. It is known that inflammation helps to grow tumor as well as development of cancer [4]. So the *TGIF2* gene might have induced inflammation during the tumourigenesis later on which turned into ovarian cancer.

3.2 *EBNA-3* gene

EBNA-3 gene involves in multiple regulation during their expression due to IR retention. For instance, a study by Kienzle et al., (1999) showed that a stop codon might be inserted into a frame shift because of IR and thus the translation process could be stopped as a premature termination of *EBNA-3* gene [81]. Moreover, it was depicted that IR can change the expression pattern of the *EBNA-3* gene in human B-lymphocyte where its protein plays a pivotal role in cell proliferation and transformation. They also play a censorious part in the development of lymphoma [82]. Patients with chronic inflammation because of autoimmune disorder have a higher risk to develop lymphoma [83]. So, herein could be a strong possibility to influence inflammation mediated lymphoma development by *EBNA-3* gene.

3.3 *APOE4*

The expression of the *APOE4* isoform shows a relation between intron retention and Alzheimer's disease (AD). The prevalence of AD was longitudinally associated with a reduced risk of cancer where the cancer incidence was associated with

Gene name	Protein name	General function	Types of cancer that is developed by IR gene	Abnormal function	References
TGIF2	TGFB Induced Factor Homeobox 2	TGF-β-induced factor homeobox 2 (*TGIF2*) is known to be transcription regulator that plays significant role in the regulation of development and cell fate decisions. Abnormal expression of TGIF family proteins has been noticed in numerous cancers which include ovarian, esophageal, and colorectal cancers.	Ovarian cancer	Over expressed	[64, 65]
EBNA-3	Epstein–Barr nuclear antigen 3	This gene plays a principle role for activation and immortalization of human B-cells. Represses transcription of viral promoters TP1 and Cp interact with RBPJ and also inhibits the *EBNA2*-mediated activation of these promoters. As Cp is known to be the promoter for all the *EBNA* mRNAs, *EBNA3A* probably provides a negative autoregulatory control loop.	Lymphoma and Epithelial cancers	Amplication	[66, 67]
APOE4	Apolipoprotein E4	This gene gives instructions to make a protein called apolipoprotein E. This protein combines with fats (lipids) in the human body to form molecules called lipoproteins. Lipoproteins in body package cholesterol and other fats and transfer them by the bloodstream.	Breast cancer	Increased frequency	[68, 69]
EGFR	Epidermal growth factor receptor	Receptor tyrosine kinase binding ligands of the EGF family. They activate a lot of signaling cascades to transform them extracellular cues into appropriate cellular responses.	Lung cancer	Mutation or cell damage	[70, 71]
ROS1	Receptor Tyrosine Kinase	*ROS1* is a proto-oncogene which encodes a type I integral membrane protein with receptor tyrosine kinase (RTK) activity. It is a member of the insulin receptor family and it is also involved in downstream signaling processes in cell growth and differentiation.	Ovarian cancer, cholangiocarcinoma, inflammatory myofibroblastic tumor, colorectal, and angiosarcoma	Mutation	[72, 73]

Gene name	Protein name	General function	Types of cancer that is developed by IR gene	Abnormal function	References
RUNX1	RUNX Family Transcription Factor 1	The protein encoded by this gene represents the alpha subunit of CBF(Core binding factor) and is thought to be involved in the development of normal hematopoiesis. Chromosomal translocations involving by this gene are well-documented and have been associated with several types of leukemia. Three transcript variants encoding different isoforms have been found for this gene	Myeloid and lymphoid	Mutation	[74, 75]
TP53	Tumor Protein 53	*TP53* gene gives instructions for making a protein called tumor protein p53. This protein acts as a tumor suppressor, which means that it regulates cell division by keeping cells from growing and dividing (proliferating) too fast or in an uncontrolled way	Breast cancer, bone and soft tissue sarcomas, brain tumors and adrenocortical carcinomas (ADC), leukemia, stomach cancer and colorectal cancer	Gene Alternation or Deletion or Mutation	[76, 77]

Table 1.
List of intron retention genes and their functions.

a reduced risk of AD [84]. Significant scientific evidence has shown that *APOE4* could able to aggravate more neurodegeneration, tau pathology and inflammation [85–87]. Liestøl et al., 2000 have observed that genotypes of *APOE4* increases the risk of cancer in patients with immunodeficiency. Interestingly, 24.6% of *APOE4* alleles have been found in variant cancer cases where 13.5% were found in noncancerous cases [88]. As the higher frequency of *APOE4* increases the risk of cancer, it also worsens inflammation. It might be possible that *APOE4* may initiate inflammation and by making it worse, it causes cancer in people with immunodeficiency.

3.4 *EGFR, ROS1, RUNX1*

It was claimed that 2340 and 1422 genes show tumor-specific and normal tissue-specific retention events respectively [89, 90]. For example, *EGFR, ROS1, RUNX1* play salient roles in carcinogenesis [72, 89]. *ROS1* gene fusion has been observed in a substantial number of malignancies which comprises ovarian cancer, cholangiocarcinoma, inflammatory myofibroblastic tumor, colorectal, and angiosarcoma [72]. Abnormal *EGFR* expression can initiate different types of respiratory diseases such as inflammation mediated lung fibrosis, cancer, and multiple hypersecretory diseases comprising COPD, asthma and cystic fibrosis [91]. Furthermore, *RUNX1* mutation has been observed in numerous malignancies in myeloid and lymphoid cell [92]. Bellissimo et al., 2020 showed that *RUNX1* regulates the signaling pathways of TLR1/2 and TLR4 and with the help of neutrophils it can produce inflammatory cytokines as well as develop inflammation mediated leukemia [74].

3.5 *TP53*

Intron retention frequency may be responsible to inactive tumor suppressor genes in many cancers cell [93]. Study revealed that in cancerous condition, retained intron transcript exits in NMD pathway and inactivates the *TP53* gene. Additionally, *TP53* gene provides instruction to code for a protein named p53 which can produce pro-inflammatory cytokines [92]. Mutation of p53 can cause inflammation mediated cancer [94].

4. Phylogenetic tree analysis of IR gene, PcGs and Ras oncogene

The evolutionary history and relationship of an organism or group of species are named phylogeny. Phylogeny depicts the connection of an organism. Phylogenetic relationships give information on shared common ancestry but not obligatory how organisms are similar or different. Phylogenic tree analysis of all genes those are performing intron retention scenario, PcGs and Ras oncogenes (**Figures 1–3**) has

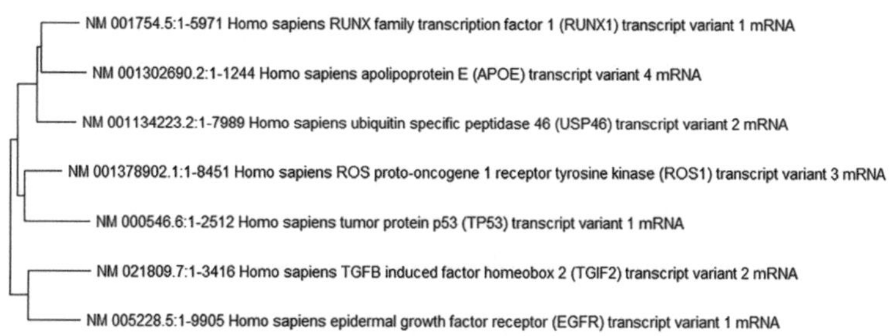

Figure 1.
Phylogenetic tree of intron retaining (IR) genes.

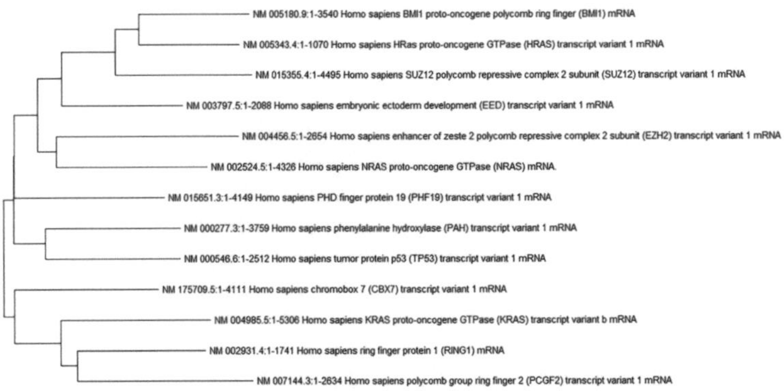

Figure 2.
Phylogenic tree between RAS oncogenes and PcGs.

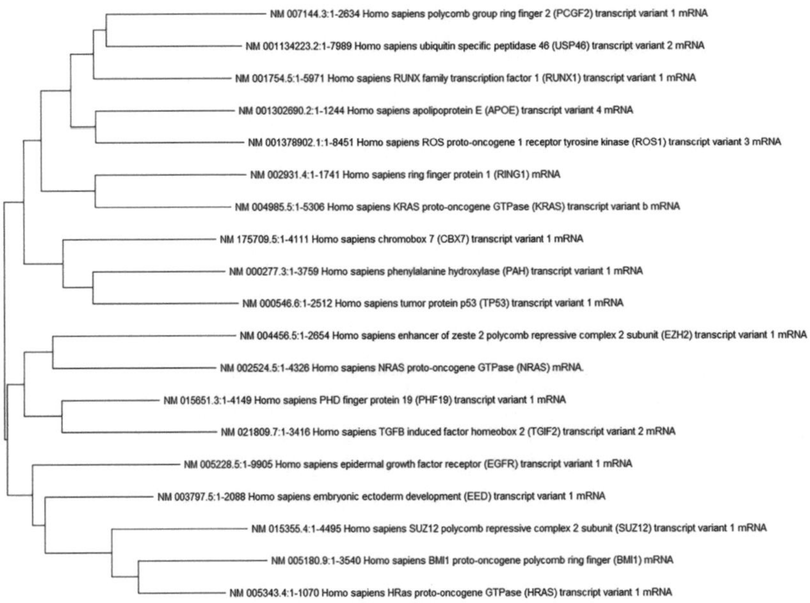

Figure 3.
Phylogenic tree among IR gene, RAS oncogenes and PcGs.

done to find out the relation among the genes. MEGA X software has been used to construct the phylogenic tree to understand the relation among all the cancers genes (**Tables 1** and **2**).

Figure 1 demonstrates that the vertical line on the left side is the common ancestor or the root of the seven gene sequences from which the genes have been evolved in a period. The evolution period can be explained through the horizontal lines near the sequences. The small length of lines before sequences means the sequences evolved in a short period whereas the long length of lines means longer time was needed for the sequences to be evolved. The common ancestor or root has been divided into two branch points. From the first branch point total of five sequences have been modified which were *RUNX1, APOE4, EBNA-3(USP46), ROS1,* and *TP53.* From the second branch point, two sequences have been evolved *TGIF2* and *EGFR.* The phylogenetic tree has three separate clades. Clade means a variety of species that include all the descendants of a common ancestor. In the first clade, the first two sequences of genes *RUNX1* and *APOE4* are closer to the ancestor than *EBNA-3* as they are from the same node. In the second clade, among *ROS1* and

Gene name	Protein name	General function	Types of cancer that is developed by IR gene	Abnormal function	References
BMI 1	B-lymphoma Moloney murine leukemia virus insertion region-1	This gene functions through chromatin remodeling as a principle epigenetic repressor of numerous regulatory genes involved in embryonic development and self-renewal in somatic stem cell and also plays a median role in DNA damage repair. It is an oncogene and abnormal expression is related with multiple cancers and resistance to certain chemotherapies.	Gastric, ovarian, breast, head and neck, pancreatic and lung cancer, primary hepatocellular carcinoma (HCC) and endometrial carcinoma	Over expression	[95, 96]
CBX7	Chromobox proteins 7	This gene encodes a protein that comprises the CHROMO (CHRomatin Organization MOdifier) domain. It is thought to control the lifespan of several normal human cells.	Breast, Thyroid, Colorectal, Pancreas, Lung carcinoma and Glioblastoma	Down regulation	[97, 98]
PH	Phenylalanine Hydroxylase	This gene gives instructions for making an enzyme called phenylalanine hydroxylase. This enzyme is responsible for the primary step in processing phenylalanine, which is a building block of proteins (an amino acid) obtained through the diet.	Liver cancer	Down regulation	[99, 100]
RING 1	Ring Finger 1A	This gene encodes proteins characterized by a RING domain, a zinc-binding motif related to the zinc finger domain. The gene product can bind DNA and can act as a transcriptional repressor. It is related with the multimericpolycomb group protein complex.	Hepatocellular and colorectal carcinomas	Down regulation	[101, 102]
MEL18	Polycomb group ring finger 2	*Mel-18* functions as a tumor suppressor via downregulation of *BMI1*. Single Nucleotide Polymorphism and down regulation of *Mel-18* is associated with prostate cancer.	Breast cancer, Prostate cancer	Loss of expression and down regulation	[103, 104]
EZH2	Enhancer of zeste homolog-2	The *EZH2*gene makes an enzyme methyltransferase. Histone methyltransferases modify proteins called histones, which are structural proteins that bind to DNA and shape chromosomes. Addition of a molecule (methyl group) to histones (methylation), histone methyltransferases can turn off (suppress) the activity of certain genes, an essential process in normal development.	Breast cancer, Colorectal cancer, Endometrial cancer, Gastric cancer, Liver cancer, Lung cancer	Over expression	[105, 106]

Gene name	Protein name	General function	Types of cancer that is developed by IR gene	Abnormal function	References
EED	Embryonic ectoderm development	This gene encodes a member of the Polycomb-group family. It maintains the transcriptional repressive state of genes over successive cell generations. This protein interacts with enhancer of zeste 2, the cytoplasmic tail of integrin beta7, immunodeficiency virus type 1 (HIV-1) MA protein, and histone deacetylase proteins. This protein mediates repression of gene activity through histone deacetylation, and may act as a specific regulator of integrin function. Two transcript variants encoding distinct isoforms have been identified for this gene.	Colorectal Cancer, acute myeloid leukemia and diffuse large B cell lymphoma	High expression	[107–109]
SUZ12	suppressor of zeste 12 homolog	This zinc finger gene has been detected at the breakpoints of a recurrent chromosomal translocation reported in endometrial stromal sarcoma. Recombination of these breakpoints results in the fusion of this gene and *JAZF1*. The protein encoded by this gene comprises a zinc finger domain in the C terminus of the coding region	Colorectal, ovarian and non-small lung cancer, head and neck squamous cell carcinoma	Over expression	[110, 111]
PCL3	PHD fing protein 19	*PHF19* promotes the proliferation, migration, and chemosensitivity of glioblastoma to doxorubicin through modulation of the SIAH1/beta-catenin axis. Human *PCL3* has an oncogenic role in hepatocellular carcinoma by activating the beta-catenin/IL6 signaling axis to promote metastasis	Hepatocellular carcinoma, glioma, and ovarian cancers, glioblastoma progression, prostate cancer	Over expression	[112, 113]
TP53	TumourProtein 53	Functions are the same as discussed in **Table 1**	Types of cancers are the same as discussed in **Table 1**	Gene alternation or deletion or mutation	[76, 77]
KRAS	Kirsten rat sarcoma viral oncogene	The *KRAS* gene gives instructions for making a protein called *K-Ras* which is a part of a signaling pathway known as the *RAS/MAPK* pathway. The protein relays signals from outside the cell to the cell's nucleus	Non-small cell lung cancer, colorectal cancer, and pancreatic cancer	Mutation	[114, 115]

Table 2.
List of PcGs genes and their functions.

TP53, ROS1 is closer to the root as its horizontal line is smaller than the *TP53* ones. In the third clade, *EGFR* is much closer to the root than *TGIF2* as its horizontal line is smaller and close to the ancestor than *TGIF2.*

Figure 2 depicts that both type of cancer genes (*RAS* oncogene and PcGs) were evolved from a common root or ancestor. The tree demonstrates that *BMI 1, HRAS, SUZ12,* and *EED* had been sharing the most recent ancestor but *BMI 1, HRAS,* and *SUZ12* remain closer than *EED* as they share the same root. Interestingly, *BMI 1 & EZH2* from *PcGs* and *HRAS & NRAS* from *Ras* oncogene are closely related to each other respectively where they are from different group's gene. The following three genes *PHF19/PCL3, PH* and *TP53* were from the same clade and they are near to one another. The last four genes *CBX7, KRAS, RING 1* and *MEL 18(PCGF2)* were from the same clade as they share the most common ancestor.

Figure 3 demonstrates that all the genes were evolved from a common ancestor. The IR gene *APOE 4* and *ROS1* are closely related each other as expected. However interestingly, IR gene *EBNA-3*shares the common ancestor with *PCGF(MEL18).* So herein might be chances for *MEL18* or *PCGF2* gene to develop inflammation mediated cancer by the influencing of IR.

5. Hypothesis: CRISPR like function might be a functioning model of intron

CRISPR-Cas9 is also known as a genome-editing tool where CRISPR stands for "Clustered Regularly Interspaced Short Palindromic Repeats and Cas9 is an enzyme that cuts foreign DNA [116]. In the 21st century, CRISPR-Cas9 is being used immensely in medical technology to edit, remove or add a gene to correct genetic defects [116]. CRISPR has conformed from the natural defense mechanism of bacteria, archaea and developed an immune system by CRISPR loci [116]. CRISPR and Cas9 enzyme serve as an immune guard and provide safety against bacteriophage, viruses, and foreign invaders [117–119]. The immunization process after invading foreign genetic elements, a small fragments of foreign DNA are integrated into the CRISPR repeat-spacer array within the host chromosome as new spacers. Thus, a genetic record of prior infection will save into the host body that enables to prevent future invasion of the same invader [120, 121] (**Figure 4**).

The nucleotide repeats and spacers are main two component of CRISPR. Repeated sequence of nucleotide is distributed in the CRISPR region and Spacers are

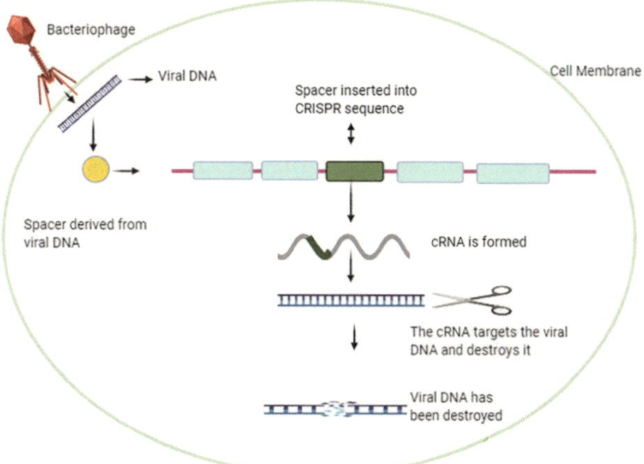

Figure 4.
CRISPR biology.

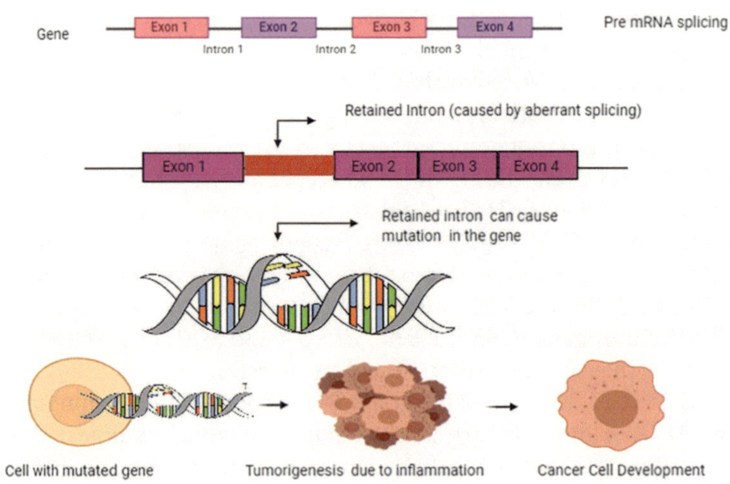

Figure 5.
Illustration of retained intron in the gene causing mutation which leads to inflammation and tumorigenesis resulting in development of cancer.

a small portion of DNA present in the CRISPR region. Destruction of foreign invading DNA or RNA occurs by Cas9 enzyme. If in future, the foreign body again attacks the organism, they fight it off as they have the virus or foreign invader's DNA from beforehand and thus they recognize it and kill it [121]. So in CRISPR biology, spacer acts as a responsible sequence to remember or decide which foreign body needs to be killed where Cas9 enzyme plays a pivotal role. According to our hypothesis, intron network might work as CRISPR like functioning model.

According to the section 3, it is confirmed that IR have the ability to influence inflammation mediated cancer development. From the CRISPR function it is clear that according to the demand of the cell, CRISPR can get activated. It might be possible that according to the demand of the abnormal cells, intron retention may form to confirm inflammation mediated malignancy state (**Figure 5**). Moreover, our phylogenetic tree analysis depicts that PcGs, *RAS* oncogenes, and intron retaining genes are related to each other and they all share a common ancestor. As all three categories of genes initiate cancer development in humans, it might be possible that PcGs and RAS oncogenes can express themselves as intron retaining genes or vice versa.

6. Conclusions

Cancer is a genetic disease and is one of the leading causes of death around the world. As a genetic event, the intron retention causes inflammation as well as the development of cancer cells. So far, it is clear that the intron is spliced away during gene expression while exons remain and express the genes. However, the retention of introns is an unlikely phenomenon that differs from the common hypothesis and appears anomalous. The genes involved in retaining intron have a carcinogenic effect. It may be speculated that some nucleotide sequence whether it is coding or non-coding region could function as a memory sequence, hence are able to remember intronic sequence as like spacer responsibility of CRISPR system and would only be functioning according to the demand of the cell. Future in depth analysis on intron retaining genes is required to explore their effect on inflammation and cancer.

Acknowledgements

We gratefully acknowledge Asian Network of Research on Antidiabetic Plants (ANRAP) and Bangladesh University of Health Sciences (BUHS) for providing all types of logistic facilities to conduct this work.

Appendices and nomenclature

VEGF	Vascular endothelium growth factor
PTC	Papillary thyroid carcinoma
CSFs	colony-stimulating factors
IL-1β	Interleukin 1β
COX2	Cyclo-oxygenase 2
PcGs	Polycomb complex target genes
AD	Alzheimer's disease
CRISPR	Clustered Regularly Interspaced Short Palindromic Repeats
AS	Alternative splicing
IR	Intron retention
COPD	Chronic obstructive pulmonary disease
MALT	Mucosa-associated lymphoid tissue

Author details

Begum Rokeya[1,2*], Mohammad Asrafuzzaman[2,3], Maliha Tabassum Rashid[2] and Shaeri Nawar[2]

1 Department of Pharmacology, Bangladesh University of Health Sciences, Dhaka, Bangladesh

2 Asian Network of Research on Antidiabetic Plants (ANRAP), Bangladesh University of Health Sciences, Dhaka, Bangladesh

3 Food Science and Technology Program, BNU-HKBU United International College, Hong Kong Baptist University, Kowloon Tong, Hong Kong

*Address all correspondence to: b_rokeya@yahoo.com

References

[1] Schmidt A, Weber OF: In Memoriam of Rudolf Virchow: A Historical Retrospective Including Aspects of Inflammation, Infection and Neoplasia. Contributions to Microbiology. 2006; 1-15. Doi: 10.1159/000092961

[2] Balkwill F, Mantovani A: Inflammation and cancer: back to Virchow?. Lancet (London, England). 2001;357(9255):539-545. DOI: https://doi.org/10.1016/S0140-6736(00)04046-0

[3] Balkwill F: Tumor necrosis factor or tumor promoting factor?. Cytokine Growth Factor Rev. 2002);13, (2):135-141. DOI: 10.1016/s1359-6101(01)00020-x

[4] Greten FR, Grivennikov SI: Inflammation and Cancer: Triggers, Mechanisms, and Consequences. Immunity. 2019;51(1):27-41. DOI:https://doi.org/10.1016/j.immuni.2019.06.025

[5] Colotta F, Allavena P, Sica A, Garlanda C, Mantovani A: Cancer-related inflflammation, the seventh hallmark of cancer: links to genetic instability. Carcinogenesis. 2009;30:1073-1081. DOI: 10.1093/carcin/bgp127

[6] Todoric J, Antonucci L, Karin M: Targeting Inflammation in Cancer Prevention and Therapy. Cancer Prevention Research . 2016;9(12):895-905. DOI: 10.1158/1940-6207

[7] Fishbein A, Wang W, Yang H, Yang J, Hallisey VM, Deng J, Verheul SML, Hwang SH, Gartung A, Wang Y, Bielenberg DR, Huang S, Kieran MW, Hammock BD, Panigrahy D: Resolution of eicosanoid/cytokine storm prevents carcinogen and inflammation-initiated hepatocellular cancer progression. Proceedings of the National Academy of Sciences. 2020;117(35):21576-21587. DOI: https://doi.org/10.1073/pnas.2007412117

[8] Song XD, Wang YN, Zhang A, Liu B: Advances in research on the interaction between inflammation and cancer. Journal of International Medical Research. 2019;48(4). DOI: https://doi.org/10.1177/0300060519895347

[9] Del Prete A, Allavena P, Santoro G, Fumarulo R, Corsi MM, Mantovani A: Molecular pathways in cancer-related inflammation. Biochemia Medica. 2011;264-275. DOI: https://doi.org/10.11613/bm.2011.036

[10] Abdulkhaleq LA, Assi MA, Abdullah R, Zamri-Saad M, Taufiq-Yap YH, Hezmee MNM: The crucial roles of inflammatory mediators in inflammation: A review. Veterinary World. 2018;11(5):627-635. DOI: https://doi.org/10.14202/vetworld.2018.627-635

[11] Allavena P, Garlanda C, Borrello MG, Sica A, Mantovani A: Pathways connecting inflammation and cancer. Current Opinion in Genetics & Development. 2008;18(1):3-10. DOI:https://doi.org/10.1016/j.gde.2008.01.003

[12] Smale ST, Natoli G: Transcriptional Control of Inflammatory Responses. Cold Spring Harbor Perspectives in Biology. 2014;6(11). DOI: https://doi.org/10.1101/cshperspect.a016261

[13] Rose AB: Introns as Gene Regulators: A Brick on the Accelerator. Frontiers in Genetics. 2019;9:1-6. DOI: https://doi.org/10.3389/fgene.2018.00672

[14] Chorev M, Carmel L: The Function of Introns. Frontiers in Genetics. 2012;3:1-15. DOI: https://doi.org/10.3389/fgene.2012.00055

[15] Zhang D, Hu Q, Liu X, Ji Y, Chao H.-P, Liu Y, Tracz A, Kirk J,

Buonamici S, Zhu P, Wang J, Liu S, Tang DG: Intron retention is a hallmark and spliceosome represents a therapeutic vulnerability in aggressive prostate cancer. Nature Communications. 2020;11(1):1-19. DOI: https://doi.org/10.1038/s41467-020-15815-7

[16] Smart AC, Margolis CA, Pimentel H, He MX, Miao D, Adeegbe D, Fugmann T, Wong KK, Van Allen EM: Intron retention is a source of neoepitopes in cancer. Nature Biotechnology. 2018;36(11): 1056-1058. DOI: https://doi.org/10.1038/nbt.4239

[17] Dvinge H, Bradley RK: Widespread intron retention diversifies most cancer transcriptomes. Genome Med. 2015;7:45. DOI: https://doi.org/10.1186/s13073-015-0168-9

[18] Jung H, Lee D, Lee J, Park D, Kim YJ, Park WY, Hong D, Park PJ, Lee E: Intron retention is a widespread mechanism of tumor-suppressor inactivation. Nature Genetics. 2015;47(11):1242-1248. DOI:https://doi.org/10.1038/ng.3414

[19] Ferrone C, Dranoff G: Dual roles for immunity in gastrointestinal cancer. J Clin Oncol. 2010;28(26):4045-4051. DOI:10.1200/JCO.2010.27.9992

[20] Wu Y, Zhou BP: TNF-alpha/NF-kappaB/Snail pathway in cancer cell migration and invasion. Br J Cancer. 2010;102(40):639-644. DOI:10.1038/sj.bjc.6605530

[21] Hold GL, El-Omar ME: Genetic aspects of inflammation and cancer. Biochemical Journal. 2008;410(2):225-235. DOI: https://doi.org/10.1042/bj20071341

[22] Multhoff G, Molls M, Radons J: Chronic Inflammation in Cancer Development. Frontiers in Immunology. 2012;2:1-17. DOI: https://doi.org/10.3389/fimmu.2011.00098

[23] Kawanishi S, Hiraku Y, Pinlaor S, Ma N. Oxidative and nitrative DNA damage in animals and patients with inflflammatory diseases in relation to inflammation-related carcinogenesis. Biol Chem . 2006;387(4):365-372. DOI: 10.1515/BC.2006.049

[24] Lechner M, Lirk P, Rieder J: Inducible nitric oxide synthase (iNOS) in tumor biology: the two sides of the same coin.Semin Cancer Biol . 2005 Aug;15(4):277-289. DOI:10.1016/j.semcancer.2005.04.004

[25] Ohshima H: Genetic and epigenetic damage induced by reactive nitrogen species: implications in carcinogenesis. Toxicol Lett. 2003;140-141:99-104. DOI: 10.1016/s0378-4274(02)00506-4

[26] Ohshima H, Tazawa H, Sylla BS, Sawa T: Prevention of human cancer by modulation of chronic inflflammatory processes. Mutat Res. 2005 ;591(1-2):110-122. DOI:10.1016/j.mrfmmm.2005.03.030.

[27] Jaiswal M, LaRusso NF, Gores GJ: Nitric oxide in gastrointestinal epithelial cell carcinogenesis: linking inflflammation to oncogenesis. Am J Physiol Gastrointest Liver Physiol. 2001;281(3):G626-G634. DOI: 10.1152/ajpgi.2001.281.3.G626.

[28] Jain RK: Tumor angiogenesis and accessibility: role of vascular endothelial growth factor. Semin Oncol. 2002;29:3-9. DOI:10.1053/sonc.2002.37265

[29] Semenza GL: Targeting HIF-1 for cancer therapy. Nat Rev Cancer. 2003;3(10):721-732. DOI: 10.1038/nrc1187.

[30] Kimbro KS, Simons JW: Hypoxia-inducible factor-1 in human breast and prostate cancer. Endocr Relat Cancer. 2006;13(3):739-749. DOI: 10.1677/erc.1.00728

[31] Matsumoto Y, Marusawa H, Kinoshita K, Endo Y, Kou T, Morisawa T,

Azuma T, Okazaki IM, Honjo T, Chiba T: Helicobacter pylori infection triggers aberrant expression of activation-induced cytidine deaminase in gastric epithelium. Nat Med. 2007;13(4):470-476. DOI: 10.1038/nm1566

[32] Komori J, Marusawa H, Machimoto T, Endo Y, Kinoshita K, Kou T, Haga H, Ikai I, Uemoto S, Chiba T: Activation-induced cytidine deaminase links bile duct inflammation to human cholangiocarcinoma. Hepatology. 2008;47(3):888-896. DOI: 10.1002/hep.22125

[33] Borrello MG, Alberti L, Fischer A, Degl'innocenti D, Ferrario C, Gariboldi M, Marchesi F, Allavena P, Greco A, Collini P, Pilotti S, Cassinelli G, Bressan P, Fugazzola L, Mantovani A, Pierotti MA: Induction of a proinflammatory program in normal human thyrocytes by the RET/PTC1 oncogene. Proc Natl Acad Sci U S A. 2005;102(41):14825-14830. DOI:10.1073/pnas.0503039102

[34] Cerutti JM, Oler G, Michaluart PJ, Delcelo R, Beaty RM, Shoemaker J, Riggins GJ: Molecular profiling of matched samples identifies biomarkers of papillary thyroid carcinoma lymph node metastasis. Cancer Res. 2007;67(16):7885-7892. DOI: 10.1158/0008-5472

[35] De Falco V, Guarino V, Avilla E, Castellone MD, Salerno P, Salvatore G, Faviana P, Basolo F, Santoro M, Melillo RM: Biological role and potential therapeutic targeting of the chemokine receptor CXCR4 in undifferentiated thyroid cancer. Cancer Res. 2007;67(24):11821-11829. DOI:10.1158/0008-5472

[36] Masih-Khan E, Trudel S, Heise C, Li Z, Paterson J, Nadeem V, Wei E, Roodman D, Claudio JO, Bergsagel PL, Stewart AK: MIP-1alpha (CCL3) is a downstream target of FGFR3 and RAS-MAPK signaling in multiple myeloma. Blood. 2006;108(10):3465-3471. DOI:10.1182/blood-2006-04-017087

[37] Wang D, Wang H, Brown J, Daikoku T, Ning W, Shi Q, Richmond A, Strieter R, Dey SK, DuBois RN: CXCL1 induced by prostaglandin E2 promotes angiogenesis in colorectal cancer. J Exp Med. 2006;203(4):941-951.DOI:10.1084/jem.20052124

[38] Yu H, Kortylewski M, Pardoll D: Crosstalk between cancer and immune cells: role of STAT3 in the tumour microenvironment. Nat Rev Immunol. 2007;7(1):41-51. DOI: 10.1038/nri1995

[39] Berget SM, Moore C, Sharp PA: Spliced segments at the 5' terminus of adenovirus 2 late mRNA. Proc Natl Acad Sci U S A. 1977;74(8):3171-3175. DOI: 10.1073/pnas.74.8.3171

[40] Chow LT, Gelinas RE, Broker TR, Roberts RJ: An amazing sequence arrangement at the 5' ends of adenovirus 2 messenger RNA. Cell. 1977;12(1):1-8. DOI; 10.1016/0092-8674(77)90180-5

[41] Long M, de Souza S J: Intron-exon structures. Advances in Genome Biology. 1998;143-178. DOI: https://doi.org/10.1016/s1067-5701(98)80020-x

[42] Baier T, Jacobebbinghaus N, Einhaus A, Lauersen KJ, Kruse O: Introns mediate post-transcriptional enhancement of nuclear gene expression in the green microalga Chlamydomonas reinhardtii. PLoS Genet. 2020;16(7):e1008944. DOI: 10.1371/journal.pgen.1008944

[43] Gallegos JE, Rose AB: An intron-derived motif strongly increases gene expression from transcribed sequences through a splicing independent mechanism in Arabidopsis thaliana. SciRep.2019;9(1):13777.DOI:10.1038/s41598-019-50389-5

[44] Jin Y, Fei M, Rosenquist S, Jin L, Gohil S, Sandström C, Olsson H,

Persson C, Höglund AS, Fransson G, Ruan Y, Åman P, Jansson C, Liu C, Andersson R, Sun C: A Dual-Promoter Gene Orchestrates the Sucrose-Coordinated Synthesis of Starch and Fructan in Barley. Mol Plant.2017;10(12):1556-1570. DOI:10.1016/j.molp.2017.10.013

[45] Akua T, Shaul O: The Arabidopsis thaliana MHX gene includes an intronic element that boosts translation when localized in a 5' UTR intron. J Exp Bot. 2013 ;64(14):4255-4270. DOI:10.1093/jxb/ert235

[46] Gromak N: Intronic microRNAs: a crossroad in gene regulation. Biochem Soc Trans. 2012;40(4):759-761. DOI:10.1042/BST20120023

[47] Kim MJ, Kim H, Shin JS, Chung CH, Ohlrogge JB, Suh MC: Seed-specific expression of sesame microsomal oleic acid desaturase is controlled by combinatorial properties between negative cis-regulatory elements in the SeFAD2 promoter and enhancers in the 5'-UTR intron. Mol Genet Genomics. 2006;276(4):351-368. DOI: 10.1007/s00438-006-0148-2.

[48] Liu Y, Gonzàlez-Porta M, Santos S, Brazma A, Marioni JC, Aebersold R, Venkitaraman AR, Wickramasinghe O: Impact of Alternative Splicing on the Human Proteome. Cell reports. 2017;20(5):1229-1241. https://doi.org/10.1016/j.celrep.2017.07.025

[49] Merkin J, Russell C, Chen P, Burge CB: Evolutionary dynamics of gene and isoform regulation in Mammalian tissues. Science. 2012;338(6114):1593-1599. DOI:10.1126/science.1228186

[50] Barbosa-Morais NL, Irimia M, Pan Q, Xiong HY, Gueroussov S, Lee LJ, Slobodeniuc V, Kutter C, Watt S, Colak R, Kim T, Misquitta-Ali CM, Wilson MD, Kim PM, Odom DT, Frey BJ, Blencowe BJ: The evolutionary landscape of alternative splicing in vertebrate species. Science. 2012;338(6114):1587-1593. DOI: 10.1126/science.1230612

[51] Braunschweig U, Barbosa-Morais NL, Pan Q, Nachman EN, Alipanahi B, Gonatopoulos-Pournatzis T, Frey B, Irimia M, Blencowe BJ. Widespread intron retention in mammals functionally tunes transcriptomes. Genome Res. 2014;24(11):1774-1786. DOI:10.1101/gr.177790.114

[52] Middleton R, Gao D, Thomas A, Singh B, Au A, Wong JJ, Bomane A, Cosson B, Eyras E, Rasko JE, Ritchie W. IRFinder: assessing the impact of intron retention on mammalian gene expression. Genome Biol. 2017;18(1):51. DOI: 10.1186/s13059-017-1184-4

[53] Niemelä EH, Oghabian A, Staals RH, Greco D, Pruijn GJ, Frilander MJ: Global analysis of the nuclear processing of transcripts with unspliced U12-type introns by the exosome. Nucleic Acids Res. 2014;42(11):7358-7369. DOI: 10.1093/nar/gku39

[54] Lejeune F, Maquat LE: Mechanistic links between nonsense-mediated mRNA decay and pre-mRNA splicing in mammalian cells. Curr Opin Cell Biol. 2005;17(3):309-315. DOI: 10.1016/j.ceb.2005.03.002

[55] Green ID, Pinello N, Song R, Lee Q, Halstead JM, Kwok CT, Wong ACH, Nair SS, Clark SJ, Roediger B, Schmitz U, Larance M, Hayashi R, Rasko JEJ, Wong JJ: Macrophage development and activation involve coordinated intron retention in key inflammatory regulators. Nucleic Acids Res. 2020;48(12):6513-6529. DOI: 10.1093/nar/gkaa435

[56] Edwards CR, Ritchie W, Wong JJ, Schmitz U, Middleton R, An X, Mohandas N, Rasko JE, Blobel GA: A dynamic intron retention program in the mammalian megakaryocyte and erythrocyte lineages. Blood.

2016;127(17):e24-e34. DOI: 10.1182/blood-2016-01-692764

[57] Llorian, M, Gooding C, Bellora N, Hallegger M, Buckroyd A, Wang X, Rajgor D, Kayikci M, Feltham J, Ule J, Eyras E, Smith CWJ: The alternative splicing program of differentiated smooth muscle cells involves concerted non-productive splicing of post-transcriptional regulators. Nucleic Acids Research. 2016;44(18):8933-8950. DOI: https://doi.org/10.1093/nar/gkw560

[58] Mauger O, Lemoine F, Scheiffele P: Targeted Intron Retention and Excision for Rapid Gene Regulation in Response to Neuronal Activity. Neuron. 2016;92(6):1266-1278. DOI: 10.1016/j.neuron.2016.11.032

[59] Naro C, Jolly A, Di Persio S, Bielli P, Setterblad N, Alberdi AJ, Vicini E, Geremia R, De la Grange P, Sette C: An Orchestrated Intron Retention Program in Meiosis Controls Timely Usage of Transcripts during Germ Cell Differentiation. Dev Cell. 2017;41(1):82-93.e4. DOI: 10.1016/j.devcel.2017.03.003

[60] Ni T, Yang W, Han M, Zhang Y, Shen T, Nie H, Zhou Z, Dai Y, Yang Y, Liu P, Cui K, Zeng Z, Tian Y, Zhou B, Wei G, Zhao K, Peng W, Zhu J: Global intron retention mediated gene regulation during CD4+ T cell activation. Nucleic Acids Res. 2016 ;44(14):6817-6829. DOI:10.1093/nar/gkw591

[61] Pimentel H, Parra M, Gee SL, Mohandas N, Pachter L, Conboy JG: A dynamic intron retention program enriched in RNA processing genes regulates gene expression during terminal erythropoiesis. Nucleic Acids Res. 2016;44(2):838-851. DOI: 10.1093/nar/gkv1168

[62] Wong JJ, Ritchie W, Ebner OA, Selbach M, Wong JW, Huang Y, Gao D, Pinello N, Gonzalez M, Baidya K, Thoeng A, Khoo TL, Bailey CG, Holst J, Rasko JE: Orchestrated intron retention regulates normal granulocyte differentiation. Cell. 2013 Aug 1;154(3):583-595. DOI: 10.1016/j.cell.2013.06.052

[63] Yap K, Lim ZQ, Khandelia P, Friedman B, Makeyev EV: Coordinated regulation of neuronal mRNA steady-state levels through developmentally controlled intron retention. Genes Dev. 2012;26(11):1209-1223. DOI:10.1101/gad.188037.112

[64] Rooney PH, Murray GI, Stevenson DA, Haites NE, Cassidy J, McLeod HL. Comparative genomic hybridization and chromosomal instability in solid tumours. Br J Cancer. 1999;80(5-6):862-873. DOI: 10.1038/sj.bjc.6690433

[65] Du R, Shen W, Liu Y, Gao W, Zhou W, Li J, Zhao S, Chen C, Chen Y, Liu Y, Sun P, Xiang R, Shi Y, Luo Y: TGIF2 promotes the progression of lung adenocarcinoma by bridging EGFR/RAS/ERK signaling to cancer cell stemness. Signal Transduct Target Ther. 2019;4:60. DOI: 10.1038/s41392-019-0098-x

[66] Ayee R, Ofori MEO, Wright E, Quaye O: Epstein Barr Virus Associated Lymphomas and Epithelia Cancers in Humans. J Cancer. 2020;11(7):1737-1750. DOI: 10.7150/jca.37282

[67] EBNA3 - Epstein-Barr nuclear antigen 3 - Epstein-Barr virus (strain B95-8) (HHV-4) - EBNA3 gene & protein. UniProt. Available from https://www.uniprot.org/uniprot/P12977 [Accessed:2021-01-14]

[68] Porrata-Doria, Matta T, Acevedo J: Apolipoprotein E Allelic Frequency Altered in Women with Early-onset Breast Cancer. Breast cancer : basic and clinical research.2010; 4: 43-48. DOI: 10.1177/117822341000400005.

[69] Huang Y, Mahley RW. Apolipoprotein E: structure and function in lipid metabolism, neurobiology, and Alzheimer's diseases. Neurobiology of disease. 2014; 72: 3-12. DOI: https://doi.org/10.1016/j.nbd.2014.08.025

[70] Lung Cancer Foundation of America. (2019, October 18). EGFR Mutation and Lung Cancer: What is it and how is it treated? Available from https://lcfamerica.org/lung-cancer-info/types-lung-cancer/egfr-mutation/. [Accessed: 2021-01-21]

[71] GeneCards -The Human Gene Database. EGFR gene (Protein Coding)-Epidermal growth factor receptor [Internet] . Available from https://www.genecards.org/cgi-bin/carddisp.pl?gene=EGFR. [Accessed: 2021-01-21]

[72] Lin JJ, Shaw AT: Recent Advances in Targeting ROS1 in Lung Cancer. J Thorac Oncol. 2017;12(11):1611-1625. DOI:10.1016/j.jtho.2017.08.002

[73] UniProt. ROS1 gene-Proto-oncogene Tyrosine Kinase receptor [Internet]. Available from https://www.uniprot.org/uniprot/P08922 . [Accessed: 2021-01-21]

[74] Bellissimo DC, Chen CH, Zhu Q, Bagga S, Lee CT, He B, Wertheim GB, Jordan M, Tan K, Worthen GS, Gilliland DG, Speck NA: Runx1 negatively regulates inflammatory cytokine production by neutrophils in response to Toll-like receptor signaling. Blood Adv. 2020;4(6):1145-1158. DOI: 10.1182/bloodadvances.2019000785

[75] GeneCards-The Human Gene Database. RUX1 gene (Protein Coding)-RUNX family transcription factor 1 [Internet]. Available from https://www.uniprot.org/uniprot/P08922 . [Accessed: 2021-01-20]

[76] Petitjean A, Achatz M, Borresen-Dale A, Hainaut P, Olivier M. TP53 mutations in human cancers: functional selection and impact on cancer prognosis and outcomes. Oncogene. 2007; 26:2157-2165. DOI: https://doi.org/10.1038/sj.onc.1210302

[77] MedlinePlus-Trusted Health Information. TP53 gene-tumor protein 53 [Internet]. Available from https://medlineplus.gov/genetics/gene/tp53/ . [Accessed: 2021-01-20]

[78] Sakabe NJ, de Souza SJ: Sequence features responsible for intron retention in human. BMC Genomics. 2007;8:59. DOI: 10.1186/1471-2164-8-59

[79] Melhuish TA, Wotton D: The Tgif2 gene contains a retained intron within the coding sequence. BMC Mol Biol. 2006;7:2. DOI: 10.1186/1471-2199-7-2

[80] ImotoI,PimkhaokhamA,WatanabeT, Saito-Ohara F, Soeda E, Inazawa J: Amplification and overexpression of TGIF2, a novel homeobox gene of the TALE superclass, in ovarian cancer cell lines. Biochem Biophys Res Commun. 2000;276(1):264-270. DOI: 10.1006/bbrc.2000.3449

[81] Kienzle N, Young DB, Liaskou D, Buck M, Greco S, Sculley TB. Intron retention may regulate expression of Epstein-Barr virus nuclear antigen 3 family genes. J Virol. 1999;73(2):1195-1204.DOI:10.1128/JVI.73.2.1195-1204.1999

[82] Bhattacharjee S, Ghosh Roy S, Bose P, Saha A: Role of EBNA-3 Family Proteins in EBV Associated B-cell Lymphomagenesis. Front Microbiol. 2016 ;7:457. DOI:10.3389/fmicb.2016.00457

[83] Lymphoma Action.Causes of lymphoma. [Internet]. Available From: https://lymphoma-action.org.uk/about-lymphoma-what-lymphoma/causes-lymphoma [Accessed:2021-01-13]

[84] Roe CM, Fitzpatrick AL, Xiong C, Sieh W, Kuller L, Miller JP,

Williams MM, Kopan R, Behrens MI, Morris JC: Cancer linked to Alzheimer disease but not vascular dementia. Neurology. 2009;74(2):106-112. DOI: https://doi.org/10.1212/wnl.0b013e3181c91873

[85] Tzioras M, Davies C, Newman A, Jackson R, Spires-Jones T: Invited Review: APOE at the interface of inflammation, neurodegeneration and pathological protein spread in Alzheimer's disease. Neuropathol Appl Neurobiol. 2019;45(4):327-346. DOI : 10.1111/nan.12529

[86] Kloske CM, Wilcock DM. The Important Interface Between Apolipoprotein E and Neuroinflammation in Alzheimer's Disease. Front Immunol. 2020;11:754. DOI:10.3389/fimmu.2020.00754

[87] Shi Y, Yamada K, Liddelow SA, Smith ST, Zhao L, Luo W, Tsai RM, Spina S, Grinberg LT, Rojas JC, Gallardo G, Wang K, Roh J, Robinson G, Finn MB, Jiang H, Sullivan PM, Baufeld C, Wood MW, Sutphen C, McCue L, Xiong C, Del-Aguila JL, Morris JC, Cruchaga C: Alzheimer's Disease Neuroimaging Initiative, Fagan AM, Miller BL, Boxer AL, Seeley WW, Butovsky O, Barres BA, Paul SM, Holtzman DM. ApoE4 markedly exacerbates tau-mediated neurodegeneration in a mouse model of tauopathy. Nature. 2017 ;549(7673):523-527. DOI: 10.1038/nature24016

[88] Liestøl K, Kvittingen EA, Rootwelt H, Dunlop O, Goplen AK, Pedersen JC, Brorson SH, Børresen-Dale AL, Myrvang B, Maehlen J: Association between apolipoprotein E genotypes and cancer risk in patients with acquired immunodeficiency syndrome. Cancer Detect Prev. 2000;24(5):496-499.

[89] Zheng JT, Lin CX, Fang ZY, Li HD. Intron Retention as a Mode for RNA-Seq Data Analysis. Frontiers in Genetics. 2020;11:1-7. DOI: https://doi.org/10.3389/fgene.2020.00586

[90] Zhang Q, Li H, Jin H, Tan H, Zhang J, Sheng S. The global landscape of intron retentions in lung adenocarcinoma. BMC Med. Genomics 2014;7:15. DOI: 10.1186/1755-8794-7-15

[91] Vallath S, Hynds RE, Succony L, Janes SM, Giangreco A: Targeting EGFR signalling in chronic lung disease: therapeutic challenges and opportunities. Eur Respir J. 2014;44(2):513-522. DOI:10.1183/09031936.00146413

[92] Sood R, Kamikubo Y, Liu P: Role of RUNX1 in hematological malignancies. Blood. 2017;129(15):2070-2082. DOI: 10.1182/blood-2016-10-687830

[93] Cooks T, Harris CC: p53 mutations and inflammation-associated cancer are linked through TNF signaling. Mol Cell. 2014;56(5):611-612. DOI: 10.1016/j.molcel.2014.11.018

[94] Uehara I, Tanaka N: Role of p53 in the Regulation of the Inflammatory Tumor Microenvironment and Tumor Suppression. Cancers (Basel). 2018;10(7):219. DOI:10.3390/cancers10070219

[95] Wang MC, Li CL, Cui J, Jiao M, Wu T, Jing LI, Nan K J. BMI-1, a promising therapeutic target for human cancer. Oncology letters. 2015; 10(2): 583-588. DOI: https://doi.org/10.3892/ol.2015.3361

[96] GeneCards-The Human Gene Database. BMI 1 Gene (Protein Coding),BMI 1 Protooncogene, Polycomb Ring Finger [Internet]. Available from https://www.genecards.org/cgi-bin/carddisp.pl?gene=BMI1 . [Accessed: 2021-01-20]

[97] Pallante P, Forzati F, Federico A, Arra C, Fusco A. Polycomb protein

family member CBX7 plays a critical role in cancer progression. American journal of cancer research. 2005; 5(5): 1594-1601.

[98] GeneCards-The Human Gene Database. CBX7 Gene (Protein Coding) Chromobox 7 [Internet]. Available from https://www.genecards.org/cgi-bin/carddisp.pl?gene=CBX7 . [Accessed: 2021-01-20]

[99] Tyagi A, Sarodaya N, Kaushal K, Chandrasekaran AP, Antao AM, Suresh B, Rhie BH, Kim KS, Ramakrishna S. E3 Ubiquitin Ligase APC/CCdh1 Regulation of Phenylalanine Hydroxylase Stability and Function. International Journal of Molecular Sciences. 2020; 21(23):9076. DOI: https://doi.org/10.3390/ijms21239076

[100] MedlinePlus-Trusted Health Information. PAH gene-phenylalaline hydroxylase [Internet]. Available from https://medlineplus.gov/genetics/gene/pah/ [Accessed: 2021-01-20]

[101] Shen J, Li P, Shao X, Yang Y, Liu X, Feng M, Yu Q, Hu R, Wang Z. The E3 Ligase RING1 Targets p53 for Degradation and Promotes Cancer Cell Proliferation and Survival. Cancer Research. 2017; 78(2): 359-371. DOI: https://doi.org/10.1158/0008-5472.can-17-1805

[102] GeneCards-The Human Gene Database. RING 1(Protein Coding) -RING Finger Protein 1 [Internet]. Available from https://www.genecards.org/cgi-bin/carddisp.pl?gene=RING1 . [Accessed:2021-01-20]

[103] Lee JY, Kong G. MEL-18, a tumor suppressor for aggressive breast cancer. Oncotarget.2015;6(18):15710-15711.

[104] GeneCards-The Human Gene Database. PCGF2 Gene(Protein Coding), Polycomb group ring finger 2 [Internet]. Available from https://www.genecards.org/cgi-bin/carddisp.pl?gene=PCGF2 [Accessed :2021-01-22]

[105] Crea F, Paolicchi E, Marquez VE, Danesi R. Polycomb genes and cancer: Time for clinical application? Critical Reviews in Oncology/Hematology. 2012; 83(2): 184-193. DOI: https://doi.org/10.1016/j.critrevonc.2011.10.007

[106] MedlinePlus-Trusted Health Information. EZH2 gene-enhancher of zeste 2 polycomb repressive complex 2 subunit [Internet]. Available from https://medlineplus.gov/genetics/gene/ezh2/ [Accessed : 2021-01-19]

[107] Seo GS, Yu JI, Chae SC, Park WC, Shin SR, Yoo ST, Choi SC, Lee SH: (2013). EED gene polymorphism in patients with colorectal cancer. The International journal of biological markers. 2013; 28(3): 274-279. DOI: https://doi.org/10.5301/JBM.5000024

[108] Yu W, Du H. Roles of Polycomb gene EED in pathogenesis and prognosis of acute myeloid leukemia and diffuse large B cell lymphoma. 2018;1-21. DOI: https://doi.org/10.1101/444745

[109] GeneCards-The Human Gene Database. EED gene-Embryonic Ectoderm Development [Internet] Available from https://www.genecards.org/cgi-bin/carddisp.pl?gene=EED [Accessed : 2021-01-21]

[110] Wu Y, Hu H, Zhang W, Li Z, Diao P, Wang D, Zhang W, Wang Y, Yang J, Cheng J. SUZ12 is a novel putative oncogene promoting tumorigenesis in head and neck squamous cell carcinoma. Journal of cellular and molecular medicine. 2018; 22(7): 3582-3594. DOI: https://doi.org/10.1111/jcmm.13638

[111] GeneCards-The Human Gene Database. SUZ12 Gene(Protein Coding), SUZ12 Polycomb Repressive Complex 2 subunit [Internet]. Available from https://www.genecards.org/cgi-bin/carddisp.pl?gene=SUZ12 . [Accessed: 2021-01-20]

[112] Jain P, Ballare C, Blanco E, Vizan P, Di Croce L. PHF19 mediated regulation of proliferation and invasiveness in prostate cancer cells. ELife. 2020; 9: 1-11. DOI: https://doi.org/10.7554/elife.51373

[113] GeneCards-The Human Gene Database. PHF19 Gene(Protein Coding), PHD Finger Protein 19 [Internet]. Available from https://www.genecards.org/cgi-bin/carddisp.pl?gene=PHF19 [Accessed: 2021-01-20]

[114] National Cancer Institute. NCI Dictionary of Cancer Terms [Internet]. Available from https://www.cancer.gov/publications/dictionaries/cancer-terms/def/kras-gene [Accessed: 2021-01-20]

[115] MedlinePlus Genetics. KRAS gene: MedlinePlus Genetics [Internet]. 2020, August 18. Available from https://medlineplus.gov/genetics/gene/kras/ [Accessed: 2021-01-19]

[116] Vidyasagar, A. What Is CRISPR? [Internet]. 2018, April 21. Available from https://www.livescience.com/58790-crispr-explained.html. [Accessed: 2021-01-19]

[117] Heler R, Marraffifini LA, Bikard D. Adapting to new threats: the generation of memory by CRISPR Cas immune systems. Mol. Microbiol. 2014; 93(1):1-9. DOI: 10.1111/mmi.12640

[118] Marraffifini LA. CRISPR-Cas immunity in prokaryotes. Nature . 2015; 526(7571):55-61. DOI: 10.1038/nature15386

[119] Mojica FJM, Rodriguez-Valera F. The discovery of CRISPR in archaea and bacteria. FEBS J. 2016; 283(17):3162-3169. DOI: 10.1111/febs.13766

[120] Jiang F, Doudna JA. CRISPR–Cas9 Structures and Mechanisms. Annual Review of Biophysics. 2017; 46(1): 505-529. DOI: https://doi.org/10.1146/annurev-biophys-062215-010822

[121] Mohamadi S, Bostanabad SZ, Mirnejad R. CRISPR Arrays: A Review on Its Mechanism. Journal of Applied Biotechnology Reports. 2020; 7(2): 81-86. DOI: 10.30491/jabr.2020.109380

Section 5

Autoimmune Diseases and Inflammation

Chapter 10

Celiac Disease

Nour Amin Elsahoryi

Abstract

Celiac disease is chronic autoimmune-mediated small intestinal enteropathy. CD caused by ingestion of the dietary gluten that found in wheat, barley, and rye, in the individual who are predisposed genetically by having leucocyte antigen, (HLA)-DQ2 or -DQ8-positive. Rigorous adherence to a gluten-free diet is the only treatment for this condition to reduce the symptoms and the consequences at the short-term and the long term. The aim of this chapter is provide updates and comprehensive overview about the celiac disease epidemiology, pathogenetic information, clinical, and diagnostic methods, updated therapeutic strategy approaches that followed as a treatment and recommendations. Its challenge to understand all the domains that causes celiac disease. Finding alternative diet and trying different lifestyle still under debates. However, complete exclusion of the gluten-containing food from the patient's diet is the only effective treatment to avoid the disease complications.

Keywords: Celiac Disease, Epidemiology, Pathophysiology, Genetics, Diagnosis, Risk Factors, Complications, Treatment

1. Introduction

In most studies and publications, coeliac disease or Celiac disease (CD) is characterized as a serological and histological immune-mediated disease caused by dietary gluten in people who are genetically predisposed to it [1, 2]. Individuals who have positive HLA-DQ2-positive and/or HLA-DQ8 and consume glute-contains diet are susceptible to have CD because they have genetic and/or environmental factors [1, 2]. Gluten is the storage protein of wheat and founds in the endosperm of other cereals (secalins in rye, hordeins in barley and avenins in oats [3]. The gluten protein is a CD trigger that could found also in that cereals hybrids such as the spelt, and the kamut [4]. This protein is composed of two main fractions: prolamin and glutelin in various proportions among the causative cereals. For example, the prolamin is about 68% and glutelin is 82% in the wheat, 52% and 71% in the rye and 62% and 71% in the barley, respectively [4]. However, the other proteins component such as albumins and the globulins are related to the IgE-mediated allergic response in the genetically susceptible individuals that have positive leukocyte antigen HLA-DQ2-and/or HLA-DQ8 [4].

The small intestinal is the primary affected organ with CD, intraepithelial lymphocytes (IELs) count increase after gluten ingestion and the immune response leads to structural changes in the gut such as villi blunting or flattening (villous atrophy) and elongation of the crypts (crypt hyperplasia) [2]. CD could lead to various extraintestinal symptoms and manifestations (Gastrointestinal and Extraintestinal) [2] as shown in **Table 1**, but also it is very important to mention that some patients remain asymptomatic.

A few decades ago, CD was hidden and underdiagnosed disease, but recently this disease was well-diagnosed sequencE by positive celiac-specific serologic tests and small intestinal biopsy specimens to ensure the true incidence and to find the true prevalence globally [5]. In 2012, Gujral et al. [6] mentioned that approximately 1% of the global prevalence is suffering from CD. Recent systematic review and meta-analysis (2018) published that the pooled global prevalence of CD was 0.7% (95% CI, 0.5%–0.9%) [5]. The seroprevalence of CD from 96 studies was 1.4% (1.1%–1.7%, 95 CI) at significant heterogeneity (97.5%). Whereas the pooled global prevalence that was confirmed by biopsy was 0.7% (0.5%–0.9%, 95%CI). The highest CD prevalence was in Europe and Oceania (0.8%), followed by Asia (0.6%), Africa (0.5%) and 0.4% in South America as shown in **Figure 1**. Prevalence among children was higher than adults (0.9% and 0.5%, respectively) higher among the females than males (0.6% and 0.4%, respectively) [5].

To date, the only effective treatment for CD is a lifelong strict gluten-free diet, which lead to recovery of the mucosal damage recovery in the small intestine. Following restricted GFD improves the clinical symptoms and reduce the short and the long term complications that associated with CD [1, 2, 7–11].

Gastrointestinal manifestations	Diarrhea, loose stools, weight loss, dyspepsia, distended abdomen, flatulence, chronic abdominal pain, anorexia, vomiting, chronic constipation, and growth retardation (in children).
Extraintestinal manifestations	Recurring headaches, Epilepsy and seizures, Peripheral neuropathy, Cerebellar ataxia, Depression and Anxiety and Chronic fatigue, Short stature, delayed puberty, hepatitis, elevated liver, transaminases, iron-deficiency anemia. Skeletal muscles: Arthralgia, osteopenia, bone fractures, osteopenia, and arthritis. In the oral cavity: Dental enamel hypoplasia, recurrent aphthous mouth ulceration.

Table 1.
The clinical gastrointestinal and extraintestinal manifestations.

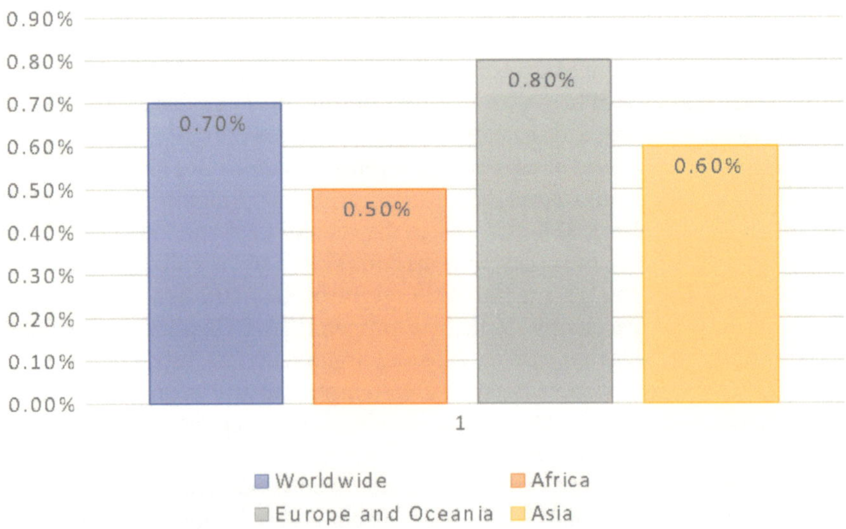

Figure 1.
The pooled prevalence of biopsy-confirmed CD worldwide [5].

2. Epidemiology

In the last decades, prevalence of CD was investigated in many countries by determining the new incidents in a specific time (cross-sectional studies mainly) [3]. According to some reports, CD prevalence has increased in some countries, such as the United States, where CD prevalence is estimated to be between 0.5 and 1 percent of the general population [3]. In Finland and Italy, however, the incidence was lower [1]. Overall, the CD prevalence was found through screening the general population which includes the serological tests. The difference in the diagnosis method led to inaccurate estimation of the prevalence and it remains greatly unrecognized [2, 12]. Numerous studies calculated the prevalence based on the positive serology test with duodenal biopsies to confirm the incident, whereas other studies diagnose the incident based on the positive serology test only [1–3, 12]. Although the differences in the CD diagnosis and cases reporting confirmation, the prevalence of CD incidents increases worldwide [1–3, 12]. Moreover, recent evidence pointed to increase the morbidity and mortality with CD [12, 13] and diminished the quality of life [12].

Recent systematic review and meta-analysis revealed that the worldwide CD seroprevalence is 1.4% based on positive IgA anti-TG2 test and/or test of anti-endomysial antibodies [5]. The pooled global prevalence based on the confirmation of the biopsy results CD was 0.7% with a different result among the countries. For example, the high prevalence was reported in Europe and Oceania (0.8%) compared with South America (0.4%), Africa (0.5%) and Asia (0.6%) [5]. The epidemiological studies of CD reported that the incidents among females are more than males and among children more than adults [2, 3, 5]. In addition, the prevalence among patients who have higher first-degree relatives is more [1]. Moreover, the prevalence of CD is higher among the patients who suffer from other chronic diseases such as diabetes Meletus type 1 (DMT1), Down syndrome, and IgA deficiency [1, 14]. Based on specific geographical areas, United States, Brazil, Italy and Russia have the highest prevalence (1.6–2.3%), but very rarely in some countries such as China, Indonesia, Pakistan and unknown in other countries such as Far East Asia and sub-Saharan Africa [2, 3]. In the Arab country, Ashraf El-Metwally et al. reported in a recent systematic review that the CD prevalence was varied and the highest estimation was in Saudi Arabia (3.2%) and the lowest prevalence was in Tunisia (0.1%) [8]. The results among the Arab population were in agreement with the other populations, the incidence was higher among females than males, among children more than adults, and it is associated with other chronic diseases mainly Down's syndrome and DMT1 [8]. Finally, some studies reported that CD prevalence is less than 0.5% such as china but Scherf et al. consider the prevalence in such countries is underdiagnosis and the remaining cases need more investigation [3].

3. Risk factors of celiac disease (CD)

Pathogenesis of CD is identified predisposing the risk factors and it is includes genetic factors and environmental exposure to the gluten protein that stimulates the autoimmunity that cause the mucosal damage and villous atrophy [1–3, 6, 12]. CD is a unique autoimmune disease in that its key genetic elements (human leukocyte antigen (HLA)-DQ2 and HLA-DQ8), the autoantigen involved (tissue transglutaminase (tTG)). In the case of CD, there is an imbalance between T helper 1 and 2 cell responses. The genetic and environmental factors are both lead to impair the function of the intestine, inappropriate immune response, and an imbalanced gut microbiome [1, 2]. Overall, susceptibility to having CD is thought to be due to a combination of genetic and environmental factors as shown in **Figure 2**.

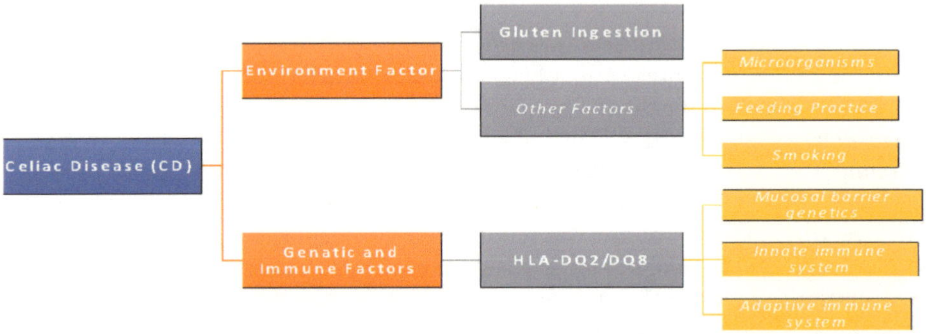

Figure 2.
Risk factors required for celiac disease development.

3.1 Genetic factor

In the heritability of CD, there is a relevant role between the incidence and HLA haplotypes class II heterodimers, specifically DQ2 and DQ8 by ~25–40% of the genetic risk. Lindfors et al. reported that class II is histocompatibility complex molecules stated on the antigen-presenting cells (APCs) surface; they consist of an α-chain and a β-chain encoded by specific variants of the HLA-DQA1 and HLA-DQB1 genes, respectively [2]. HLA-DQ2 is encoded by the HLADQA1*05:01 and HLADQB1*02:01 (also called HLA-DQ2.5) alleles, whereas HLA-DQ8 is encoded by the HLADQA1*03 and HLADQB1*03:02 alleles [2]. Most CD patients (around 90%) have positive-HLA-DQ2 and the rest of them carry HLA-DQ8 [2]. HLA-DQ2 homozygosis form a higher risk of the early appearance of the disease in the children within the first relatives [1] and the average prevalence of CD among the first degree is more than the general population. It's important to mention that HLADQ2 and HLA-DQ8 are common among the general peoples (25–35%), and only 3% of this HLA compatible person have CD [1]. Most studies reported that the other HLA-DQ variants form a fairly modest risk effect (~15%) on CD because they are infrequently associated with this condition [1, 2, 12].

3.2 Environmental factor

Pro-autoimmune genetic background, viral infections not only the factors that could lead to the incident of CD [1–3, 12]. Ingestion gluten protein and early termination feeding practices are considered viral in CD development, autoimmunity, and then damage the mucosal tissue [1–3, 12]. Gluten is the storage protein in wheat that gives the dough viscoelastic properties [2]. Gluten is composed of alcohol-soluble constituents (gliadins) that consist of α-gliadins, γ-gliadinsand ω-gliadins, whereas the alcohol-insoluble glutenin consists of high-molecular-mass and low-molecular-mass glutenins [2]. Both segments (Gliadins and glutenins) are high in proline and glutamine amino acids which are resistant to proteolytic processing by gastric and pancreatic enzymes as well as mammalian small intestinal brush-border membrane enzymes [2]. Gluten is called CD trigger; it is a harmful dietary factor for CD patients, but to date, it is not clear why not all peoples who are genetically predisposed have CD and why some cases are diagnosed later in life [12]. The prevalence of CD is higher among the population that is characterized by higher consumption of wheat [12]. The recent epidemiological studies show the difference in the prevalence based on the region [12]. The effect of the environmental factor still varies among the studies. For example, three systematic reviews and meta-analysis [15–17] reported that is no association between timing of gluten introduction and CD and the age of the patient, whereas other studies reported conflicting data [18, 19]. Incomplete digestion of the gluten in the human gut led to producing the gluten peptide that accesses the lamina propria through the epithelial barrier via the transcellular or paracellular route. Among CD patients, gluten peptides activate both adaptive and innate immune responses [1, 2]. Small intestinal mucosal gluten specific CD4+ T cell is an immune response in CD patients in addition to producing antibodies towards wheat gliadin and the enzyme TG2 (encoded by *TGM2*). The amino acids that available in the gluten peptide at key positions are selectively deamidated by TG2 [2].

3.3 Feeding practice

Numerous studies indicated that CD is associated with feeding practice, time of gluten introduction to the infant (age of gluten intake) and the infant diet type [1–3, 6, 12]. Consuming gluten-containing food in the first three months of the infant age is significantly associated with CD autoantibodies development compared with the latest months [2, 12, 20]. On the other hand, recent meta-analyses reported that there is no association between CD and breastfeeding [15]. Regards the time of the gluten intake, large prospective studies show that no association between CD and gluten introduction time among the high-risk populations [17, 18]. One study reported that high gluten doses in the infancy stage associated with CD [19]. The results still contradictory in this regard and more research is required.

3.4 Infection

An increased risk of CD has been linked to repeated rotavirus infection in a previous longitudinal prospective study [21]. Therefore, a recently study reported that rotavirus vaccination could have a protective effect on developing CD [22]. Furthermore, early childhood infections with enterovirus A and B, especially those with a high titer and a long duration, were linked to later CD, while adenovirus infections were not. Surprisingly [3, 23]. The prevalence of acute respiratory infections seems to be a factor as well [3, 23].

3.5 Microorganisms

CD is like all autoimmune diseases, reducing the risk of microorganisms, decrease exposure to various microorganisms and increase the hygiene aspects which could be related to reducing the autoimmune disorders [1, 2, 12]. Many studies supported the abundance of specific bacterial types with CD patients such as *Clostridium*, *Prevotella* and *Actinomyces and* specific microbial virulence genes such as viruses, including rotavirus and reovirus [2, 12]. In addition, a recent study reported that infants who carrying a high-risk genotype characterized by a low number of Bifidobacterium; *B. longus* [24]. The presence of these microorganisms and changing their function lead to an increase the autoimmune and inflammatory diseases [12]. Therefore, a number of recent studies supported the role of these microorganisms in CD development as a secondary cause with remains the direct cause proved [2, 12]. On the other hand, some studies suggested that some microorganism such as *Helicobacter pylori* or cytomegalovirus) may delay CD development, but the mechanism still unknown [2]. Some epidemiological studies focused on modulating the intestinal microbiota but still, the evidence is limited [25]. Furthermore, smoking is another environmental factor that mentions in some old studies. Snook et al. mentioned that the prevalence of CD was higher among smokers [26]. Lower economic status as well as and it is worthy to mention under the risk factors of CD because it is the inferior hygienic environment [27]. Overall, explaining the development of CD requires deep and accurate evidence related to the patient's characteristics, genetic and environmental factors together that is currently not fully understood.

4. Classification of variants of CD

4.1 Potential CD

Potential CD characterized by positive antibody (IgA EmA and anti-tTG) for CD with HLA-DQ2/HLA-DQ8, positive genetic markers, a normal intestinal mucosa, and few inflammation signs [28]. The intestinal mucosa in the potential CD is normal or inflamed slightly due to an increase in Els number [29]. Patients with potential CD could be asymptomatic or they may have extraintestinal symptoms [29]. Most children (80%) who suffer from the potential CD are asymptomatic and the other 20% have intestinal symptoms and extraintestinal signs such as delay in the anthropometrics [30, 31]. In CD adults, the symptomatic phenotype is common than in children and mostly extraintestinal symptoms [30–32]. Regarding the treatment, the current studies suggested that symptomatic potential patients only should follow GFD [30–32] . However, only a small percentage of patients with potential CD stick to the GFD and they suffer from villous atrophy [29, 30, 32]. The villous atrophy in the CD cases happen normally due to many causes as shown in **Figure 3**, but the restricted GFD reduce the probability of most causes and consequently reduce the small intestinal villi damage [33, 34].

4.2 Seronegative CD

A CD genetic test is also important because a negative outcome definitively rules out the disorder and leads doctors to look for other causes of villous atrophy. Morphology of the intestinal mucosal and serology testing is the basics tool for CD diagnosis [1]. The endoscopy is performed after the serological tests that including EmAs TG2-Ab assays [2]. The serological tests are very accurate and sensitive, its sensitivity arrived at (90–100%) and 100% specificity for coeliac CD [35]. EmA

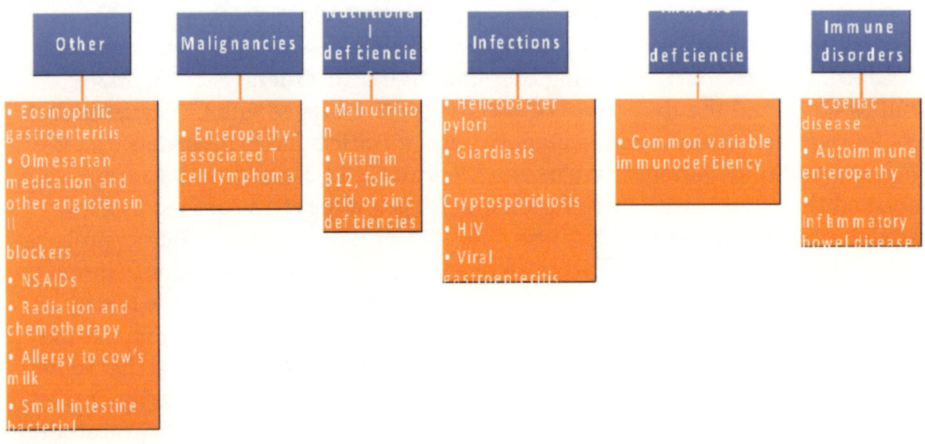

Figure 3.
Causes of small intestinal villous atrophy.

testing has long been considered the gold-standard tool for detecting the autoantibodies of CD [2]. On the other hand, the serological tests are considered a subjective test, indirect immunofluorescence, expensive and low throughput. Whereas the operator-independent enzyme is more common and operated on automated instruments by linking the immunosorbent assay (ELISA) and radio binding assay for TG2-Abs. the last method depends on the TG2 antigen quality, this means some of these tests could reveal negative and false-positive results negative and false-positive results. However, low TG2-Ab may be associated with other autoimmune diseases such as infectious disease and DMT1 [36]. Furthermore, approximately 10% of CD patients are seronegative, meaning they are undetectable by any of the existing serological methods [37]. After one year of GFD adherence, patients performed seronegative which assure improvement in the disease symptoms and the histology, because the diagnosis in the seronegative case depends on detection of small intestinal mucosa injury [37].

5. Diagnosis and screening of celiac disease (CD)

Currently, the clinically diagnosed cases are reported the epidemiological studies, but most research reported that there are heavily underestimated cases in every country [2]. In the high knowledge countries, the prevalence of CD is closer to the real estimation, whereas the other country still has the submerged CD iceberg. Working on increasing the diagnostic rate of CD is still a point of contention [3, 38, 39]. The current findings reported that there is growth in CD diagnosis. Mucosal changes detected by duodenal biopsy and serological test positivity (antitTG antibodies, anti-endomysium antibodies (EmA), and deamidated gliadin peptide (DGP) antibodies) are the gold standard, according to the most recently updated data. Intestinal biopsy is a critical assistant to assure a correct diagnosis because there is no antibody test that can provide perfect accuracy of sensitivity and specificity [1]. Commonly, the Pediatrics skipped the duodenal biopsy if they have high anti-tTG antibodies, positive EmA, HLA-DQ2/HLA-DQ8 and CD symptoms CD based on the recent recommendations of the European Society for Pediatric Gastroenterology Hepatology and Nutrition (ESPGHAN) [1, 40]. However, not all the world countries followed ESPGHAN recommendations such as the USA due to weakness in anti-tTG assays [41]. Despite this, duodenal biopsy remains an important part of the diagnosis of adult patients with suspected CD. The common clinical signs and symptoms of CD have evolved from childhood malabsorption symptoms to milder multi-organ manifestations that can occur in both childhood and adulthood [2, 12]. Loose stools, stomach pain, and flatulence are the most common signs, although in certain instances, no gastrointestinal disorders could be discovered [2]. In addition, there are some common clinical symptoms among CD patients. For instant, 10% of CD adults have Dermatitis herpetiformis and the iron deficiency anemia is also common [2, 8, 12, 42, 43]. Moreover, CD could be asymptomatic in specific cases for those who are screening with the high-risk group such as first-degree relative CD, DMT1 and down syndrome [2, 41, 42]. The current gold standard of care stated that four out of five of the following conditions are sufficient to diagnose CD [1, 45]: observe the typical signs and symptoms which include diarrhea and malabsorption; positive antibody test; positive HLA-DQ2 and/or HLA-DQ8, villous atrophy and damage in the intestine and clinical improvement resulted from following GFD. Most of these rules are used by the physicians to identify the other CD forms. Absence of intestinal damage point guides them to the potential CD, absence of the antibody positivity guids them to the seronegative CD, absence of the typical signs and symptoms guide them to a non-classic CD while absence of the response to GFD guide them to non-responsive CD [1].

5.1 Hematologic and blood biochemistry tests

CD could be suspectable by routine blood tests [46]. Low albumin, hemoglobin and micronutrients such as potassium, calcium, vitamin D and magnesium are associated with classical CD. Concerning iron and ferritin values, low ferritin and microcytic anemia values are very common among CD patients. Dimorphic anemia, macrocytic and non-macrocytic is not popular among patients with CD [47]. Numerous micronutrients deficiency was detected among CD that leads to important symptoms and diseases such as vitamin D3 deficiency that causes osteopenia and osteoporosis [48]. Even in the absence of other relevant symptoms, a cryptogenic increase in transaminases may signal the onset of CD. Transaminases return to normal range within 6–12 months after following a GFD [49]. Among the adults, Corazza et al. reported that the blood smear has the ability to identify changes in the membrane and cytoplasm of red blood cells, whereas, Nomarski phase contrast microscopy could detect the pitted red cells [50]. However, autoimmune diseases and their complications such as refractory CD, ulcerative jejunoileitis, and lymphoma are associated with macroscopically apparent or even functional hyposplenism, which is a predisposing factor for the development of infectious diseases caused by encapsulated bacteria such as Meningococcus and Pneumococcus [51].

5.2 Serology tests

A CD genetic test is also important because a negative outcome definitively rules out the disorder and leads doctors to look for other causes of villous atrophy [1]. Morphology of the intestinal mucosal and serology testing is the basics tool for CD diagnosis [1]. The endoscopy is performed after the serological tests that including EmAs TG2-Ab assays [2]. The serological tests are very accurate and sensitive, its sensitivity arrived at (90–100%) and 100% specificity for coeliac CD [35]. EmA testing has long been considered the gold-standard tool for detecting the autoantibodies of CD [2]. On the other hand, the serological tests are considered a subjective test, indirect immunofluorescence, expensive and low throughput. Whereas the operator-independent enzyme is more common and operated on automated instruments by linking the immunosorbent assay (ELISA) and radio binding assay for TG2-Abs. the last method depends on the TG2 antigen quality, this means some of these tests could reveal negative and false-positive results negative and false-positive results. However, low TG2-Ab may be associated with other autoimmune diseases such as infectious disease and DMT1 [36]. Furthermore, approximately 10% of CD patients are seronegative, meaning they are undetectable by any of the existing serological methods [37]. After one year of GFD adherence, patients performed seronegative which assure improvement in the disease symptoms and the histology, because the diagnosis in the seronegative case depends on detection of small intestinal mucosa injury [37].

The diagnosis of CD is not simple as its overlaps with different conditions of villous atrophy such as *Giardia lamblia* (parasitic infections), Crohn's disease, autoimmune enteropathy, immunodeficiency, HIV enteropathy, tropical sprue, and Whipple disease [1, 52, 53]. However, CD patients with seronegative are associated more with autoimmune diseases compared with classical CD patients. This association the morbidity due to the late diagnosis of a specific condition [52]. Deamidated Gliadin Peptide (DGP) antibodies test is the recent test that suggested in the CD diagnosis for cases the not detected by the EmA and TG2-Ab tests, but this method is not popular in the clinical practice [54]. In addition, number of commercial point-of-care rapid tests are available currently. For anti-DGPs and TG2-Abs detection [55]. Although there is little data on the performance of rapid tests, they provide immediate results in a primary care setting and may be useful in resource-constrained settings [55].

5.3 Duodenal biopsy

The duodenal biopsy still a cornerstone in the Morphological evaluation in CD confirmation and Histology still the gold standard choice of CD diagnosis [52]. With the addition of mild villous atrophy and minimal lesions as potential expressions of gluten-related intestinal injury, the histological requirements for CD have drastically modified [56]. Currently, four biopsies on the second duodenal portion are recommended and additional two biopsies at the bulb [57]. Based on Marsh classification (modified by Oberhüber), the different types of lesions of the intestinal mucosa are classified into five stages. This classification is used as a reference for CD diagnosis in all CD centres [58]. Lesion's types one and two described high IELs (with or without crypt hyperplasia) and standard villi. The potential CD is characterized by minimal intestinal lesions and positive anti-tTG and EmA. Moreover, this case (minimal intestinal lesions) is consistent with other causes such as allergies of some types of food as cow milk proteins, Crohn's disease, lymphocytic colitis. In lymphocytic enteritis, IEL cytometric pattern is more precise than subepithelial deposits of anti-TG2 IgA for CD diagnosis [59]. For CD patients, the recent evidence approved that the normal cut-off of IEL is ≥25 lymphocytes over 100 epithelial cells. The typical lesion (type 3) of CD demonstrates villous atrophy with a change in the villi-to-crypt ratio and an increase in IEL. Type three lesions are divided into three subdivided based on the severity of the atrophy as following: 3a means mild atrophy, 3b means partial atrophy, 3c means subtotal atrophy [58]. The diagnostic algorithm for CD diagnosis was illustrated by [1] in **Figures 4** and 5.

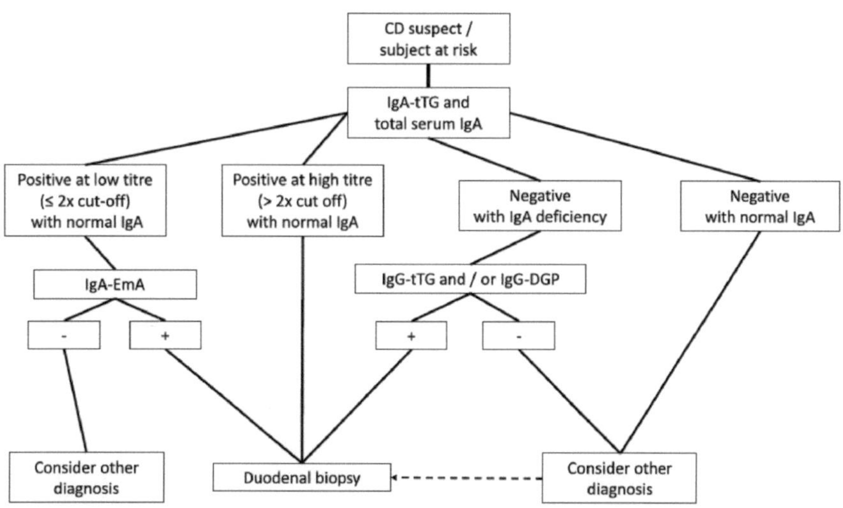

Figure 4.
The diagnostic algorithm for celiac disease diagnosis. Figure source [1].

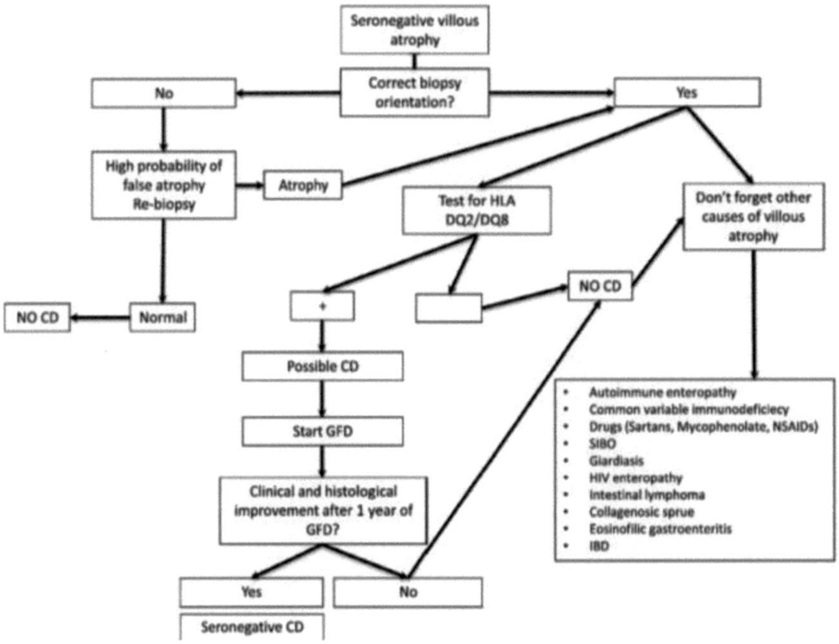

Figure 5.
The diagnostic algorithm for seronegative villous atrophy. Figure source [1].

6. Complications and consequences of CD

Most evidence suggests that having a late diagnosis of CD and/or not adhering to a strict GFD increase the mortality rate than the general population [60]. The most common complications of CD among elderly patients include Hyposplenism, Refractory CD, Hyposplenism and ulcerative jejunoileitis [1]. Around 30% of the CD adults have hyposplenism and it is associated with bacterial infections and other autoimmune diseases [61]. The refractory CD is associated with malabsorption, BMI reduction and diarrhea but it is from a small percentage of the CD cases (around 1–1.5%). Refractory CD is classified into two categories (type 1 and type 2). However, both categories are depending on the symptoms, improvement level and the CD patients response after following GFD [62]. Commonly the diagnosis of refractory CD takes place after one year of GFD by the negative serology tests [62].

Furthermore, the CD is correlated with malabsorption which resulted from villous atrophy [2]. Nutrition malabsorption leads to multiple deficiencies in the macronutrients such as the calories and micronutrients such as the vitamins and the minerals deficiencies [63, 64]. Following the GFD, on the other hand, was linked to adverse effects such as improvements in food delivery, insufficient fortification of gluten-free foods items, and individual dietary habits. The most common nutritional consequences of CD include Iron deficiency, Vitamin B12 deficiency, Vitamin D & calcium deficiencies, Folic acid deficiency, micronutrient and mineral deficiencies [63, 64]. All these nutrients deficiencies are linked with the traditional symptoms as diarrhea and BMI fluctuation [2]. Few studies have been assessed the nutritional value of the GFD, but most studies concluded that GFD has an imbalance of nutrients and could be associated with vitamins and minerals deficiencies such as calcium and vitamin and non-starch polysaccharides [2, 63, 64]. Therefore, the ideal treatment contains balanced GFD and the nutrients deficiencies should be diagnosed and treated by dietary supplement intake [63, 64].

7. Celiac disease (CD) prevention and management

7.1 Prevention

Inconsistent results were published regarding the prevention intervention for CD. The old study suggested starting early feeding wheat during breastfeeding to the infant [65]. In contrast, other intervention and cohort studies concluded that early wheat feeding practice did not prevent CD [3, 17]. Moreover, a number of systematic reviews and meta-analyses were approved that the infant practice such as duration of the breastfeeding not associated with CD prevention [15, 66]. Another Swedish cohort data reported that increasing the gluten consumption above five grams daily during the first two years is associated with an increase in the risk of CD among the study population [67]. From another side of view, some studies link intestinal infection and increase the CD risk factor [27, 68]. Therefore, the association between CD prevention effect and the environmental practice still needs further evaluation. Overall, the primary strategies of CD are the early and the correct diagnosis by screening diagnosis or by case finding [2]. Whereas secondary prevention reducing the symptom and the complications by following the recommended treatment [3, 17].

7.2 CD management

To date, the only effective treatment for CD is consuming gluten-free food such as fruit, vegetables, legumes, and gluten-free cereals. According to Codex Alimentarius (Codex Standard 118-1979) the recommended amount of gluten for CD patients does not exceed 20 mg/kg of gluten [69]. The researchers now are trying to improve the quality of gluten-free products by developing new analysis methods for gluten detection [3]. The safety of the gluten-free diet is an important aspect for CD patients because the contaminated products could have an illegal amount of gluten. In addition, the tolerable level varies among the CD patients.

The compliance rate of CD patients to the GFD is very poor. In general, children have more adherence to the GFD than adults because they are diagnosed in early childhood [3]. Patients compliance is affected by the age, gender, socioeconomic status of the patients [70]. Many studies were conducted on the CD patients compliance to the GFD to improve adherence [70–73]. However, some of these studies result was based on the symptoms diagnosis after following GFD and other studies used Anti-TG2 serology test to check the compliance rate. In general, the antibody titers decrease gradually after following a strict GFD, sometimes it takes a longer time in the case if it was high at diagnosis [70]. However, the best test is performing duodenal biopsies to check the compliance and the adherence of the CD patients. Comino et al. reported that detection of the gluten immunogenic peptides (GIP) in patient's feces urine was used as a biomarker for the patients gluten intake and consequently to the GFD adherence [74]. However, the last method is non-invasive as duodenal biopsies and it is relatively simple but it has weakness point in the relation of the antibody levels and with the dietary assessment questionnaires [74].

Following GFD is the only treatment to date and efficacious for most patients but following strict GFD is not easy. On the other hand, Most CD patients prefer any non-dietary treatments like vaccination, supplements, or medications [75].

Therefore, studies are making a great effort to find alternative treatments for CD patients [12]. A number of studies reported the availability of proteolytic enzymes (glutenases) of microbial or plant origins that could degrade gluten proteins quickly in similar conditions to the human stomach (low pH). These glutenases enzymes are promising drugs to eliminate the immunogenic capacity of dietary gluten due to their effectiveness in cleaving proline-and glutamine-rich gluten sequences [76–78]. Vitro and pre-clinical studies indicated that the glutenase leads to reduce the number of gluten epitopes in wheat-containing food [76–78]. Bethune believes that using glutenases as an oral enzymatic therapy for CD is a good idea [79]. These enzymes can be produced by the germination of wheat and it could be used to eliminate residual gluten from the food, but it is not enough to use as oral supplements [80]. Alternative treatment for CD patients is still being researched in vitro and in vivo, either as an add-on therapy to the GFD, as a rescue therapy after accidental gluten exposure, or as a substitute for the GFD [3].

8. Gluten-free diet (GFD)

The recommended and the documented treatment for CD patients, to date, is lifelong strict adherence to GFD [3, 8, 9, 44, 81–83]. Catassi et al. revealed that consuming 50 mg of gluten for three months could destroy the small intestine [84]. However, there is no documented recommended dose for the threshold dose for CD especially for the children [12]. While good adherence to the GFD leads to better intestinal healing and consequently improves the symptoms compared with patients who consumed gluten-contaminated food [12]. Using GFD led to avoid the gluten peptide sources located in the wheat, rye, barley and all cross-breeds of these cereals [85]. Wheat varieties such as kamut, einkorn, spelt also should be avoided because it is derived from wheat and many cereals are still in debate because it is contaminated by the wheat as oat [12]. However, wheat is the main component of the main food items such as bread and pasta. In addition, it is used in food processing as a thickening and stabilizing agent. Therefore, it exists in many food products. Following GFD leads to improve the symptoms which are considered as the first key sign of GFD adherence [86]. In addition, the small intestinal histology assessment and the inflammation tests, serology tests and dietary history assessment are the clinical checkpoints that are used to confirm the GFD adherence [87]. However, patients who are following GFD notes improvements in all the previous symptoms. Furthermore, some studies reported that following restricted GFD among CD patients is associated positively with the intelligence and education level [88]. In contrast, untreated patients and poor adherence to the GFD could lead to intestinal mucosa destruction and consequently suffer from nutrients deficiencies such as iron-deficiency anemia, malnutrition, malabsorption such as calcium and vitamin D, bone disorders [64]. Improvement the symptoms, malabsorption adjustment and health status recovery could be observed gradually after following GFD [89]. On the other hand, following GFD is a common trend worldwide as some peoples consider omitting wheat from the diet to support the health status [90]. Furthermore, patients with gluten intolerance that caused or Non-celiac gluten sensitivity follow GFD without proof of CD [91].

WHO codex [92] FDA define the gluten-free term in (2013) that food contains <20 parts per million (ppm) of gluten which equivalent to 20 mg of gluten per kg of food [12]. The starch of gluten contains little amounts of residual gluten, therefore, most factories nowadays are trying to purify the starch based on the standard to meet the Codex requirements in the US [12]. In other countries such as Australia and New Zealand, the guidelines are different. The rule is zero gluten in gluten-free food [12]. Currently, the most common analysis method to measuring the gluten in the food is R5 ELISA (Mendez) [93]. Despite the current use of this assay, it is not accurate to detect the contaminated product such as the oats and the barely as they contain different -molecular-weight peptides unlike that found in the wheat [94]. Therefore, improve more accurate analysis methods to detect the gluten in the food is still under enhancement [12].

Overall, following GFD is the ideal treatment for CD patients, but this diet includes a number of considerations as it contains a high amount of carbohydrates and a lower amount of fibers compared to the normal diet [12]. The ideal GFD should include balanced nutrients besides deity supplements if needed in the case of the nutrients deficiencies [63, 64]. The nutrient recommendations (based on age and gender) revealed that the carbohydrates should cover 55% of total calories with adequate dietary fiber (20–35 g daily). Around 25–30% or less of the total caloric should come from the monounsaturated and polyunsaturated fatty acids. In addition, five servings of fruit or vegetables daily at least are also recommended [63, 64].

9. Follow-up CD patients

Consult a dietitian is strongly recommended for CD patients after confirming the diagnosis [63, 64]. The dietitian can help the patient how to balance the GFD to improve the symptoms through six main principles that have been recommended for CD patients by NIH guidelines [95]. As well as follow of the CD patients is very important to confirm the patent's adherence to GFD and to check the consequences and the complications [2]. Analysis of the serum antibodies used to detect the GFD although other tests such as serological testing are also recommended [2]. The only reliable tool now is repeating the biopsy during the GFD but it is challenging [96].

10. Conclusions

Based on the most recent research, the prevalence of CD is increasing over time CD and it is starting to become emerge in some countries such as Africa and Asia. Many factors were suggested by a large number of studies that include mainly; Genetic predisposition, exposure to gluten, loss of intestinal barrier function, a pro-inflammatory innate immune response triggered by gluten; inappropriate adaptive immune response is the main reason for CD. The imbalanced gut microbiome has an indirect cause that could enhance disease development. Economic status and smoking are considered as other risk factors that could be related to CD. To date, there is still a gap in the scientific evidence regards the relationship between all the suggested factors that could lead to the CD. Therefore, more data should be collected to estimate the prevalence of CD in the world. In addition, further research is needed to identify the factors that influence the progression of CD autoimmunity to mucosal damage, as well as the biomarkers that predict this progression, so that preventive measures and non-dietary treatments can be developed. Following GFD is the effective treatment until now. Raise awareness level of CD regards the early diagnostic, effective diet, and other related issues are the most appropriate policy to be implemented to improve the diagnostic rate of CD.

11. Recommendations

- Biopsy remains the main and the essential tool for CD diagnosis and the serology cannot substitute for biopsy in the diagnosis of adult CD.

- When a patient is on a GFD, a duodenal biopsy is needed, as well as positive serology in the vast majority of adult patients.
- Patients should adhere to a GFD and have an intake of less than 10 mg gluten per day and the aim of the follow-up is to ensure strict adherence to the GFD.
- At the time of diagnosis, patients may begin eating gluten-free oats.
- In patients with CD, a GFD is advised to reduce the risk of adverse foetal outcome and lymphoma.
- When adherence is challenged, patients with CD should be followed up by a dietitian and/or clinician with an experience or expertise in this area.
- Patients with symptoms should be evaluated more closely than those with no symptoms.
- Patients should be encouraged to join their local coeliac support group as soon as they are diagnosed.
- Duodenal biopsy should be considered in people who have an upper endoscopy and have laboratory tests, signs, or endoscopic features that indicate CD.
- To rule out CD, HLA typing should be used. A positive DQ2.5 or DQ8 result will never be enough to validate the diagnosis.
- Individuals who are self-treating on a GFD who have never had adequate CD testing before changing their diet can use HLA typing.
- In high-risk individuals with CD, such as first-degree kin, HLA typing may be used to rule out CD and reduce potential testing.
- The diagnosis of CD requires duodenal biopsy when the patient is on a gluten-containing diet and for the vast majority of adult patients also positive serology.
- Duodenal biopsy should be retained as the mainstay for the diagnosis of adult CD and cannot be replaced by serology.
- If CD is suspected during endoscopy, at least four biopsy specimens, including a duodenal bulb biopsy, should be collected.
- A duodenal biopsy should be considered in serologically negative patients who exhibit symptoms of malabsorption (such as anemia or diarrhea) or have a family history of CD.
- Follow-up biopsies may be considered in patients with CD and are potentially helpful in identifying patients at increased risk of lymphoma.
- Follow-up biopsies are not mandatory if the patient with CD is asymptomatic on a GFD and has no other features that suggest an increased risk of complications.

- Follow-up biopsies should be undertaken in patients with CD whose condition does not respond to a GFD.
- Although there is insufficient evidence to suggest community screening for CD, according to National Institute for Health and Care Excellence recommendations, there should be a low threshold for case finding in clinical practice.
- CD tests should be done on symptomatic first-degree relatives of CD patients.
- Patients that have additional risk factors for osteoporosis or who are over the age of 55 should have a Pneumococcus vaccine.
- Bone density should be assessed after 1 year of diet in patients that have additional risk factors for osteoporosis or who are over the age of 55.
- Adult patients with CD should have a calcium intake of at least 1000 mg per day.
- Patients can have annual hematological and biochemical profiles, and a GFD is the mainstay of CD patients' osteoporosis prevention plan.

Conflict of interest

The authors declare no conflict of interest.

Acronyms and abbreviations

CD	Celiac Disease.
DMT1	Diabetes Meletus Type 1.
ELISA	The enzyme-linked immunosorbent assay.
GFD	Gluten Free Diet.
IELs	Intraepithelial Lymphocytes.
WHO	World Healthcare Organization.

Author details

Nour Amin Elsahoryi
Department of Nutrition, Faculty of Pharmacy and Medical Sciences,
The University of Petra, Amman, Jordan

*Address all correspondence to: nour.elsahoryi@uop.edu.jo

References

[1] Caio G, Volta U, Sapone A, Leffler DA, Giorgio R De, Catassi C, et al. Celiac disease: a comprehensive current review. BMC medicine. 2019;17(142).

[2] Lindfors K, Ciacci C, Kurppa K, Lundin KEA, Makharia GK, Mearin ML, et al. Coeliac disease. Nature Reviews Disease Primers. 2019 Dec 10;5(1):3. Available from: http://www.nature.com/articles/s41572-018-0054-z

[3] Scherf KA, Catassi C, Chirdo F, Ciclitira PJ, Feighery C, Gianfrani C, et al. Recent Progress and Recommendations on Celiac Disease From the Working Group on Prolamin Analysis and Toxicity. Frontiers in Nutrition. 2020 Mar 17;7(March):1-14. Available from: https://www.frontiersin.org/article/10.3389/fnut.2020.00029/full

[4] Rallabhandi P, Sharma GM, Pereira M, Williams KM. Immunological Characterization of the Gluten Fractions and Their Hydrolysates from Wheat, Rye and Barley. Journal of Agricultural and Food Chemistry. 2015 Feb 18;63(6):1825-1832. Available from: https://pubs.acs.org/doi/10.1021/jf505716p

[5] Singh P, Arora A, Strand TA, Leffler DA, Catassi C, Green PH, et al. Global Prevalence of Celiac Disease: Systematic Review and Meta-analysis. Clinical Gastroenterology and Hepatology. 2018 Jun;16(6):823-836.e2. Available from: https://linkinghub.elsevier.com/retrieve/pii/S1542356517307838

[6] Naiyana Gujral, Hugh J Freeman ABT. Celiac disease: Prevalence, diagnosis, pathogenesis and treatment. World Journal of Gastroenterology. 2012; 18(42):6036. Available from: http://www.wjgnet.com/1007-9327/full/v18/i42/6036.htm

[7] Husby S, Koletzko S, Korponay-Szabó I, Kurppa K, Mearin ML, Ribes-Koninckx C, et al. European Society Paediatric Gastroenterology, Hepatology and Nutrition Guidelines for Diagnosing Coeliac Disease 2020. Journal of Pediatric Gastroenterology and Nutrition. 2020 Jan;70(1):141-156. Available from: http://journals.lww.com/10.1097/MPG.0000000000002497

[8] El-Metwally A, Toivola P, AlAhmary K, Bahkali S, AlKhathaami A, AlSaqabi MK, et al. The Epidemiology of Celiac Disease in the General Population and High-Risk Groups in Arab Countries: A Systematic Review. BioMed Research International. 2020 Jun 4;2020:1-13. Available from: https://www.hindawi.com/journals/bmri/2020/6865917/

[9] Odeh R, Alassaf A, Gharaibeh L, Ibrahim S, Khdair Ahmad F, Ajlouni K. Prevalence of celiac disease and celiac-related antibody status in pediatric patients with type 1 diabetes in Jordan. Endocrine Connections. 2019 Jun;8(6): 780-787. Available from: https://ec.bioscientifica.com/view/journals/ec/8/6/EC-19-0146.xml

[10] Billerbeck NC, Borges LP, Silva MEA. Nível De Atividade Física E Tabagismo. International Journal of Movement Science and Rehabilitation. 2019;01:24-32.

[11] Dowd AJ, Kronlund L, Parmar C, Daun JT, Wytsma-Fisher K, Reimer RA, et al. A 12-Week Pilot Exercise Program for Inactive Adults With Celiac Disease: Study Protocol. Global Advances in Health and Medicine. 2019;8:216495611985377.

[12] Tye-Din JA, Galipeau HJ, Agardh D. Celiac Disease: A Review of Current Concepts in Pathogenesis, Prevention, and Novel Therapies. Frontiers in Pediatrics. 2018 Nov 21;6. Available from: https://www.frontiersin.org/article/10.3389/fped.2018.00350/full

[13] Anderson RP. Editorial: towards an understanding of increased mortality in coeliac disease. Alimentary Pharmacology and Therapeutics. 2021;53(5):654-655.

[14] Alessio Fasano, Catassi C. Clinical practice. Celiac disease. N Engl J Med. 2012;20(367(25)):2419-26.

[15] Szajewska H, Shamir R, Chmielewska A, Pieścik-Lech M, Auricchio R, Ivarsson A, et al. Systematic review with meta-analysis: early infant feeding and coeliac disease - update 2015. Alimentary Pharmacology & Therapeutics. 2015 Jun;41(11):1038-1054. Available from: http://doi.wiley.com/10.1111/apt.13163

[16] Chmielewska A, Pieścik-Lech M, Szajewska H, Shamir R. Primary Prevention of Celiac Disease: Environmental Factors with a Focus on Early Nutrition. Annals of Nutrition and Metabolism. 2015;67(Suppl. 2):43-50. Available from: https://www.karger.com/Article/FullText/440992

[17] Lionetti E, Castellaneta S, Francavilla R, Pulvirenti A, Tonutti E, Amarri S, et al. Introduction of Gluten, HLA Status, and the Risk of Celiac Disease in Children. New England Journal of Medicine. 2014 Oct 2;371(14): 1295-1303. Available from: http://www.nejm.org/doi/10.1056/NEJMoa1400697

[18] Vriezinga SL, Auricchio R, Bravi E, Castillejo G, Chmielewska A, Crespo Escobar P, et al. Randomized Feeding Intervention in Infants at High Risk for Celiac Disease. New England Journal of Medicine. 2014 Oct 2;371(14):1304-1315. Available from: http://www.nejm.org/doi/10.1056/NEJMoa1404172

[19] Andrén Aronsson C, Lee H-S, Koletzko S, Uusitalo U, Yang J, Virtanen SM, et al. Effects of Gluten Intake on Risk of Celiac Disease: A Case-Control Study on a Swedish Birth Cohort. Clinical Gastroenterology and Hepatology. 2016 Mar;14(3):403-409.e3. Available from: https://linkinghub.elsevier.com/retrieve/pii/S1542356515013324

[20] Norris JM. Risk of Celiac Disease Autoimmunity and Timing of Gluten Introduction in the Diet of Infants at Increased Risk of Disease. JAMA. 2005 May 18;293(19):2343. Available from: http://jama.jamanetwork.com/article.aspx?doi=10.1001/jama.293.19.2343

[21] Stene LC, Honeyman MC, Hoffenberg EJ, Haas JE, Sokol RJ, Emery L, et al. Rotavirus Infection Frequency and Risk of Celiac Disease Autoimmunity in Early Childhood: A Longitudinal Study. The American Journal of Gastroenterology. 2006 Oct;101(10):2333-2340. Available from: http://www.nature.com/doifinder/10.1111/j.1572-0241.2006.00741.x

[22] Bouziat R, Biering SB, Kouame E, Sangani KA, Kang S, Ernest JD, et al. Murine Norovirus Infection Induces TH1 Inflammatory Responses to Dietary Antigens. Cell Host & Microbe. 2018 Nov;24(5):677-688.e5. Available from: https://linkinghub.elsevier.com/retrieve/pii/S1931312818305420

[23] Bouziat R, Hinterleitner R, Brown JJ, Stencel-Baerenwald JE, Ikizler M, Mayassi T, et al. Reovirus infection triggers inflammatory responses to dietary antigens and development of celiac disease. Science. 2017 Apr 7;356(6333):44-50. Available from: https://www.sciencemag.org/lookup/doi/10.1126/science.aah5298

[24] Olivares M, Walker AW, Capilla A, Benítez-Páez A, Palau F, Parkhill J, et al. Gut microbiota trajectory in early life may predict development of celiac disease. Microbiome. 2018 Dec 20;6(1): 36. Available from: https://microbiomejournal.biomedcentral.com/articles/10.1186/s40168-018-0415-6

[25] Koletzko S, Lee H-S, Beyerlein A, Aronsson CA, Hummel M, Liu E, et al.

Cesarean Section on the Risk of Celiac Disease in the Offspring: The Teddy Study. Journal of Pediatric Gastroenterology & Nutrition. 2018 Mar;66(3):417-424. Available from: https://journals.lww.com/00005176-201803000-00014

[26] Snook JA, Dwyer L, Lee-Elliott C, Khan S, Wheeler DW, Nicholas DS. Adult coeliac disease and cigarette smoking. Gut. 1996 Jul 1;39(1):60-62. Available from: https://gut.bmj.com/lookup/doi/10.1136/gut.39.1.60

[27] Kemppainen KM, Lynch KF, Liu E, Lönnrot M, Simell V, Briese T, et al. Factors That Increase Risk of Celiac Disease Autoimmunity After a Gastrointestinal Infection in Early Life. Clinical Gastroenterology and Hepatology. 2017 May;15(5):694-702.e5. Available from: https://linkinghub.elsevier.com/retrieve/pii/S1542356516310436

[28] Ludvigsson JF, Leffler DA, Bai JC, Biagi F, Fasano A, Green PHR, et al. The Oslo definitions for coeliac disease and related terms. Gut. 2013 Jan;62(1):43-52. Available from: https://gut.bmj.com/lookup/doi/10.1136/gutjnl-2011-301346

[29] Volta U, Caio G, Giancola F, Rhoden KJ, Ruggeri E, Boschetti E, et al. Features and Progression of Potential Celiac Disease in Adults. Clinical Gastroenterology and Hepatology. 2016 May;14(5):686-693.e1. Available from: https://linkinghub.elsevier.com/retrieve/pii/S1542356515014913

[30] Tosco A, Salvati VM, Auricchio R, Maglio M, Borrelli M, Coruzzo A, et al. Natural History of Potential Celiac Disease in Children. Clinical Gastroenterology and Hepatology. 2011 Apr;9(4):320-325. Available from: https://linkinghub.elsevier.com/retrieve/pii/S1542356510008657

[31] Rodríguez-Almagro J, Hernández-Martínez A, Lucendo AJ, Casellas F, Solano-Ruiz MC, Siles-González J. Health-related quality of life and determinant factors in celiac disease. A population-based analysis of adult patients in Spain. Revista Espanola de Enfermedades Digestivas. 2016; 108(4):181-189.

[32] Zanini B, Caselani F, Magni A, Turini D, Ferraresi A, Lanzarotto F, et al. Celiac Disease With Mild Enteropathy Is Not Mild Disease. Clinical Gastroenterology and Hepatology. 2013 Mar;11(3):253-258. Available from: https://linkinghub.elsevier.com/retrieve/pii/S1542356512011421

[33] Owen DR, Owen DA. Celiac Disease and Other Causes of Duodenitis. Archives of Pathology & Laboratory Medicine. 2018 Jan 1;142(1):35-43. Available from: http://meridian.allenpress.com/aplm/article/142/1/35/65558/Celiac-Disease-and-Other-Causes-of-Duodenitis

[34] DeGaetani M, Tennyson CA, Lebwohl B, Lewis SK, Abu Daya H, Arguelles-Grande C, et al. Villous Atrophy and Negative Celiac Serology: A Diagnostic and Therapeutic Dilemma. American Journal of Gastroenterology. 2013 May;108(5):647-653. Available from:https://journals.lww.com/00000434-201305000-00004

[35] Giersiepen K, Lelgemann M, Stuhldreher N, Ronfani L, Husby S, Koletzko S, et al. Accuracy of Diagnostic Antibody Tests for Coeliac Disease in Children. Journal of Pediatric Gastroenterology & Nutrition. 2012 Feb;54(2):229-241. Available from: https://journals.lww.com/00005176-201202000-00015

[36] Ferrara F, Quaglia S, Caputo I, Esposito C, Lepretti M, Pastore S, et al. Anti-transglutaminase antibodies in non-coeliac children suffering from infectious diseases. Clinical & Experimental Immunology. 2010 Feb;159(2):217-223. Available from:

http://doi.wiley.com/10.1111/j.1365-2249.2009.04054.x

[37] Aziz I, Peerally MF, Barnes J-H, Kandasamy V, Whiteley JC, Partridge D, et al. The clinical and phenotypical assessment of seronegative villous atrophy; a prospective UK centre experience evaluating 200 adult cases over a 15-year period (2000-2015). Gut. 2017 Sep;66(9):1563-1572. Available from: https://gut.bmj.com/lookup/doi/10.1136/gutjnl-2016-312271

[38] Rubio–Tapia A, Kyle RA, Kaplan EL, Johnson DR, Page W, Erdtmann F, et al. Increased Prevalence and Mortality in Undiagnosed Celiac Disease. Gastroenterology. 2009 Jul;137(1):88-93. Available from: https://linkinghub.elsevier.com/retrieve/pii/S001650850900523X

[39] Hujoel IA, Van Dyke CT, Brantner T, Larson J, King KS, Sharma A, et al. Natural history and clinical detection of undiagnosed coeliac disease in a North American community. Alimentary Pharmacology & Therapeutics. 2018 May;47(10):1358-1366. Available from: http://doi.wiley.com/10.1111/apt.14625

[40] Husby S, Koletzko S, Korponay-Szabó IR, Mearin ML, Phillips A, Shamir R, et al. European Society for Pediatric Gastroenterology, Hepatology, and Nutrition Guidelines for the Diagnosis of Coeliac Disease. Journal of Pediatric Gastroenterology & Nutrition. 2012 Jan;54(1):136-160. Available from: https://journals.lww.com/00005176-201201000-00028

[41] Egner W, Shrimpton A, Sargur R, Patel D, Swallow K. ESPGHAN Guidance on Coeliac Disease 2012. Journal of Pediatric Gastroenterology & Nutrition. 2012 Dec;55(6):733-735. Available from: https://journals.lww.com/00005176-201212000-00017

[42] Parzanese I, Qehajaj D, Patrinicola F, Aralica M, Chiriva-Internati M, Stifter S, et al. Celiac disease: From pathophysiology to treatment. World Journal of Gastrointestinal Pathophysiology. 2017;8(2):27.

[43] Pudasaini S. Celiac disease and its histopathology. Journal of Pathology of Nepal. 2017 Mar 30;7(1):1118-1123. Available from: https://www.nepjol.info/index.php/JPN/article/view/16948

[44] Singh P, Arora S, Lal S, Strand TA, Makharia GK. Risk of Celiac Disease in the First- and Second-Degree Relatives of Patients With Celiac Disease: A Systematic Review and Meta-Analysis. American Journal of Gastroenterology. 2015 Nov;110(11):1539-1548. Available from:https://journals.lww.com/00000434-201511000-00010

[45] Catassi C, Fasano A. Celiac Disease Diagnosis: Simple Rules Are Better Than Complicated Algorithms. The American Journal of Medicine. 2010 Aug;123(8): 691-693. Available from: https://linkinghub.elsevier.com/retrieve/pii/S0002934310003591

[46] Kostopoulou O, Devereaux-Walsh C, Delaney BC. Missing Celiac Disease in Family Medicine: The Importance of Hypothesis Generation. Medical Decision Making. 2009 May 6;29(3):282-290. Available from: http://journals.sagepub.com/doi/10.1177/0272989X08327493

[47] Baydoun A, Maakaron JE, Halawi H, Abou Rahal J, Taher AT. Hematological manifestations of celiac disease. Scandinavian Journal of Gastroenterology. 2012 Dec 6;47(12):1401-1411. Available from: http://www.tandfonline.com/doi/full/10.3109/00365521.2012.706828

[48] Zanchetta MB, Longobardi V, Bai JC. Bone and Celiac Disease. Current Osteoporosis Reports. 2016 Apr 13; 14(2):43-48. Available from: http://link.springer.com/10.1007/s11914-016-0304-5

[49] Volta U, Franceschi L De, Lari F, Molinaro N, Zoli M, Bianchi FB. Coeliac disease hidden by cryptogenic hypertransaminasaemia. The Lancet. 1998 Jul;352(9121):26-29. Available from: https://linkinghub.elsevier.com/retrieve/pii/S0140673697112223

[50] Corazza GR, Zoli G, Di Sabatino A, Ciccocioppo R, Gasbarrini G. A Reassessment of Splenic Hypofunction in Celiac Disease. American Journal of Gastroenterology. 1999 Feb;94(2):391-397. Available from: https://journals.lww.com/00000434-199902000-00023

[51] Caio G, Riegler G, Patturelli M, Facchiano A, DE Magistris L, Sapone A. Pathophysiology of non-celiac gluten sensitivity: where are we now? Minerva gastroenterologica e dietologica. 2017 Mar;63(1):16-21. Available from: http://www.ncbi.nlm.nih.gov/pubmed/27808487

[52] Volta U, Caio G, Boschetti E, Giancola F, Rhoden KJ, Ruggeri E, et al. Seronegative celiac disease: Shedding light on an obscure clinical entity. Digestive and Liver Disease. 2016 Sep;48(9):1018-1022. Available from: https://linkinghub.elsevier.com/retrieve/pii/S1590865816304601

[53] Greenson JK. The biopsy pathology of non-coeliac enteropathy. Histopathology. 2015 Jan;66(1):29-36. Available from: http://doi.wiley.com/10.1111/his.12522

[54] Farahid OH, Khawaja N, Shennak MM, Batieha A, El Khateeb M, Ajlouni K. Prevalence of coeliac disease among adult patients with autoimmune hypothyroidism in Jordan. Eastern Mediterranean Health Journal. 2014 Jan 1;20(1):51-55. Available from: http://applications.emro.who.int/emhj/v20/01/EMHJ_2014_20_1_51_55.pdf

[55] Singh P, Arora A, Strand TA, Leffler DA, Mäki M, Kelly CP, et al. Diagnostic Accuracy of Point of Care Tests for Diagnosing Celiac Disease. Journal of Clinical Gastroenterology. 2019 Aug;53(7):535-542. Available from: https://journals.lww.com/00004836-201908000-00016

[56] Corazza GR. Coeliac disease. Journal of Clinical Pathology. 2005 Jun 1;58(6):573-574. Available from: http://jcp.bmj.com/cgi/doi/10.1136/jcp.2004.023978

[57] Oxentenko AS, Murray JA. Celiac Disease: Ten Things That Every Gastroenterologist Should Know. Clinical Gastroenterology and Hepatology. 2015 Aug;13(8):1396-1404. Available from: https://linkinghub.elsevier.com/retrieve/pii/S1542356514010532

[58] Oberhuber G, Granditsch G, Vogelsang H. The histopathology of coeliac disease: time for a standardized report scheme for pathologists. European Journal of Gastroenterology & Hepatology. 1999 Oct;11(10):1185. Available from: http://journals.lww.com/00042737-199910000-00019

[59] Fernández-Bañares F, Carrasco A, García-Puig R, Rosinach M, González C, Alsina M, et al. Intestinal Intraepithelial Lymphocyte Cytometric Pattern Is More Accurate than Subepithelial Deposits of Anti-Tissue Transglutaminase IgA for the Diagnosis of Celiac Disease in Lymphocytic Enteritis. D'Auria S, editor. PLoS ONE. 2014 Jul 10;9(7):e101249. Available from: https://dx.plos.org/10.1371/journal.pone.0101249

[60] Rubio-Tapia A, Ludvigsson JF, Choung RS, Brantner TL, Rajkumar SV, Landgren O, et al. Increased mortality among men aged 50 years old or above with elevated IgA anti-transglutaminase antibodies: NHANES III. BMC Gastroenterology. 2016 Dec 3;16(1):136. Available from: https://bmcgastroenterol.biomedcentral.com/articles/10.1186/s12876-016-0547-8

[61] Caraceni P, Benazzi B, Caio G, Zaccherini G, Domenicali M, Volta U.

Hyposplenism as a cause of pneumococcal meningoencephalitis in an adult patient with coeliac disease. Italian Journal of Medicine. 2013 Mar 7;124-127. Available from: https://italjmed.org/index.php/ijm/article/view/itjm.2011.124

[62] Collin P, Thorell L, Kaukinen K, Mäki M. The safe threshold for gluten contamination in gluten-free products. Can trace amounts be accepted in the treatment of coeliac disease? Alimentary Pharmacology & Therapeutics. 2004 Jun;19(12):1277-1283. Available from: http://doi.wiley.com/10.1111/j.1365-2036.2004.01961.x

[63] Theethira TG, Dennis M, Leffler DA. Nutritional consequences of celiac disease and the gluten-free diet. Expert Review of Gastroenterology & Hepatology. 2014 Feb 13;8(2):123-129. Available from: http://www.tandfonline.com/doi/full/10.1586/17474124.2014.876360

[64] Kohout P. Nutrition in celiac disease. International Journal of Celiac Disease. 2014;2(3):115-117.

[65] Ivarsson A, Myleus A, Norstrom F, van der Pals M, Rosen A, Hogberg L, et al. Prevalence of Childhood Celiac Disease and Changes in Infant Feeding. PEDIATRICS. 2013 Mar 1;131(3):e687–e694. Available from: http://pediatrics.aappublications.org/cgi/doi/10.1542/peds.2012-1015

[66] Silano M, Agostoni C, Sanz Y, Guandalini S. Infant feeding and risk of developing celiac disease: a systematic review. BMJ Open. 2016 Jan 25;6(1):e009163. Available from: https://bmjopen.bmj.com/lookup/doi/10.1136/bmjopen-2015-009163

[67] Mariné M, Farre C, Alsina M, Vilar P, Cortijo M, Salas A, et al. The prevalence of coeliac disease is significantly higher in children compared with adults. Alimentary Pharmacology & Therapeutics. 2011 Feb;33(4):477-486. Available from: http://doi.wiley.com/10.1111/j.1365-2036.2010.04543.x

[68] Mårild K, Kahrs CR, Tapia G, Stene LC, Størdal K. Infections and Risk of Celiac Disease in Childhood: A Prospective Nationwide Cohort Study. American Journal of Gastroenterology. 2015 Oct;110(10):1475-1484. Available from: https://journals.lww.com/00000434-201510000-00021

[69] Dieterich W, Ehnis T, Bauer M, Donner P, Volta U, Riecken EO, et al. Identification of tissue transglutaminase as the autoantigen of celiac disease. Nature Medicine. 1997 Jul;3(7):797-801. Available from: http://www.nature.com/articles/nm0797-797

[70] Leffler DA, Dennis M, Edwards George JB, Jamma S, Magge S, Cook EF, et al. A Simple Validated Gluten-Free Diet Adherence Survey for Adults With Celiac Disease. Clinical Gastroenterology and Hepatology. 2009 May;7(5):530-536.e2. Available from: http://dx.doi.org/10.1016/j.cgh.2008.12.032

[71] Saadah OI. Effect of gluten-free diet and adherence on growth and diabetic control in diabetics with coeliac disease. Archives of Disease in Childhood. 2004 Sep 1;89(9):871-876. Available from: https://adc.bmj.com/lookup/doi/10.1136/adc.2002.012799

[72] Hall NJ, Rubin G, Charnoch A. Systematic review: adherence to a gluten-free diet in adult patients with coeliac disease. Alimentary Pharmacology & Therapeutics. 2009 Aug;30(4):315-330. Available from: http://doi.wiley.com/10.1111/j.1365-2036.2009.04053.x

[73] Elsahoryi NA, Altamimi E, Subih HS, Hammad FJ, Woodside J V. Educational Intervention Improved Parental Knowledge, Attitudes, and Practices (KAP) and Adherence of Patients with Celiac Disease to Gluten-Free Diet. International Journal of Food

Science. 2020 Sep 21;2020:1-9. Available from: https://www.hindawi.com/journals/ijfs/2020/8850594/

[74] Comino I, Fernández-Bañares F, Esteve M, Ortigosa L, Castillejo G, Fambuena B, et al. Fecal Gluten Peptides Reveal Limitations of Serological Tests and Food Questionnaires for Monitoring Gluten-Free Diet in Celiac Disease Patients. American Journal of Gastroenterology. 2016 Oct;111(10):1456-1465. Available from: https://journals.lww.com/00000434-201610000-00024

[75] Rabinowitz LG, Zylberberg HM, Levinovitz A, Stockwell MS, Green PHR, Lebwohl B. Skepticism Regarding Vaccine and Gluten-Free Food Safety Among Patients with Celiac Disease and Non-celiac Gluten Sensitivity. Digestive Diseases and Sciences. 2018 May 14;63(5):1158-1164. Available from: http://link.springer.com/10.1007/s10620-017-4879-1

[76] Wolf C, Siegel JB, Tinberg C, Camarca A, Gianfrani C, Paski S, et al. Engineering of Kuma030: A Gliadin Peptidase That Rapidly Degrades Immunogenic Gliadin Peptides in Gastric Conditions. Journal of the American Chemical Society. 2015 Oct 14;137(40):13106-13113. Available from: https://pubs.acs.org/doi/10.1021/jacs.5b08325

[77] Mitea C, Havenaar R, Drijfhout JW, Edens L, Dekking L, Koning F. Efficient degradation of gluten by a prolyl endoprotease in a gastrointestinal model: implications for coeliac disease. Gut. 2007 May 14;57(1):25-32. Available from: https://gut.bmj.com/lookup/doi/10.1136/gut.2006.111609

[78] Cavaletti L, Taravella A, Carrano L, Carenzi G, Sigurtà A, Solinas N, et al. E40, a novel microbial protease efficiently detoxifying gluten proteins, for the dietary management of gluten intolerance. Scientific Reports. 2019 Dec 11;9(1):13147. Available from: http://www.nature.com/articles/s41598-019-48299-7

[79] Bethune MT, Khosla C. Oral Enzyme Therapy for Celiac Sprue. In 2012. p. 241-271. Available from: https://linkinghub.elsevier.com/retrieve/pii/B9780124160392000136

[80] Knorr V, Wieser H, Koehler P. Production of gluten-free beer by peptidase treatment. European Food Research and Technology. 2016 Jul 21;242(7):1129-1140. Available from: http://link.springer.com/10.1007/s00217-015-2617-5

[81] Dennis M, Lee AR, McCarthy T. Nutritional Considerations of the Gluten-Free Diet. Gastroenterology Clinics of North America. 2019 Mar;48(1):53-72. Available from: https://linkinghub.elsevier.com/retrieve/pii/S0889855318300785

[82] Irvine AJ, Chey WD, Ford AC. Screening for Celiac Disease in Irritable Bowel Syndrome: An Updated Systematic Review and Meta-analysis. American Journal of Gastroenterology. 2017 Jan;112(1):65-76. Available from: http://journals.lww.com/00000434-201701000-00017

[83] Ludvigsson JF, Card T, Ciclitira PJ, Swift GL, Nasr I, Sanders DS, et al. Support for patients with celiac disease: A literature review. United European Gastroenterology Journal. 2015 Apr 9;3(2):146-159. Available from: http://journals.sagepub.com/doi/10.1177/2050640614562599

[84] Catassi C, Fabiani E, Iacono G, D'Agate C, Francavilla R, Biagi F, et al. A prospective, double-blind, placebo-controlled trial to establish a safe gluten

threshold for patients with celiac disease. The American Journal of Clinical Nutrition. 2007 Jan 1;85(1):160-166. Available from: https://academic.oup.com/ajcn/article/85/1/160/4649352

[85] Simell S, Kupila A, Hoppu S, Hekkala A, Simell T, Stahlberg M-R, et al. Natural history of transglutaminase autoantibodies and mucosal changes in children carrying HLA-conferred celiac disease susceptibility. Scandinavian Journal of Gastroenterology. 2005 Jan 1;40(10): 1182-1191. Available from: https://www.tandfonline.com/doi/full/10.1080/00365520510024034

[86] Moreno M, Rodríguez-Herrera A, Sousa C, Comino I. Biomarkers to Monitor Gluten-Free Diet Compliance in Celiac Patients. Nutrients. 2017 Jan 6;9(1):46. Available from: http://www.mdpi.com/2072-6643/9/1/46

[87] Taavela J, Koskinen O, Huhtala H, Lähdeaho M-L, Popp A, Laurila K, et al. Validation of Morphometric Analyses of Small-Intestinal Biopsy Readouts in Celiac Disease. Sestak K, editor. PLoS ONE. 2013 Oct 11;8(10):e76163. Available from: https://dx.plos.org/10.1371/journal.pone.0076163

[88] Biagi F, Bianchi PI, Marchese A, Trotta L, Vattiato C, Balduzzi D, et al. A score that verifies adherence to a gluten-free diet: a cross-sectional, multicentre validation in real clinical life. British Journal of Nutrition. 2012 Nov 28;108(10):1884-1888. Available from: https://www.cambridge.org/core/product/identifier/S0007114511007367/type/journal_article

[89] Diamanti A, Capriati T, Basso M, Panetta F, Di Ciommo Laurora V, Bellucci F, et al. Celiac Disease and Overweight in Children: An Update. Nutrients. 2014 Jan 2;6(1):207-220. Available from: http://www.mdpi.com/2072-6643/6/1/207

[90] Biesiekierski JR, Muir JG, Gibson PR. Is Gluten a Cause of Gastrointestinal Symptoms in People Without Celiac Disease? Current Allergy and Asthma Reports. 2013 Dec 12;13(6):631-638. Available from: http://link.springer.com/10.1007/s11882-013-0386-4

[91] Verdu EF, Armstrong D, Murray JA. Between Celiac Disease and Irritable Bowel Syndrome: The "No Man's Land" of Gluten Sensitivity. The American Journal of Gastroenterology. 2009 Jun 19;104(6):1587-1594. Available from: http://www.nature.com/articles/ajg2009188

[92] Codex Alimentarius International Food Standards. Standard for foods for special dietary use for persons intolerant to gluten. Codex Stan 118-1979. 2008;

[93] Mendez E, Vela C, Immer U, Janssen FW. Report of a collaborative trial to investigate the performance of the R5 enzyme linked immunoassay to determine gliadin in gluten-free food. European Journal of Gastroenterology & Hepatology. 2005 Oct;17(10):1053-1063. Available from: http://journals.lww.com/00042737-200510000-00008

[94] See JA, Kaukinen K, Makharia GK, Gibson PR, Murray JA. Practical insights into gluten-free diets. Nature Reviews Gastroenterology & Hepatology. 2015 Oct 22;12(10):580-591. Available from: http://www.nature.com/articles/nrgastro.2015.156

[95] Rubio-Tapia A, Hill ID, Kelly CP, Calderwood AH, Murray JA. ACG Clinical Guidelines: Diagnosis and Management of Celiac Disease. American Journal of Gastroenterology. 2013 May;108(5):656-676. Available

from: https://journals.lww.com/00000434-201305000-00007

[96] Taavela J, Popp A, Korponay-Szabo IR, Ene A, Vornanen M, Saavalainen P, et al. A Prospective Study on the Usefulness of Duodenal Bulb Biopsies in Celiac Disease Diagnosis in Children: Urging Caution. American Journal of Gastroenterology. 2016 Jan;111(1):124-133. Available from: https://journals.lww.com/00000434-201601000-00029

Chapter 11

Sialoendoscopy in Juvenile Recurrent Parotitis That Could Be Primary Pediatric Sjogren's Syndrome

Brigida Iorio, Roberto De Luca, Gianpaolo Tartaro and Giuseppe Colella

Abstract

Parotid swelling often is encountered in the pediatric population, essentially acute and self-limiting, which usually represents viral or bacterial infections. Less common etiologies include juvenile recurrent parotitis (JRP) or pneumoparotid or anatomic abnormalities. Sjögren's syndrome is common in JRP (40% almost). Levels of suspicion for an autoimmune disorder should be maintained for children affected by JRP, particulary in bilateral glands involvement in order to optimize diagnoses and facilitate treatment. Cytological examination of saliva, which is normally in children is acellular, shows granulocytes, lymphocytes, and in some cases 50% of bacteria. Sialoendoscopy typically shows whitish ductal walls and the presence of stenosis without evidence of solid obstructions and/or mucous membranes. Sialoendoscopic treatment can improve symptoms thanks to local anti-inflammatory therapy and sialoendoscopic washing.

Keywords: juvenile recurrent parotitis (JRP), Sjögren's syndrome (SS), sialoendoscopy, pediatric parotitis, sialoadenitis

1. Introduction

Juvenile recurrent parotitis (JRP) was firstly described by Rose in 1953 [1]. The prevalence of JRP in children is 10 times lower than in adults, yet it is the second leading cause of inflammatory salivary gland disease in children after mumps, and the differential diagnosis between them is difficult in young children [2].

JRP is defined when a minimum of 2 and maximum of 30 episodes per year of painful parotid inflammation occur, usually associated with fever, swelling, and erythema of the overlying skin gland [3, 4].

Sjögren's syndrome (SS) is an idiopathic systemic autoimmune disease affecting exocrine glands with classic symptom complex of dry eyes (xerophthalmia) and dry mouth (xerostomia). Extraglandular involvement in SS may affect many systems such as renal, central nervous system, and vascular and hematological ones. Primary SS (pSS) occurs with a prevalence of 0.1-0.4% in the Caucasian population with a female predominance in the fourth and fifth decades. Conversely, in childhood and early adulthood SS is an extremely rare autoimmune condition (only 147 cases described in literature) [5, 6].

We hypothesized a higher prevalence of pSS in our young patients and we adopted a protocol with clinical, laboratory, and endoscopic examination. Sialoendoscopy has gained an increasing role in both diagnosis and treatment of JRP in a pediatric age. After its introduction in 1991 for the treatment of salivary disorders in adults, sialoendoscopy has also been validated as a safe technique in JRP treatment by Nahieli and Marchal [2, 7].

2. Clinical findings

2.1 JRP

JRP clinical symptoms include intermittent, usually unilateral swelling of the parotid gland, which occurs suddenly (over minutes or hours) and may persist for days or weeks [8]. The first episode typically occurs in scholar age, between 3 and 6 years, more often in males [9].

The etiopathology of JRP remains obscure; many factors have been suggested for the development of JRP including retrograde infection of the duct, viral or bacterial infection, autoimmune disease [10], disrupted enzyme activity [11], dental occlusion disorders [8, 12, 13], hypogammaglobulinemia, immunoglobulin A deficiency, and immunoglobulin G3 deficiency [14, 15]. These theories subtend a phagocyte dysfunction and humoral immunodeficiency. Another hypothesis considers JRP as mucosa-associated lymphoid tissue disorder, hyperplastic cells surrounding the ducts in a manner similar to chronic inflammatory disorders. The recurrent nonsuppurative ductal inflammation in JRP leads to a squamous ductal metaplasia, progressive parotid atrophy, and insufficient salivary outflow throughout the ductal system [16].

Histologically, there are intraductal cystic dilatations of peripheral ducts with periductal lymphocytic infiltration, called sialectasis [2]. The ecstatic ducts are usually 1–2 mm in diameter and typically have a white appearance of the ductal layer without the healthy blood vessel coverage, when compared with a normal gland [9]. This aspect is believed to be the characteristic of JRP.

The diagnosis is based on the clinical history, and clinical examination shows parotidomegaly with or without mucopurulent salivary secretion from the Stensen's duct with papilla hyperemia. Diagnosis is confirmed by ultrasound and sialography [17, 18]. Some studies also describe the use of magnetic resonance (MR), MR-sialography, characterized by T1-weighted hypointensity and T2-weighted hyperintensity; MR and MR-sialography, and CT and sialo-CT are reserved for special cases in which expansionary diseases may be suspected [19].

Thanks to reproducible, safe, and economic rule salivary gland ultrasonography in the most used imaging, especially in childrens. Choi [20], Blatt [21], and Xie [17] proposed classification on sialographic images: Glandular homogeneity and the presence of hypoechogenic areas were evaluated and graded (range 0–3).

Grades 0–1 were considered to correspond to normal/nonspecific changes and grades 2–3 to correspond to pathologic changes.

Treatments in acute are based on antibiotics and anti-inflammatory corticosteroid therapy; rule of low-dose preventive corticosteroid was not confirmed. Chronic management intercurrent periods are based on massage, warmth, chewing gum use, and sialogogues. Sialography reduces frequency of acute episodes but also sialoendoscopy is useful in diagnostic and treatment of JRP. Many authors underline a reduction of episodes [2, 22, 23]. In summary, JRP is a clinical condition characterized by parotid gland recurrent episodes of pain and swelling, usually accompanied by fever and malaise determined by inflammation. This condition affects infants and children between 3 and 6 years old, with a clear preference for the male, and usually disappears at puberty. It is associated with not obstructive parotid gland sialectasis. Although the affected gland demonstrates distal duct sialectasis, it seems there is evidence of obstruction in most cases. Symptoms are generally unilateral, when bilaterals are always marked on one side. The number of occurrences individually varies but is more commonly repeated every 3–4 months. Some recent studies (Houghton et al.) suggest that some symptoms, including recurrent conjunctivitis and mumps, if added to the diagnostic criteria encoded by AECG greatly increase the sensitivity of the latter in the diagnosis of pSS in the child. In the pSS population, misclassification is especially problematic at disease onset and early in disease course, when classic symptoms and signs are often not manifested [24].

2.2 Juvenile Sjögren's syndrome

Juvenile Sjögren's syndrome is extremely rare; the average presentation time is around 10 years and affects 77% of girls. Juvenile Sjögren's syndrome begins with major salivary gland swelling but can involve in 50% of patient many organ systems with neurologic, dermatologic, musculoskeletal, vascular, gastrointestinal, respiratory manifestations. There are no criteria for Juvenile Sjögren's syndrome and the use of adult criteria has not been validated. Recently, ultrasound criteria were developed compared with promising results both with salivary gland biopsy and with seroprevalence of antibodies anti-Ro/SSA and anti-La/SSB. Homogenity and the presence of hypoechogenic zones and cystic areas were evaluated by ultrasound of the parotid and submandibular glands on a scale from 0 to 3 where the degree 0–1 corresponds to normal and degrees 2 and 3 to the pathological changes [25]. Primary SS is a difficult diagnosis in childhood because of different presentation of symptoms. There are specific laboratory findings as lymphocytic infiltration of exocrine glands, hypergammaglobulinemia, anti-Ro/SSA, and anti-La/SSB antibodies but the manifestations of oral dryness are rarer and appear later, mainly concerning dry and cracked lips and tongue depapillation [26].

There are several proposed sets of diagnostic criteria for adult pSS. The revised European Community Study Group classification criteria proposed by the American-European consensus group (AECG) [24] have been validated for adults and include six items: ocular symptoms, oral symptoms, evidence of keratoconjunctivitis sicca, focal sialoadenitis by minor salivary gland biopsy, instrumental evidence of salivary gland involvement, and presence of SSA or SSB autoantibodies. In adults, the presence of four of the criteria, with the exclusion of patients who have negative autoantibodies or minor salivary gland biopsy, was found to have a sensitivity of 89.5% and specificity of 95.2%. The proposed diagnostic criteria for Sjogren's syndrome in adults (formulated by the European Community Study Group and later revisited by the American-European Consensus Group Criteria) cannot be applied for the diagnosis in children because they have an unacceptably low sensitivity. Further, the criteria for the diagnosis of juvenile pSS suggested by Bartunkova et al. [27] were not validated because pediatric patients rarely have sicca syndrome or xerophthalmia at presentation (almost always present in the adult with pSS) and autoantibodies often appear late in the course of the disease but often present with parotid symptomatology (mainly intended as swelling and pain) as evidenced by studies carried out by Baszis et al. and by our clinical experience. According to our opinion, levels of suspicion for an autoimmune disorder should be maintained for children affected by recurrent parotitis, particularly bilateral involvement in order to timely recognize this disease and to facilitate treatment and screening for complications.

Treatment of pSS is based on anti-inflammatory and immunosuppressive drugs especially in patients with muscle and joint pain; salivary substitutes and cholinergic stimulators can be applied locally through oral dry [26].

2.3 Clinical experience

We reported our experience in the sialoendoscopic management of JRP that represents a valid and effective treatment.

We enrolled 16 consecutive patients aged between 5 and 17 years (mean 7.5), 10 males and 6 females, referred to Multidisciplinary Department of Medical and Dental Specialities, Division of Oral and Maxillofacial Surgery (Università degli Studi della Campania Luigi Vanvitelli, Naples, Italy) in the last 5 years. They were subjected to clinical, serological, microbiological and ultrasound screening for excluding tumors or infectious diseases. We have therefore included children with remitting unilateral or bilateral swelling of the parotid region that may last from a few days to months; with the presence or absence of autoantibodies suggestive of autoimmune disease, we analyzed typical SS antibodies (SS-A, SS-B, anti-dsDNA, anti-Sm, anti-RNP), antinuclear antibody (ANA), rheumatoid factor (RF). Ultrasound images were characterized by areas of ectasia and hypoechoic spots or sialoendoscopic features of whitish ductal walls, ectasia, and stenosis. Seven of 16 patients, 4 males and 3 females, with a mean age of 9.57 years, reported SS clinical and laboratories signs.

Exclusion criteria were the presence of viral markers, neoformations detectable with methods of imaging, the acclaimed presence of autoimmune disease, sarcoidosis, graft-versus-host disease (GVHD), past head and neck radiation, and known human immunodeficiency virus infection or hepatitis C infection.

Patients thus selected were diagnosed with JRP and were treated with sialoendoscopy (intraductal wash of saline solution and steroids) or other anti-inflammatory drugs (**Figures 1** and **2**).

From the formulation of diagnosis, patients were subjected to careful follow-up checks with 6, 12, and 18 months during which they proceeded to repeat initial serological screening if the endoscopic or systemic therapy became ineffective.

The endoscopic-assisted procedures were performed in the ambulatory operating suite. After detection of the impaired gland, a local anesthesia with lidocaine 2% to the orifice region and a gradual dilatation of the duct orifice were performed, (thanks to increasing diameter lacrimal probes from 0000 to 0 size) and also with a standard salivary dilator. In this way, we reached 1.3 mm diameter, matching the outer diameter of the sialoendoscope diagnostic unit (Erlangen Sialoendoscope—Karl Storz). The larger (1.6 mm diameter) scopes were introduced as needed. The diagnostic unit 0.8 mm was introduced into the duct and was advanced forward, until reaching the ductal system and thanks to continuous lavage with isotonic saline solution. The plaques were washed out, and any structures were dilated. Mucous plugs and debris were removed with irrigation or with a forceps if necessary. At the end of the procedure, the ductal system was irrigated with a steroid- solution of Besamethasone, under direct vision while withdrawing the scope in order to treat the inflammation of the ductal epithelium (sialodochitis) and to promote the dilatation of ductal structures. In the post-operatory, we prescribed Rovamycine 3000 U.I. every 12 hours for one week. The follow-up period was at least 12 months to 5 years. In all 16 patients, sialoendoscopic treatment was effective. We reported only 2 patients with a recurrence at 5 and 3 years, respectively. Seven of 16 patients (43,75%) presented SS features. In contrast to other cases of JRP resolution, the symptoms were not immediate, but an average of three sialoendoscopic treatments; the patients identified had the following characteristics (**Table 1**).

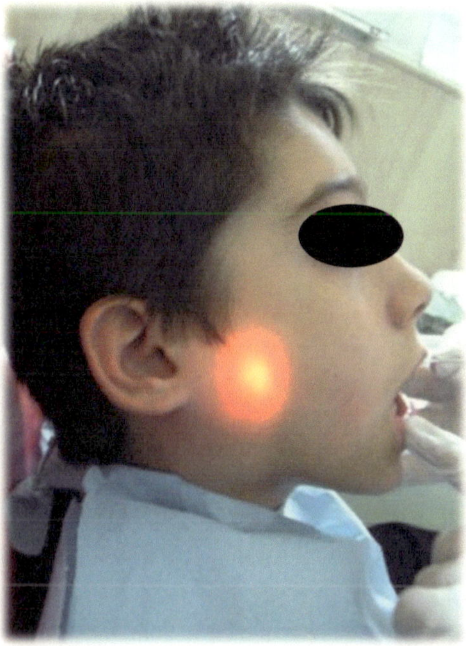

Figure 1.
Sialoendoscopic treatment in young patient.

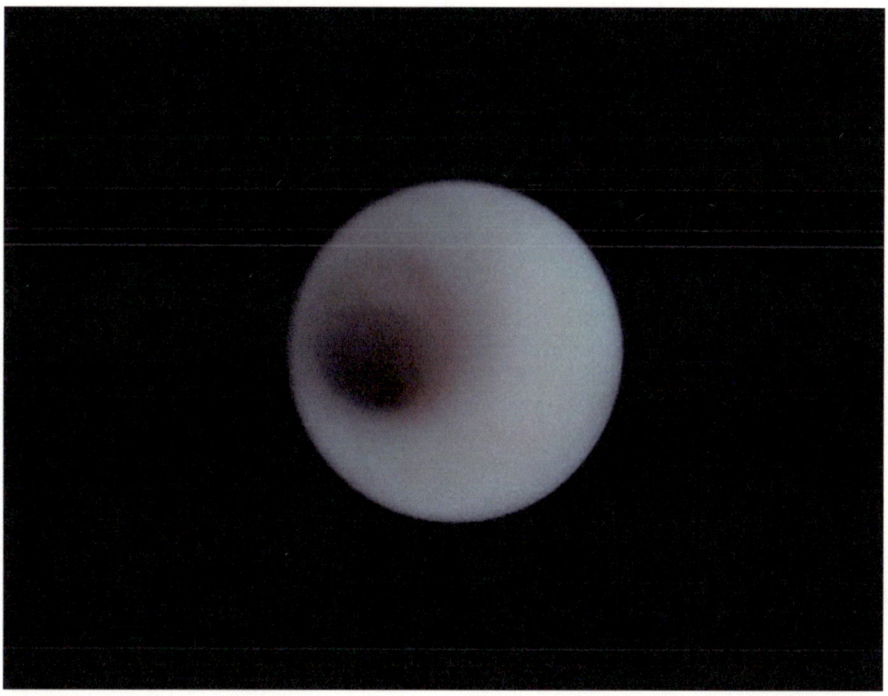

Figure 2.
Sialoendoscopic image of duct.

pSS is probably underdiagnosed in childhood, as the mode of presentation can be large and are not rare long delays in diagnosis. And likely that some patients diagnosed with PSS in adulthood have experienced the onset of symptoms during

Pat	Age	Sex	Onset age (Months)	Symptoms	US	Endoscopic findings	Antibodies	Follow-up
1	6	M	6	Right parotid swelling dry eyes, dry mouth, dysphagia	inhomogeneous parenchyma, multiple hypoechoic areas, and hypoechoic spots	whitish ductal walls, moderate stenosis, mucous fibrinous material in the main duct	negative RF, ANA, SSA, SSB, Sm, and RNP	Success at 18 months
2	9	M	12	Right parotid swelling, dry eyes, dry mouth, or dysphagia	inhomogeneous parenchyma, multiple hypoechoic areas, and hypoechoic spots	whitish ductal walls, moderate stenosis, mucous fibrinous material in the main duct	negative RF, ANA, SSA, SSB, Sm, and RNP	Success at 18 months
3	12	F	84	Left parotid swelling, fever, intermittent headaches. Sicca syndrome symptoms, dysphagia.	inhomogeneous parenchyma, multiple hypoechoic areas, and intraglandular adenopathy	parenchymal inflammation, fibrosing footprint, ectasia of the duct system	positive RF; positive ANA; high-titer antibodies to SSA and SSB; negative anti-dsDNA, Sm, and RNP	Immediate success
4	12	M	24	Bilateral parotid swelling dry eyes, dry mouth, dysphagia	inhomogeneous parenchyma	whitish ductal walls, mucous fibrinous material in the main duct.	negative RF, ANA, SSA, SSB, Sm, and RNP	Success at 18 months
5	13	F	12	Right parotid swelling dry mouth; dysphagia	inhomogeneous parenchyma, multiple hypoechoic areas, and intraglandular adenopathy	whitish ductal walls, mucous fibrinous material in the main duct	positive ANA; elevated SSA and SSB; negative anti-dsDNA, Sm, and RNP	Success at 12 months
6	8	F	12	Bilateral parotid swelling dry eyes, dry mouth, dysphagia	parenchyma, multiple hypoechoic areas, and hypoechoic spots	whitish ductal walls, moderate stenosis, mucous fibrinous material in the main duct	negative RF, ANA, SSA, SSB, Sm, and RNP	Success at 18 months
7	7	M	4	Left parotid swelling dry eyes, dry mouth, dysphagia	inhomogeneous parenchyma, multiple hypoechoic areas, and hypoechoic spots	whitish ductal walls, moderate stenosis, mucous fibrinous material in the main duct	negative RF, ANA, SSA, SSB, Sm, and RNP	Success at 18 months

Table 1.
Clinical, ultrasound, endoscopic, and laboratory features of patients with suspected SS.

Adult	Children
Classic symptoms: xerostomia, xerophthalmia, and glans swelling	Atypical symptoms: gland swelling, tongue depapillation, dry and cracked lips
	Our experience: Swelling 7/7100% Dry mouth 7/7100% Dry eyes 4/7 57,14% SS antibodies 2/7 28,57%

Table 2.
Presentation differences in adults and children.

childhood. In fact, the clinical presentation of pSS in childhood may differ from the clinical presentation in adulthood (**Table 2**). The cases of pediatric PSS are reported to have a higher incidence of recurrent parotitis and a lower incidence of xerostomia and xerophthalmia. We found dry eyes in four patients. Laboratory and pathological findings in children with SS are positive antinuclear antibody (ANA) of 80% and autoantibodies to nuclear antigens Ro/SSA and La/SSB2 of only 70–75% [27]. In our experience, we have detected the presence of specific antibodies in only two patients.

In pediatric recurrent parotitis, laboratory evaluation and sialoendoscopy may be very helpful. A combination of positive ANA, RF, SS-A, and SS-B; hypergammaglobulinemia; elevated amylase (parotid or pancreatic); elevated ESR and suggestive chronic inflammatory endoscopic patterns are suspicious for SS (however, the presence of anti-double-stranded DNA antibodies or hypocomplementemia raises the concern for other systemic autoimmune disorders, such as systemic lupus erythematosus, SLE, or another connective tissue disease) [5].

3. Conclusion

In summary, parotitis is a frequently encountered pediatric problem. Although infection, recurrent juvenile parotitis, and anatomic abnormalities are more common etiologies, primary pediatric SS should be considered when encountering a patient with recurrent parotitis, especially no responsive to sialoendoscopic treatment. We have to consider pSS when JRP is assessed, despite the rareness of condition. Typical sign of sialectasis is the same in JRP and in pSS as ultrasonography ones. Antibodies are not in all patients: anti-Ro/SSA 29% seronegativity and anti-La/SSB 33%; similarly, eye dryness is present in just over half of patients.

These patients typically exhibit a distinctive laboratory and autoantibody profile and will benefit from early referral to a pediatric rheumatologist for treatment and monitoring for disease complications. Accurate diagnosis of pSS in the pediatric population is difficult. Recurrent parotitis should alert the clinician to the possibility of pSS especially if it does not respond to treatment with anti-inflammatory therapy and sialoendoscopic washing. The proposed pediatric criteria lack sensitivity and clinical utility. Until validated diagnostic criteria are available, clinical acumen will prevail as the gold standard. Reid et al.'s theory of ascending infections from the upper respiratory tract would merit a multicenter study of prevalence in patients undergoing adenotonsillectomy that should slow down the frequency of the disease. Our intention is to verify this deduction in the near future. Prospective multicenter studies are needed to further characterize pSS in the pediatric population, and to better define and develop appropriate classification criteria.

Consideration should be given to inclusion of specific obligatory criteria such as the presence of SSA or SSB autoantibodies or classic histopathology changes on minor salivary gland biopsy. The development of an international database would enable epidemiologic and clinical study.

In the majority of our patients, it is suggested that sialoendoscopy can offer a minimally invasive and gland-preserving approach to obstructive salivary glands diseases; this technique is proven to be safe, suitable in children under local anesthesia and able to improve swelling, pain, and social life.

Conflict of interest

The authors declare no conflict of interest. Neither author nor any member of their families received any material or financial gain or personal advancement in the production of this manuscript. We have read the Helsinki Declaration and have followed the guidelines in this investigation. For each patients, we have written parent's contents.

Notes/thanks/other declarations

Thanks to our young patients.

Author details

Brigida Iorio[1*], Roberto De Luca[1], Gianpaolo Tartaro[2] and Giuseppe Colella[2]

1 Maxillofacial Surgery Unit, Department of Medical, Surgical and Dental Speciality, Campania University "Luigi Vanvitelli" Naples, and Department of Neuroscience, Reproductive and Odontostomatologic Sciences, University of Naples Federico II, Naples, Italy

2 Maxillofacial Surgery Unit, Department of Medical, Surgical and Dental Speciality, Campania University "Luigi Vanvitelli" Naples, Italy

*Address all correspondence to: brigida.iorio@libero.it; brigida.iorio82@gmail.com

References

[1] S.S. Rose, A clinical and radiological survey of 192 cases of recurrent swellings of the salivary glands; Hunterian lecture delivered at the Royal College of Surgeons of England on 26th March 1953, Ann. R. Coll. Surg. Engl. 15 (1954) 374-401.

[2] Nahlieli O., Shacham R, Shlesinger M, et al. Juvenile recurrent parotitis: a new method of diagnosis and treatment. Pediatrics. 2004;114:9-12. DOI: 10.1542/peds.114.1.9

[3] L.B. Kaban, J.B. Mulliken, J.E. Murray, Sialadenitis in childhood, Am. J. Surg. 135 (1978) 570-576.

[4] G. Grevers, Chronic recurrent parotitis in childhood, Laryngorhinootologie 71 (1992) 649-652.

[5] Houghton K, Malleson P, Cabral D, Petty R Primary Sjögren's syndrome in children and adolescents: are proposed diagnostic criteria applicable?J Rheumatol. 2005 Nov;32(11):2225-32.

[6] Schuetz C, Prieur AM, Quartier P. *sicca* syndrome and salivary gland infiltration in children with autoimmune disorders: when can we diagnose Sjögren syndrome? Clin Exp Rheumatol. 2010 May-Jun;28(3):434-9. Epub 2010 Jun 23.

[7] Quenin S, Plouin-Gaudon I, Marchal F, Froehlich P, Disant F, Faure F. Juvenile recurrent parotitis: sialendoscopic approach. Arch Otolaryngol Head Neck Surg. 2008 Jul;134(7):715-9.

[8] Leerdam CM, Martin HC, Isaacs D. Recurrent parotitis of childhood. J Paediatr Child Health 2005;41:631-4

[9] Ericson S, Zetterlund B, Ohman J. Recurrent parotitis and sialectasis in childhood. Clinical, radiologic, immunologic, bacteriologic and histologic study. Ann Otol Rhinol Laryngol 1991;100:527-35

[10] E. Reid, F. Douglas, Y. Crow, A. Hollman, J. Gibson, Autosomal dominant juvenile recurrent parotitis, J. Med. Genet. 35 (1998) 417-419.

[11] K.-L. Kolho, R. Saarinen, A. Paju, J. Stenman, U.-H. Stenman, A. Pitkäranta, New insights into juvenile parotitis, Acta Paediatr. Oslo Nor. 94 (2005) 1566-1570 1992

[12] V.V. Chitre, D.J. Premchandra, Recurrent parotitis, Arch. Dis. Child. 77 (1997) 359-363.

[13] E. Bernkopf, G.C. De Vincentiis, Parotite (o paroditite) ricorrente giovanile e malocclusione dentaria, Medico e Bambino pagine elettroniche 11 (2008) 9.

[14] M.S. Giglio, M. Landaeta, M.E. Pinto, Microbiology of recurrent parotitis, Pediatr. Infect. Dis. J. 16 (1997) 386-390.

[15] P. Katz, D.M. Hartl, A. Guerre, Treatment of juvenile recurrent parotitis, Otolaryngol. Clin. 42 (2009) 1087-1091.

[16] A. Gallo, M. Benazzo, P. Capaccio, et al., Sialoendoscopy: state of the art, challenges and further perspectives. Round Table, 101(st) SIO National Congress, Catania 2014, Acta Otorhinolaryngol. Ital. 35 (2015) 217-233.

[17] L. Xie, Y. Pu, L. Zheng, C. Yu, Z. Wang, H. Shi, Function of the parotid gland in juvenile recurrent parotitis: a case series, Br. J. Oral Maxillofac. Surg. 54 (2016) 270-274.

[18] V. Narsimha Rao, J.S. Putta Buddi, A. Kurthukoti, Juvenile recurrent parotitis in children: diagnosis and treatment

using sialography, J. Indian Soc. Pedod. Prev. Dent. 32 (2014) 262.

[19] A. Gadodia, A. Seith, R. Sharma, A. Thakar, MRI and MR sialography of juvenile recurrent parotitis, Pediatr. Radiol. 40 (2010) 1405-1410.

[20] J.-W. Choi, S.-S. Lee, K.-H. Huh, W.-J. Yi, M.-S. Heo, S.-C. Choi, The relationship between sialographic images and clinical symptoms of inflammatory parotid gland diseases, Oral Surg. Oral Med. Oral Pathol. Oral Radiol. Endod. 107 (2009) e49-56.

[21] I.M. Blatt, On sialectasis and benign lymphosialdenopathy. (the pyogenic parotitis, gougerot-sjoegren's syndrome, mikulicz's disease complex.) a ten-year study, The Laryngoscope 74 (1964) 1684-1746.

[22] . S. Quenin, I. Plouin-Gaudon, F. Marchal, P. Froehlich, F. Disant, F. Faure, Juvenile recurrent parotitis: sialendoscopic approach, Arch. Otolaryngol. Head Neck Surg. 134 (2008) 715-719.

[23] J.E. Strychowsky, D.D. Sommer, M.K. Gupta, N. Cohen, O. Nahlieli, Sialendoscopy for the management of obstructive salivary gland disease: a systematic review and meta-analysis, Arch. Otolaryngol. Head Neck Surg. 138 (2012) 541-547, https://doi.org/10.1001/archoto.2012.856.

[24] Vitali C, Bombardieri S, Moutsopoulos HM, et al. Assessment of the European classification criteria for Sjögren's syndrome in a series of clinically defined cases: results of a prospective multicentre study. The European Study Group on Diagnostic Criteria for Sjögren's Syndrome. Ann Rheum Dis 1996;55: 116-21.

[25] Hammenfors D. S., Valim V., Bica B. E. R. G. et al. Juvenile Sjögren's Syndrome: clinical characteristics with focus on salivary gland ultrasonography. Arthritis care & Research vol 72 n° 1 January 2020 pp 78-87.

[26] De Oliveira M. A., Medeiros de Rezende N. P. et al. Primary Sjögren's syndrome in a 2-years-old patient: role of the dentist in diagnosis and dental management with a 6-years follow-up. International Journal of pediatric dentistry 2011; 21:471-478.

[27] Bartunkova J, Sediva A, Vencovsky J, Tesar V. Primary Sjögren's syndrome in children and adolescents: proposal for diagnostic criteria. Clin Exp Rheumatol 1999;17: 381-6

Chapter 12

Inflammation in the Pathogenesis of Rheumatoid Arthritis and in Experimental Arthritis: Evaluation of Combinations of Carnosic Acid and Extract of *Rhodiola rosea* L. with Methotrexate

Silvester Ponist, Katarina Pruzinska and Katarina Bauerova

Abstract

The host immune response generates the pro-inflammatory immune response as a protective measure against invading pathogens, allergens, and/or trauma. However, dysregulated and chronic inflammation may result in secondary damage to tissues and immune pathology to the host. Rheumatoid arthritis (RA) is a chronic systemic autoimmune disease which primarily involves synovial inflammation, joint pain, immobility, and stiffness. Increased infiltration of inflammatory immune cells and fibroblast-like synoviocytes into joints, form pannus and small blood vessels that lead to synovium and cartilage destruction. In this chapter we will focus on the role of inflammatory cytokines (IL-1β, IL-6 and IL-17), chemokine monocyte chemotactic protein-1 and matrix metalloproteinase-9 in the pathogenesis of experimental arthritis in animals and in human RA. Further, we will be discussing about methotrexate's (cornerstone of anti-rheumatic therapy) immune suppressing activity, anti-inflammatory properties of carnosic acid and extract of *Rhodiola rosea* L., and their innovative combination treatments with methotrexate in rat adjuvant arthritis.

Keywords: arthritis, IL-1β, IL-6, IL-17, monocyte chemotactic protein-1, matrix metalloproteinase-9, carnosic acid, *Rhodiola rosea* L

1. Introduction

Inflammation is an inherent defensive mechanism against damage of tissues, infection and is quickly stopped in physiological state of organism. In chronic diseases, the inflammation continues and is able to cause substantial organ and tissue damage. A lot of evidence showed that pathological inflammatory response is closely related with different chronic diseases, particularly autoimmune ones, such as systemic lupus erythematosus, rheumatoid arthritis (RA), inflammatory bowel disease, diabetes, and gout [1–3]. Although the key feature of inflammatory dysregulation in many chronic diseases has been supported by plenty of studies,

 IntechOpen

the pathogenesis of this dysregulation in the autoimmune diseases is not well understood yet. Knowledge about the signaling and mechanism of regulation of inflammation will bring noticeable clinical benefits for the therapy of autoimmune disease.

In this chapter we will present our preliminary results from new original combination treatments of methotrexate with carnosic acid and with extract of *Rhodiola rosea* L and discuss about the role of IL-1β, IL-6 and IL-17, chemokine monocyte chemotactic protein-1 and matrix metalloproteinase-9 in the pathogenesis of experimental arthritis in animals and in human RA.

2. Cytokines involved in rheumatoid arthritis

To fully understand a complex disease like a RA, animal models are indispensable due to their ability to mimic the conditions and demonstrate the similarity to the human RA. Rodent models are essential for further knowledge of the pathogenic processes of RA in humans and therefore are important in the process of testing new and already existing drugs for their efficiency and safety. There are many animal models used for the research of RA, but each model varies in the similarities to the human RA. The most frequently used animal models are collagen-induced arthritis and adjuvant-induced arthritis models. Less often are used animal models with proteoglycan-induced arthritis and streptococcal cell wall-induced arthritis [4].

The adjuvant-induced arthritis (AIA) model has been used widely for testing novel drugs for inflammatory arthritis and for studies of the disease pathogenesis. After administering an injection with complete adjuvant, it was possible to induce polyarthritis [5]. AA is inducible in susceptible rat strains, for example, Lewis rat strain, by a single subcutaneous injection of heat-killed *Mycobacterium tuberculosis* H37Ra in oil. Following the induction, the inflammation begins in 8–10 days, the symptoms are the most apparent on the 15th or 16th day, and then undergo spontaneous recovery. Autoimmune inflammation of the paws starts with the infiltration of mononuclear cells, mostly lymphocytes, macrophages, and monocytes [6]. The severity of the RA could lead to chronic malformation of affected joints, together with ankylosis. Adjuvant-induced arthritis exhibit similar symptoms to human RA, such as joint swelling, invasion of lymphocytes, and destruction of cartilage [4].

The difference between AIA in rats and human RA seems to be in the rapid onset of the erosive polyarthritis in the AIA model, Rheumatoid Factor is not present, the disease seems to have a monophasic course. There is also an involvement of axial skeleton seen in the model of AIA, affected gastrointestinal, genitourinary tract and skin, periostitis, ankylosis, and extra-articular manifestations not typical of RA [7]. Inflamed joints of rats with AIA contain activated T-cells. T-cells infiltrating joints originate from several compartments, such as the spleen, Peyer's patches, lymph nodes, and T-cell pool that recirculates [8]. Specific antigen heat shock protein (Hsp65) has been shown to activate the immune response, with peptide 180–186 being the responsible epitope [9]. The cytokines that are expressed in the joint during the early stages of inflammation include IL-17, IFN, and TNF-α, as well as cytokines implicated in macrophage stimulation. Increased levels of IL-4, IL-6, monocyte chemotactic protein 1 (MCP-1), and TGF-β can be observed as inflammation progresses in the joint. TNF-α, IL-1β, IL-21, and IL-17 all contribute to the pathology of this disorder [8]. The main source of the irreversible tissue damage is in an area rich in macrophages, called the pannus, which is located at the junction of the synovium lining of the joint capsule together with the cartilage and a bone. Pannus cells migrate over the cartilage and into the subchondral bone, subsequently causing the erosion of these tissues [10]. The activity of matrix metalloproteinases (MMPs) seems to be the reason for the irreversible destruction of the cartilage seen in RA. MMPs are enzymes produced as a response to proinflammatory cytokines as IL-1 and TNFα by activated macrophages and fibroblasts [11]. MMPs can be further divided into three main groups. Collagenase MMP-1 (interstitial) and MMP-8 (neutrophil), whose major substrates are collagen forms I, II, and III, belong to the first group. The second group consists of the gelatinase/type IV collagenases such as MMP-2, the 72kD gelatinase A, and 92-kD gelatinase B (MMP-9). The main function of these matrix metalloproteinases from the second group is to degrade gelatin and collagen type IV in the basement membrane. Group 3 consists of the stromelysins, stromelysin 1 (MMP-3), stromelysin 2 (MMP-10), and pump-1 (MMP-7). These stromelysins have activity against a range spectrum of substrates, mainly proteoglycans, fibronectin, laminin, and some collagens [11]. During arthritis, especially MMP-1 and MMP-3 play an important role in the pathophysiology of the disease, and what is worse, the destruction of the connective tissue they cause is largely irreversible [12–14]. Fibroblasts from a healthy organism produce very low levels of both enzymes [12–14]. On the other hand, during RA and osteoarthritis levels of these enzymes rapidly increase in response to various stimuli [12–14]. Potent inducers of collagenases and stromelysins could be cytokines such as IL-1α and IL-1β, epidermal growth factor (EGF), platelet-derived growth factor, and tumor necrosis factor α. Inducers of these two enzymes could also be crystals of monosodium urate monohydrate, debris phagocytosis, and formulation of multinucleated giant cells. In an environment of stimulated synovial fibroblast cells, which resembles proliferating rheumatoid synovial tissue, collagenase and stromelysin becomes major gene product of these synovial fibroblasts [14]. Patients with RA and OA also have higher levels of collagenase and stromelysin in cartilage and the synovial fluid, especially patients with RA [15, 16]. The level of enzymatic activity is increased concordantly with the severity of the disease [17]. Apart from MMPs, there are other enzymes synthesized by cells within cartilage and bone as well as infiltrating inflammatory cells. These enzymes include aspartic, serine, and cysteine endopeptidases such as cathepsin B, which are capable of cleaving and therefore destructing the main components of cartilage and bone (such as proteoglycan and collagen type I, II, IX, X, and XI) [18].

2.1 Interleukin-1β

Interleukin-1β (IL-1β) is a cytokine belonging to the same family of cytokines as IL-1α, yet they show different features and are produced by two different genes [19]. IL-1β is mainly produced by macrophages as an inactive precursor (pro-IL-1β) and then cleaved by cysteine protease caspase-I into its mature form (IL-1β) [20]. The major distinction between IL-1β and IL-1α is that pro-IL-1β is biologically inactive, while pro-IL-1α and mature IL-1α can bind to their receptors and therefore stimulate cellular responses. Most IL-1α also stays coupled with the plasma membrane and stimulates cells by direct cell–cell interaction, which can induce its functions [21]. IL-1β is produced by blood monocytes, tissue macrophages, and dendritic cells by direct cellular contact with stimulated T-lymphocytes, a mechanism related to chronic inflammation [22]. IL-1β mRNA requires an extra signal for synthesis so transcription of IL-1β is a rate-limiting step of its synthesis. The extra signal to induce the production of IL-1β can be a microbial product or cytokines as TNF-α, IL-1α, IL-18, or IL-1β itself [23]. By binding to the same receptors as IL-1α and IL-1β, yet not inducing any consequent cellular responses, IL-1 receptor antagonist (IL-I Ra) acts as a naturally occurring inhibitor [24]. IL-1β seems to be not present in healthy individuals, or its levels are hard to detect by standard assays. Such low levels are needed to be maintained due to the potency of IL-1β to induce inflammatory responses [25]. During RA, serum levels of IL-1β are higher in patients with RA compared to healthy individuals, and the concentrations of IL-1β increase during the acute phase of the disease [26].

2.2 Interleukin-6

IL-6 has been suggested to be a major player in the pathological changes during RA because of the broad spectrum of activities IL-6 participates in. Il-6 is recognized as an endogenous pyrogen [27], and also as an inducer of acute phase response genes [28]. IL-6 stimulates B- and T-cells activity and promotes proliferation of plasmablast into mature immunoglobulin-producing plasma cells [29]. IL-6 acts stimulatory on the immune system's cells, vascular endothelial cells, synovial fibroblasts, and osteoclasts upon coupling with its soluble IL-6 receptor (sIL-6Rα). Activated sIL-6Rα complex stimulates the production of a subset of chemokines by endothelial cells and subsequently upregulates the expression of adhesion molecules, resulting in direct recruitment of leukocytes to the sites of inflammation [30]. Apart from that, by having stimulatory effects on synovial fibroblast and osteoclast activation, IL-6 contributes to the formation of synovial pannus and bone resorption in inflamed joints [31, 32]. Interestingly, patients with various forms of arthritis have high levels of IL-6 in serum and synovial fluids, but on the other hand, their structural cells from joints (chondrocytes, fibroblasts, synoviocytes, and endothelial cells) lack expression of IL-6R [33]. These cells are also not responsive to IL-6 itself. The complex of IL-6 bound to its receptor might, therefore, represents the mechanism behind the action of IL-6 during arthritis. In a synovial fluid of RA patients, it has been shown that an increase in sIL-6Rα correlates with the extent of the joint destruction which coincides with more advanced stages of RA [32].

2.3 Interleukin-17

IL-17 is another cytokine possibly contributing to the pathogenesis of RA. IL-17 is produced by CD4+ CD45RO+ memory T cells in synovium during RA, upon activation with phorbolmyristate acetate/ionomycin or CD3/CD28 Abs [34, 35]. IL-17A is relatively homologous to IL-17F (~50%) with which it can form heterodimers (IL-17A/F). Activated human CD4+ T cells produce IL-17A/F heterodimers along with IL-17A and IL-17F homodimers [36]. The signaling is based on the coupling of IL-1A and IL-1F to a multimeric receptor composed of two subunits IL-17RA and IL-17RC [37]. Cytokines from the IL-17 family activate pro-inflammatory pathways through activating NF-κB or inducing signaling through MAPK and the C/EBP transcription factors. It seems IL-17A signaling intends to activate a gene expression of an innate-type inflammatory effector program that mediates potent inflammation and plays a critical role in a defense of a host [38]. It has been shown that IL-17 can trigger the production of IL-6, IL-8, GM-CSF, and also prostaglandin E2 (PGE2), a strong mediator of inflammation, in human synoviocytes [34, 35, 39]. Additionally, IL-17 showed stimulating effect on granulopoiesis in a murine model [40], on osteoclastogenesis [41], up-regulated synthesis of NO in cultured human cartilage [42], stimulated the synthesis of proinflammatory mediators as TNF-α, IL-1β, IL-10, IL-12, stromelysin, and IL-1Ra in human peripheral blood macrophages [43]. Furthermore, levels of IL-17 in synovial fluid and serum from RA patients are high in contrast to OA patients [44].

2.4 Monocyte chemoattractant protein-1

The rheumatoid synovial environment suggests a possible role for leukocyte chemoattractant molecules such as chemokines. Chemokines form a superfamily consisting of low molecular weight peptides (7–15 kDa) with conserved four-cysteine motif and consist of at least two subfamilies: first are the C-X-C (α) chemokines which all majorly attract neutrophils. Here belong IL-8, melanoma growth stimulating activity, and epithelial neutrophil-activating peptide 78. Secondly, C-C (β) chemokines are RANTES (regulated upon activation normal T cell expressed and secreted), monocyte chemoattractant protein 1 (MCP-1), and macrophage inflammatory protein 1α (MIP-1α), which chiefly recruit T cells and monocytes [45]. Many of the cells present in RA joints, such as endothelial cells, macrophages, fibroblasts, and lymphocytes can release chemokines. In the pathogenesis of RA, members of both subclasses of chemokines have been implicated. The production of MCP-1 is enhanced in human RA patients compared to osteoarthritis patients [46]. In the murine model of collagen-induced arthritis the earliest detectable levels of MIP-1α, MCP-1, and MIP-2 expression were observed 4 weeks after the initial collagen challenge [47].

2.5 Matrix metalloproteinase 9

Degradation of articular cartilage is important feature of RA and is caused by elevated activity of proteolytic enzymes [48]. In RA, synovial fibroblasts are extensively producing the matrix-degrading enzymes [49] known as matrix metalloproteinases (MMPs). MMPs are a zinc-dependent peptidases, which are degrading the components of extracellular matrix. MMPs are the key proteases associated with the degradation and invasion through anatomical barriers [50]. The MMP-9 (gelatinase B) and MMP-2 (gelatinase A), are very important in the degradation of collagen by cleaving the denatured collagen, produced by collagenases. Moreover, these MMPs degrade other substrates, such as collagen I and II [51] and aggrecan, which is abundant in cartilage [50].

MMP-9 has a posttranscriptional regulation on multiple levels. Its activity is inhibited in tissues by inhibitors of metalloproteinase (TIMP-1 to TIMP-4) with strongest binding between TIMP-1 and MMP-9 [52]. MMPs (including MMP-9) are produced and secreted in latent soluble form of enzyme, which needs activation extra-celullarly. In tissues the mast cell-derived tryptase and chymase are effective activators of MMPs [53, 54]. Regulation of MMPs is situated at the level of their transcription. Expression of MMPs is modulated by different stimuli including also cytokines [55] and growth factors [56].

MMP-9 was first discovered in neutrophils [57]. MMP-9 is also present in other leukocytes including T cells, macrophages, and eosinophils [58]. MMP-9 cleaves IL-8 and increases its activity as a chemoattractant for neutrophil more than 10-fold according to acute and chronic inflammatory processes [59]. The evidence is now growing that along with the storage of serine proteases, mast cells are secreting significant amount of MMPs such as MMP-9 [60, 61]. Although there is limited evidence for the expression of MMP-9 in mast cells in rheumatoid synovium [62], its regulation in RA is poorly understood. MMP-9 expression in rheumatoid synovial mast cells is via its regulation by TNF-α and IFN-γ in cord blood-derived human mast cell and the human mast cell line-1 (HMC-1). MMP-9 is not a product which is permanently stored in mast cells, but this enzyme is secreted under inflammatory conditions. MMP-9 may help in the migration of mast cell progenitors to inflammatory sites and could also promote the local damage of tissues [63]. In RA, MMP-9 is markedly elevated in serum and joint synovial fluid and positively correlates with disease progression and severity [64]. MMP-9 knockout mice show decreased severity of antibody-induced arthritis [65].

3. Innovative combination treatments of methotrexate with natural compounds in experimental arthritis

Current drugs for rheumatoid arthritis (RA) are: corticosteroids, disease-modifying anti-rheumatic drugs (DMARDs), non-steroidal anti-inflammatory drugs (NSAIDs), and biological response modifiers [66]. However, these antirheumatics have several adverse effects. NSAIDs are dangerous to patients due to the adverse effects such as bleeding of upper gastrointestinal tract, liver, and kidney adverse reactions [67]. Moreover, cognitive disorders, headaches, allergic reactions often force the patients to stop the treatment. This behavior is greatly limiting the use of NSAIDs. The long-term administration of corticosteroids can induce hypersplenism, hypertension, infection, osteoporosis and fractures [68]. DMARDs often cause diarrhea, rashes, vomiting, decreased white blood cell levels, and impaired kidney and liver functions [69]. Biological agents with high target specificity and less side effects are the new agents for therapy of RA [70]. However, these biological agents are expensive and not available for many patients [71]. Thus, development of novel anti-rheumatic drugs and strategies for RA therapy is a high priority. The combination treatments of low-dose methotrexate (MTX) with natural substances, which have the potential to improve the efficacy and to reduce adverse side effects of drugs, could be one possible direction in these strategies for RA therapy. Extract or phytochemical selected for combination therapy with MTX is expected to have anti-inflammatory and antioxidant activity to treat the inflammation and oxidative stress, occurring during RA development. Many chronic diseases with inflammatory pathology are abundant in elderly population. The widely administered anti-inflammatory drugs have many side effects and are expensive (biologic drugs). Alternative option are natural extracts and substances used in traditional medicine. These natural products offer a possibility to identify the bioactive compounds and for the development of new inflammatory drugs. Traditional remedies and phytochemicals are being used for the treatment of inflammatory and other disorders since ancient times [72] and with proper scientific research background can be more extensively used for treatment also in the present.

3.1 Methotrexate

MTX is still for decades a primary antirheumatic drug and the cornerstone of the RA treatment. MTX has an acceptable safety profile, efficacy, and low cost as well as many years of clinical experience make it the gold standard of RA treatment and the key drug for combination with different biological drugs [73]. MTX is usually effective in RA treatment and patients are usually administered for several years with MTX, thus information about long-term safety is very important. However, administration of MTX is in some cases limited because of its toxic adverse effects. During long treatment period by MTX, often adverse reactions occur such as mucous ulceration, cytopenia, nausea, liver damage and serious infections. Some studies showed that due to toxic manifestations, the interruption of MTX treatment in RA patients is in the range from 10–37% [74].

Despite the introduction of numerous biologic agents for the treatment of RA, low-dose MTX therapy remains still the gold standard in the RA therapy. MTX is generally the first-line drug for the treatment of RA, psoriatic arthritis, and it enhances the effect of most biologic agents in RA. Methotrexate inhibits polyglutamates inhibit aminoimidazole-4-carboxamide ribonucleotide (AICAR) transformylase (ATIC), leading to intracellular accumulation of AICAR and increased adenosine release; adenosine binds to cell surface receptors and suppresses many inflammatory and immune reactions [75].

The activity of MTX has also been studied in monocyte cell lines. Different from fibroblast like synoviocytes and T-lymphocytes, monocytes trigger apoptosis as a response to MTX treatment. Moreover, MTX activates a dose-dependent elevation in the expression of inflammatory cytokines, such as TNF, IL-1 and IL-6, in monocytic cell lines [76]. Adenosine (AS) via its receptors regulates monocyte activity, and hence MTX may influence monocytes indirectly by increasing AS release by other immune cells. AS binds to its A_1 receptor on peripheral blood monocytes and activates the formation of giant cells with multiple nuclei [77]. Moreover, the binding of AS to A_{2a} receptors and A_3 receptors on monocytes decreases the production and release of IL-6 and TNF and initiates the transformation of inflammatory M1 phenotype of monocytes to anti-inflammatory M2 phenotype.

Macrophages with M2 phenotype have are responsible for termination of inflammation, clearing the apoptotic cells and support wound healing by secreting profibrotic and angiogenic cytokines. Adenosine, binding on A_{2a} receptors, inhibits the production of inflammatory cytokines and promotes the expression of anti-inflammatory mediators such as vascular endothelial growth factor and IL-10 [78]. A_{2a} receptor stimulation triggers a switching from an M1 (pro-inflammatory phenotype) to a modified macrophage M2 phenotype [79]. One way by which A_{2a} receptor binding affects macrophage function is by stimulating the expression of the NR4A - orphan nuclear receptor, which is inhibiting the activation of NFκB-dependent nuclear gene expression [80]. A_{2b} receptor also induces the switching from a M1 macrophage phenotype to a M2 phenotype [81]. Cultivating synovial fibroblasts and T cells from RA patients triggered T cell TNF-α, IL-17, and IFNγ expression, which resulted in increased fibroblast IL-6, IL8 and IL-15 expression [82]. Methotrexate inhibited the upregulation of IL-6, IL8 and IL-15 by stimulated RA synovial fibroblasts. MTX also decreased IFNγ and IL-17 expression in T cells co-cultured with RA synovial fibroblasts (**Table 1**).

3.2 Combination of methotrexate and carnosic acid

In our previous study, we have selected the carnosic acid for combination with methotrexate for its anti-inflammatory and antioxidative properties, to reduce the development of rat adjuvant arthritis.

3.2.1 Carnosic acid

Carnosic acid (CA) was discovered first by Linde in *Salvia officinalis* L. [83]. Carnosic acid (C20H28O4, **Figure 1**), is a phenolic diterpene that belongs to the terpene class of secondary metabolites [84], is localized in rosemary leaves, more precisely in chloroplasts of trichome cells. CA and carnosol have been reported to display beneficial effects against acute and chronic inflammation, cardiovascular diseases, obesity, and cancer [85, 86], inhibition of prostaglandin synthesis [87], skin inflammation [88], inhibition of NF-κB [89], inhibition of 5-lipoxygenase [90] and antioxidant activity *in vivo* [91].

CA prevented cartilage degeneration though induction of hemeoxygenase-1 (HO-1) in cell culture with human chondrocytes. The results showed that CA increased enzyme levels in a dose-dependent manner. Moreover, it was able to restore HO-1 levels under IL-1β treatment, which specifically inhibits the antioxidant effects of this enzyme. CA induced HO-1 and miR-140 expression in human

Cell type	Methotrexate action
Monocyte	Inhibition of IL-1β, IL-6, and TNF-α production; downregulation of receptors FcγRI and IIa; increases ROS synthesis and apoptosis
Macrophage	Inhibition of IL-1β, IL-6, and TNF-α production;
Th-1 lymphocyte	Decreases IL-2, IFN-γ and IL-17 gene expression; increases ROS synthesis and apoptosis
Th-2 lymphocyte	Increases IL-4 and IL-10 gene expression
Neutrophil	Increases ROS synthesis
Synovial fibroblast	Inhibition of IL-15, IL-6, and IL-8 expression; inhibitory effect on prostaglandin E2 production; inhibition of COX-2 and MMP expression

ROS, reactive oxygen species; COX-2, cyclooxygenase 2; MMP, synovial matrix metalloproteinase.

Table 1.
Immune regulatory action of low dose MTX in the RA synovial tissue (according to Miranda-Carús et al. [82]).

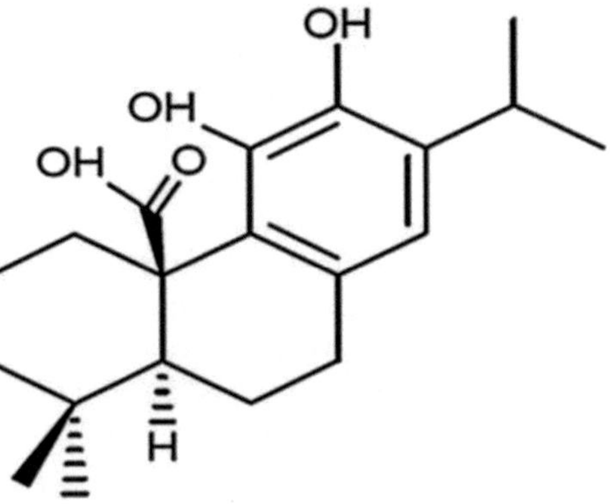

Figure 1.
Chemical structure of carnosic acid.

articular chondrocytes, thus cartilage degeneration was attenuated by CA treatment [92]. The activation of macrophages triggered by exogenous infection or endogenous stress stimuli is thought to be implicated in the pathogenesis of various inflammatory diseases. In a study of Wang et al. [93], authors applied an integrated approach based on unbiased proteomics and bioinformatics analysis to elucidate the anti-inflammatory property of CA. CA significantly inhibited the increase of NO and TNF-α, downregulated cyclooxygenase-2 (COX-2) protein expression and decreased the transcriptional level of inflammatory genes including NOS-2, TNF-α, COX-2, in LPS-stimulated RAW264.7 macrophages. The liquid chromatography-based assessment showed CA negatively regulated 217 proteins elicited by lipopolysaccharide (LPS), which are responsible for multiple inflammatory pathways including nuclear factor (NF)-κB, MAPK and FoxO signaling. A following analysis showed that CA effectively inhibited ERK/JNK/p38 MAPKs, IKKβ/IκB-α/NF-κB and FoxO1/3 signaling. These results illustrate the ability of CA to regulate the inflammatory signaling triggered by LPS [93].

In another study by de Oliveira [94] authors have found that activation of cell antioxidant defense is mediated via transcription factor nuclear factor erythroid 2-related factor (Nrf2). Therefore, authors investigated whether CA is able to block paraquat (PQ)-induced inflammatory alterations in SH-SY5Y neuroblastoma cells. CA reduced the PQ-induced changes on the levels of TNF-α, IL-1β, and COX-2 via signaling responsible for the activation of the Nrf2/HO-1 pathway. Furthermore, they observed a crosstalk between the Nrf2/HO-1 signaling pathway and the activation of the nuclear factor-κB [94]. Two Rosemary extracts and their main components - CA and carnosol affected the cell migration. Monocyte chemoattractant protein-1 (MCP-1) and matrix metalloproteinase-9 (MMP-9) were determined by Western blot and gelatin zymography, respectively, in RAW 264.7 macrophages and vascular smooth muscle cells (VSMCs). MMP-9 and MCP-1 levels were significantly diminished with methanol extract (RM), n-hexane fraction (RH), and CA in RAW 264.7 macrophages. RM, RH, CA, and carnosol suppressed TNF-α induced VSMC migration by inhibiting MMP-9 expression. Rosemary, especially its CA component, has potential anti-atherosclerotic effects related to cell migration [95].

Liu and colleagues [96] studied the anti-inflammatory activity of CA on destruction of osteoclasts, fibroblast-like synoviocytes in the collagen-induced arthritis model. Abovementioned *in vitro* and *in vivo* experiments showed that CA inhibited the expression of pro-inflammatory cytokines such as IL-1β, IL-6, TNF-α, IL-17, IL-8 and MMP-3, and suppressed the secretion of RANKL. Moreover, authors determined that CA reduced osteoclastogenesis and resorption of the bone *in vitro* and had therapeutic protective activity against joint damage *in vivo*. Further results showed that CA inhibited RANKL-induced activations of MAPKs (JNK and p38) and NF-κB resulting in the suppressing of NFATc1 [96].

3.2.2 Effect of the combination therapy of methotrexate and carnosic acid in rat adjuvant arthritis

In this section we will present our preliminary results from combination therapy of methotrexate (MTX) and carnosic acid in rat adjuvant arthritis.

Hind paw volume (HPV) was significantly increased on days 14, 21 and 28 during the development of AA. CA in monotherapy was without a significant effect on this parameter. The administration of methotrexate in sub-therapeutic dose markedly reduced HPV on days 14 and 21, but not on day 28. The combination of MTX and CA was more effective in decreasing the HPV on days 14, 21 and 28 than MTX in monotherapy. The most effective reduction of HPV was on day 21 (**Table 2**).

MCP-1 is responsible for recruiting monocytes on the sites of inflammation, and it is involved in the pathogenesis of human [46] and also in experimental arthritis [47]. AA caused a significant increase in the levels of MCP-1 on days 14, 21 and 28. Neither CA nor MTX administered in monotherapy were able to significantly reduce the elevated MCP-1 levels on days 14, 21 and 28. On day 21, only the combination of MTX and CA significantly decreased the level of MCP-1 in plasma of AA animals (**Table 3**).

3.3 Combination of methotrexate and ethanol extract of *Rhodiola rosea*

Rhodiola rosea L. is known as an adaptogen and has been confirmed to possess protective effects against inflammatory diseases, including cardiovascular diseases, neurodegenerative diseases, diabetes, sepsis, and cancer [97]. Less is known about the anti-inflammatory activity of Rhodiola extract in the experimental arthritis, thus we decided to select this extract for our study in monotherapy and in combination with methotrexate.

3.3.1 Rhodiola rosea *L.*

In this section we will focus on the anti-inflammatory effect of *Rhodiola rosea* L. (RhR). RhR has been found to possess anti-inflammatory properties in diseases

Changes in hind paw volume (%)	Day 7	Day 14	Day 21	Day 28
CO	4.66 ± 1.83	8.14 ± 3.23	9.79 ± 2.27	12.35 ± 1.95
AA	6.82 ± 2.13	35.90 ± 5.40*	71.79 ± 5.45**	54.81 ± 5.56***
AA-CA	4.73 ± 1.56	43.59 ± 9.70	72.63 ± 4.80	55.79 ± 5.11
AA-MTX	8.26 ± 1.85	11.63 ± 2.58+	30.47 ± 7.85+++	34.40 ± 9.74
AA-CA-MTX	3.84 ± 1.30	7.41 ± 1.53++	8.43 ± 0.81+++/#	12.33 ± 1.90+++

CO: healthy control animals, AA: untreated arthritic animals, AA-CA: arthritic animals treated with carnosic acid, AA-MTX: arthritic animals treated with methotrexate, AA-CA-MTX: arthritic animals treated combination of methotrexate and carnosic acid.
Values are expressed as average ± standard error of mean, statistical significance was calculated using ANOVA-Tukey–Kramer post hoc test.
*$p < 0.05$.
**$p < 0.01$.
***$p < 0.001$ vs. CO.
+$p < 0.05$.
++$p < 0.01$.
+++$p < 0.001$ vs. AA.
#$p < 0.05$ vs AA-MTX.

Table 2.
Effect of carnosic acid, methotrexate and their combination on hind paw swelling.

MCP-1 (pg/mL)	Day 14	Day 21	Day 28
CO	306.43 ± 7.91	337.27 ± 17.06	137.36 ± 20.61
AA	395.68 ± 19.20**	516.31 ± 22.00***	183.96 ± 12.48*
AA-CA	431.30 ± 21.14	510.00 ± 21.92	174.75 ± 18.45
AA-MTX	410.44 ± 9.75	491.74 ± 20.25	181.87 ± 25.07
AA-CA-MTX	411.82 ± 17.71	429.94 ± 13.38+	165.21 ± 13.95

CO: healthy control animals, AA: untreated arthritic animals, AA-CA: arthritic animals treated with carnosic acid, AA-MTX: arthritic animals treated with methotrexate, AA-CA-MTX: arthritic animals treated combination of methotrexate and carnosic acid.
Values are expressed as average ± standard error of mean, statistical significance was calculated using ANOVA-Tukey–Kramer post hoc test.
*$p < 0.05$.
**$p < 0.01$.
***$p < 0.001$ vs. CO.
+$p < 0.05$ vs AA.

Table 3.
Effect of carnosic acid, methotrexate and their combination on levels of monocyte chemotactic protein-1 in blood plasma.

such as sepsis, endotoxemia, asthma *in vivo* and *in vitro*. Pu et al. [97] have found that seven compounds (Ferulic acid, Kaempferol, Salidroside, Tyrosol, Catechin, Gallic acid and Caffeic acid phenethyl ester) isolated from RhR showed protective activity against LPS-induced sepsis in mice via decreasing TNF-α, nitric oxide and lactate dehydrogenase [97]. By many scientists, salidroside (SAL) was reported to possess protective ability in many disease models through particularly regulating different inflammatory mediators.

SAL decreased the inflammatory injury via reducing inflammatory cytokines (IL-1β, TNFα, IL-6), small molecules (mainly nitric oxide), chemokines (monocyte chemo-attractant protein (MCP)-1 and macrophage inflammatory protein (MIP)-1α) and COX-2 in animal models, such as LPS induced endotoxemia in mice [98], LPS induced murine acute lung injury [99], ovalbumin induced asthma in mice [100], and ethanol triggered acute gastric ulceration [101]. Further *in vitro* experiment confirmed the protective effects of SAL in neuro-inflammation. In murine microglial BV2 cells treated by LPS, Lee et al. showed that the main compounds of RhR (salidroside and rosarin) reduced the production of nitric oxide and inflammatory cytokines such as IL-6, IL-1β, and TNF-α via the NF-κB and MAPK signaling pathways [102]. Another *in vitro* study showed that SAL may inhibit the synthesis of inflammatory mediators. Authors found that in mice macrophages (J774.1 and RAW264.7) activated by LPS, SAL pre-treatment can reduce the levels of IL-1β, TNFα, IL-6, NO and MCP-1 via NF-κB pathway [103]. Further experiment showed that the mechanism might also be associated with down regulation of STAT3 and JAK2, and with translocation of STAT3 in nucleus [99]. STAT3 belongs to STAT (Signal Transducers and Activators of Transcription) family and has a key role in inflammatory processes. Many cytokines bind to GP130, which is a IL-6-type cytokines receptor, and activate Janus kinases (JAKs), what leads to the phosphorylation of STAT3. The phosphorylated STAT3 is translocated into the nucleus and regulates the expression of different target genes including also pro-inflammatory mediators [104].

Osteoarthritis (OA) is the most common disease, which seriously affects the daily life of the elderly. Currently, no drug therapy has been shown to explicitly block the progression of OA. The study by Gao et al. [105] showed that salidroside could significantly promote the proliferation of chondrocytes in OA rats induced by an anterior cruciate ligament transection and renew the OA-induced changes of cartilage. Salidroside increased the levels of aggrecan and collagen II and reduced the MMP-13 level. Moreover, salidroside reduced Th-17 cells and the levels of IKBα and p65, and IL-17, while elevated the count of CD4 + IL-10+ cells and IL-10. The reduction of IL-17 levels further diminished the dissociation of IKBα to p65, what resulted in the reduction of the release of VCAM-1 and TNF-α. Salidroside decreases the cartilage degradation via promoting proliferation of chondrocytes, reducing collagen fibrosis, and regulating the inflammatory processes and immune responses through NF-κB pathway in anterior cruciate ligament transection-induced OA in rats [105]. Another study involving chondrocytes by Wu et al. [106] showed that salidroside suppressed IL-1β-induced apoptosis in chondrocytes. Salidroside stimulated proliferation of chondrocytes, reduced IL-1ß-triggered inflammation and apoptosis, and scavenged NO and reactive oxygen species generated by chondrocytes. Salidroside upregulated the level of B-cell lymphoma 2 protein and downregulated the level of apoptosis regulator Bax. Salidroside also inhibited the production of caspase 3/9 and suppressed the phosphorylation of phosphoinositide-3-kinases (PI3K) and protein kinase B (AKT). These results indicate that salidroside prevents osteoarthritis by its anti-inflammatory, anti-apoptotic and pro-proliferating activities by suppressing the PI3K/AKT pathway [106].

3.3.2 *Effect of the combination therapy of methotrexate and extract of* Rhodiola rosea *in rat adjuvant arthritis*

Hind paw volume (HPV) was significantly increased on days 14 and day 21 during the development of AA. Administration of *Rhodiola rosea* ethanol extract (RS) in monotherapy markedly decreased HPV on day 14, but it had no effect on HPV on day 21. MTX and the combination of MTX with RS administered in monotherapy significantly decreased the HPV on days 14 and 21 (**Table 4**).

AA caused significant increase in the levels of IL-6 on days 14 and 21. Administration of MTX in monotherapy significantly decreased the plasmatic level of IL-6 only on day 14. Administration of RS in monotherapy had no effect on

Changes in hind paw volume (%)	Day 7	Day 14	Day 21
CO	0.55 ± 1.05	7.14 ± 1.33	11.99 ± 1.01
AA	3.16 ± 1.63	21.34 ± 3.70***	55.38 ± 2.76***
AA-MTX	3.95 ± 0.91	5.40 ± 0.86+++	14.79 ± 2.66+++
AA-RS	3.79 ± 1.88	8.35 ± 2.12++	48.62 ± 5.34
AA-RS-MTX	6.13 ± 1.66	7.77 ± 2.49++	12.10 ± 4.24+++

CO: healthy control animals, AA: untreated arthritic animals, AA-RS: arthritic animals treated with extract of Rhodiola rosea, AA-MTX: arthritic animals treated with methotrexate, AA-RS-MTX: arthritic animals treated combination of methotrexate and extract of Rhodiola rosea.
Values are expressed as average ± standard error of mean, statistical significance was calculated using ANOVA-Tukey–Kramer post hoc test
***$p < 0.001$ *vs. CO.*
++$p < 0.01$.
+++$p < 0.001$ *vs. AA.*

Table 4.
Effect of Rhodiola rosea *ethanol extract, methotrexate and their combination on hind paw swelling.*

IL-6 (pg/mL)	Day 14	Day 21
CO	62,67 ± 4,30	51,50 ± 4,77
AA	141,45 ± 14,66*	88,33 ± 5,74*
AA-MTX	82,10 ± 18,95+	70,19 ± 7,12
AA-RS	148,92 ± 10,44	77,99 ± 5,44
AA-RS-MTX	70,05 ± 6,84+	43,13 ± 3,05+

CO: healthy control animals, AA: untreated arthritic animals, AA-RS: arthritic animals treated with extract of Rhodiola rosea, AA-MTX: arthritic animals treated with methotrexate, AA-RS-MTX: arthritic animals treated combination of methotrexate and extract of Rhodiola rosea.
Values are expressed as average ± standard error of mean, statistical significance was calculated using ANOVA-Tukey–Kramer post hoc test.
*$p < 0.05$ *vs. CO.*
+$p < 0.05$, *vs. AA.*

Table 5.
Effect of Rhodiola rosea *ethanol extract, methotrexate and their combination on levels of IL-6 in blood plasma.*

levels of IL-6. However, the combination treatment of MTX and RS significantly decreased the levels of IL-6 on both measured days (**Table 5**).

4. Conclusions

Animal models of rheumatoid arthritis (RA) are used widely in research on pathogenesis of inflammatory arthritis and in the testing of potential anti-arthritic agents. In this chapter we highlighted the importance of inflammatory mediators IL-1β, IL-6, IL-17, MCP-1 and MMP-9 in experimental arthritis and RA. We have demonstrated, that MTX is a therapeutic standard for human arthritis as well as for adjuvant arthritis in rats, which make this model suitable for studying the pharmacotherapy of RA. Our preliminary results with combination treatments of MTX with carnosic acid and *Rhodiola rosea* ethanol extract showed, that these combinations are more effective in reducing hind paw volume, and the levels of MCP-1 and IL-6 than MTX in monotherapy. Thus, natural compounds with anti-inflammatory activities could be also a perspective candidate for combination treatments with MTX to treat human autoimmune diseases.

Acknowledgements

This work was supported by grants: VEGA 2/0115/19, VEGA 2/0136/20, APVV-15-0308, APVV SK-PT-18-0022 and SAS-BAS project: Anti-inflammatory effect of astaxanthin, sulforaphane and crocus sativus extract evaluated in two rodent models of age related diseases.

Conflict of interest

Authors have no conflict of interests.

Notes/thanks/other declarations

Authors thanks to colleagues Jana Urgosova, Danica Mihalova, MSc. Martin Chrastina, MSc., Frantisek Drafi, PharmDr., PhD. and Karol Svik, MSc., PhD for their support and assistance in performing experiments of rat adjuvant arthritis.

Author details

Silvester Ponist[1,3], Katarina Pruzinska[1,2] and Katarina Bauerova[1*]

1 Center of Experimental Medicine, Institute of Experimental Pharmacology and Toxicology, Slovak Academy of Sciences, Bratislava, Slovak Republic

2 Jessenius Faculty of Medicine in Martin, Comenius University in Bratislava, Slovak Republic

3 Slovak Medical University in Bratislava, Bratislava, Slovak Republic

*Address all correspondence to: katarina.bauerova@savba.sk

References

[1] Chen Z, Bozec A, Ramming A, Schett G. Anti-inflammatory and immune-regulatory cytokines in rheumatoid arthritis. Nat Rev Rheumatol. 2019;15:9-17. https://DOI.org/10.1038/s41584-018-0109-2.

[2] Shen HH, Yang YX, Meng X, Luo XY, Li XM, Shuai ZW, Ye DQ, Pan HF. NLRP3: A promising therapeutic target for autoimmune diseases. Autoimmun Rev. 2018;17:694-702. DOI: 10.1016/j.autrev.2018.01.020.

[3] Nikoopour E, Schwartz JA, Singh B. Therapeutic benefits of regulating inflammation in autoimmunity. Inflamm Allergy Drug Targets. 2008;7:203-210. DOI: 10.2174/187152808785748155.

[4] Choudhary N, Bhatt LK, Prabhavalkar KS. Experimental animal models for rheumatoid arthritis. Immunopharmacol Immunotoxicol. 2018;40:193-200. DOI: 10.1080/08923973.2018.1434793.

[5] Pearson CM, Waksman BH, Sharp JT. Studies of arthritis and other lesions induced in rats by injection of mycobacterial adjuvant. V. Changes affecting the skin and mucous membranes. Comparison of the experimental process with human disease. J Exp Med. 1961;113:485-510. DOI: 10.1084/jem.113.3.485.

[6] Pearson CM, Wood FD. Studies of arthritis and other lesions induced in rats by the injection of mycobacterial adjuvant. VII. Pathologic details of the arthritis and spondylitis. Am J Pathol. 1963;42:73-95.

[7] Joe B, Wilder RL. Animal models of rheumatoid arthritis. Mol Med Today. 1999;5:367-369. DOI: 10.1016/s1357-4310(99)01528-2.

[8] Roy T, Ghosh S. Animal models of rheumatoid arthritis: correlation and usefulness with human rheumatoid arthritis. Indo American Journal of Pharm Research. 2013;3:6131-6142.

[9] Billingham ME, Carney S, Butler R and Colston MJ. A mycobacterial 65-kD heat shock protein induces antigen-specific suppression of adjuvant arthritis, but is not itself arthritogenic. J Exp Med 1990;171:339-344.

[10] Allard SA, Muirden KD, Camplejohn KL, Maini RN. Chondrocyte-derived cells and matrix at the rheumatoid cartilage-pannus junction identified with monoclonal antibodies. Rheumatol Int. 1987;7:153-159. DOI: 10.1007/BF00270363.

[11] Vincenti MP, Clark IM, Brinckerhoff CE. Using inhibitors of metalloproteinases to treat arthritis. Easier said than done? Arthritis Rheum. 1994;37:1115-1126. DOI: 10.1002/art.1780370802.

[12] Harris ED Jr. Rheumatoid arthritis. Pathophysiology and implications for therapy. N Engl J Med. 1990;322:1277-1289. DOI: 10.1056/NEJM199005033221805.

[13] Werb Z. Proteases and matrix degradation. In: Kelley WN, Harris ED Jr, Ruddy S, Sledge CB, editors. Textbook of Rheumatology. 3th ed. Philadelphia: WB Saunders; 1989. p. 300-321.

[14] Brinckerhoff CE, Auble DT. Regulation of collagenase gene expression in synovial fibroblasts. Ann N Y Acad Sci. 1990;580:355-374. DOI: 10.1111/j.1749-6632.1990.tb17944.x.

[15] Walakovits LA, Moore VL, Bhardwaj N, Gallick GS, Lark MW. Detection of stromelysin and collagenase in synovial fluid from patients with rheumatoid arthritis and

posttraumatic knee injury. Arthritis Rheum. 1992;35:35-42. DOI: 10.1002/art.1780350106.

[16] Clark IM, Powell LK, Ramsey S, Hazleman BL, Cawston TE. The measurement of collagenase, tissue inhibitor of metalloproteinases (TIMP), and collagenase-TIMP complex in synovial fluids from patients with osteoarthritis and rheumatoid arthritis. Arthritis Rheum. 1993;36:372-379. DOI: 10.1002/art.1780360313.

[17] Dean DD, Martel-Pelletier J, Pelletier JP, Howell DS, Woessner JF Jr. Evidence for metalloproteinase and metalloproteinase inhibitor imbalance in human osteoarthritic cartilage. J Clin Invest. 1989;84:678-685. DOI: 10.1172/JCI114215.

[18] Buttle DJ, Saklatvala J. Lysosomal cysteine endopeptidases mediate interleukin 1-stimulated cartilage proteoglycan degradation. Biochem J. 1992;287:657-661. DOI: 10.1042/bj2870657.

[19] Dinarello CA, Ikejima T, Warner SJ, Orencole SF, Lonnemann G, Cannon JG, Libby P. Interleukin 1 induces interleukin 1. I. Induction of circulating interleukin 1 in rabbits in vivo and in human mononuclear cells in vitro. J Immunol. 1987;139:1902-1910.

[20] Black RA, Kronheim SR, Cantrell M, Deeley MC, March CJ, Prickett KS, Wignall J, Conlon PJ, Cosman D, Hopp TP, et al. Generation of biologically active interleukin-1 beta by proteolytic cleavage of the inactive precursor. J Biol Chem. 1988;263: 9437-9442.

[21] Niki Y, Yamada H, Kikuchi T, Toyama Y, Matsumoto H, Fujikawa K, Tada N. Membrane-associated IL-1 contributes to chronic synovitis and cartilage destruction in human IL-1 alpha transgenic mice. J Immunol. 2004;172:577-584. DOI: 10.4049/jimmunol.172.1.577.

[22] Burger D, Dayer JM. The role of human T-lymphocyte-monocyte contact in inflammation and tissue destruction. Arthritis Res. 2002;4:169-176. DOI: 10.1186/ar558.

[23] Dinarello CA. Biologic basis for interleukin-1 in disease. Blood. 1996;87:2095-2147.

[24] Eisenberg SP, Brewer MT, Verderber E, Heimdal P, Brandhuber BJ, Thompson RC. Interleukin 1 receptor antagonist is a member of the interleukin 1 gene family: evolution of a cytokine control mechanism. Proc Natl Acad Sci U S A. 1991;88:5232-5236. DOI: 10.1073/pnas.88.12.5232.

[25] Burger D, Dayer JM, Palmer G, Gabay C. Is IL-1 a good therapeutic target in the treatment of arthritis? Best Pract Res Clin Rheumatol. 2006;20:879-896. DOI: 10.1016/j.berh.2006.06.004.

[26] Altomonte L, Zoli A, Mirone L, Scolieri P, Magaró M. Serum levels of interleukin-1b, tumour necrosis factor-a and interleukin-2 in rheumatoid arthritis. Correlation with disease activity. Clin Rheumatol. 1992;11:202-205. DOI: 10.1007/BF02207957.

[27] Chai Z, Gatti S, Toniatti C, Poli V, Bartfai T. Interleukin (IL)-6 gene expression in the central nervous system is necessary for fever response to lipopolysaccharide or IL-1 beta: a study on IL-6-deficient mice. J Exp Med. 1996;183:311-316. DOI: 10.1084/jem.183.1.311.

[28] Streetz KL, Wüstefeld T, Klein C, Manns MP, Trautwein C. Mediators of inflammation and acute phase response in the liver. Cell Mol Biol (Noisy-le-grand). 2001;47:661-673.

[29] Van Snick J. Interleukin-6: an overview. Annu Rev Immunol.

1990;8:253-278. DOI: 10.1146/annurev.iy.08.040190.001345.

[30] Romano M, Sironi M, Toniatti C, Polentarutti N, Fruscella P, Ghezzi P, Faggioni R, Luini W, van Hinsbergh V, Sozzani S, Bussolino F, Poli V, Ciliberto G, Mantovani A. Role of IL-6 and its soluble receptor in induction of chemokines and leukocyte recruitment. Immunity. 1997;6:315-325. DOI: 10.1016/s1074-7613(00)80334-9.

[31] Tamura T, Udagawa N, Takahashi N, Miyaura C, Tanaka S, Yamada Y, Koishihara Y, Ohsugi Y, Kumaki K, Taga T, et al. Soluble interleukin-6 receptor triggers osteoclast formation by interleukin 6. Proc Natl Acad Sci U S A. 1993;90:11924-11928. DOI: 10.1073/pnas.90.24.11924.

[32] Mihara M, Moriya Y, Kishimoto T, Ohsugi Y. Interleukin-6 (IL-6) induces the proliferation of synovial fibroblastic cells in the presence of soluble IL-6 receptor. Br J Rheumatol. 1995;34:321-325. DOI: 10.1093/rheumatology/34.4.321.

[33] Desgeorges A, Gabay C, Silacci P, Novick D, Roux-Lombard P, Grau G, Dayer JM, Vischer T, Guerne PA. Concentrations and origins of soluble interleukin 6 receptor-alpha in serum and synovial fluid. J Rheumatol. 1997;24:1510-1516.

[34] Yao Z, Painter SL, Fanslow WC, Ulrich D, Macduff BM, Spriggs MK, Armitage RJ. Human IL-17: a novel cytokine derived from T cells. J Immunol. 1995;155:5483-5486. PMID: 7499828.

[35] Fossiez F, Djossou O, Chomarat P, Flores-Romo L, Ait-Yahia S, Maat C, Pin JJ, Garrone P, Garcia E, Saeland S, Blanchard D, Gaillard C, Das Mahapatra B, Rouvier E, Golstein P, Banchereau J, Lebecque S. T cell interleukin-17 induces stromal cells to produce proinflammatory and hematopoietic cytokines. J Exp Med. 1996;183:2593-2603. DOI: 10.1084/jem.183.6.2593.

[36] Wright JF, Guo Y, Quazi A, Luxenberg DP, Bennett F, Ross JF, Qiu Y, Whitters MJ, Tomkinson KN, Dunussi-Joannopoulos K, Carreno BM, Collins M, Wolfman NM. Identification of an interleukin 17F/17A heterodimer in activated human CD4+ T cells. J Biol Chem. 2007;282:13447-13555. DOI: 10.1074/jbc.M700499200.

[37] Gaffen SL. Structure and signalling in the IL-17 receptor family. Nat Rev Immunol. 2009;9:556-567. DOI: 10.1038/nri2586.

[38] Shen F, Gaffen SL. Structure-function relationships in the IL-17 receptor: implications for signal transduction and therapy. Cytokine. 2008;41:92-104. DOI: 10.1016/j.cyto.2007.11.013.

[39] Yao Z, Fanslow WC, Seldin MF, Rousseau AM, Painter SL, Comeau MR, Cohen JI, Spriggs MK. Herpesvirus Saimiri encodes a new cytokine, IL-17, which binds to a novel cytokine receptor. Immunity. 1995;3:811-821. DOI: 10.1016/1074-7613(95)90070-5.

[40] Schwarzenberger P, La Russa V, Miller A, Ye P, Huang W, Zieske A, Nelson S, Bagby GJ, Stoltz D, Mynatt RL, Spriggs M, Kolls JK. IL-17 stimulates granulopoiesis in mice: use of an alternate, novel gene therapy-derived method for in vivo evaluation of cytokines. J Immunol. 1998;161:6383-6389.

[41] Kotake S, Udagawa N, Takahashi N, Matsuzaki K, Itoh K, Ishiyama S, Saito S, Inoue K, Kamatani N, Gillespie MT, Martin TJ, Suda T. IL-17 in synovial fluids from patients with rheumatoid arthritis is a potent stimulator of osteoclastogenesis. J Clin Invest. 1999;103:1345-1352. DOI: 10.1172/JCI5703.

[42] Attur MG, Patel RN, Abramson SB, Amin AR. Interleukin-17 up-regulation of nitric oxide production in human osteoarthritis cartilage. Arthritis Rheum. 1997;40:1050-1053. DOI: 10.1002/art.1780400609.

[43] Jovanovic DV, Di Battista JA, Martel-Pelletier J, Jolicoeur FC, He Y, Zhang M, Mineau F, Pelletier JP. IL-17 stimulates the production and expression of proinflammatory cytokines, IL-beta and TNF-alpha, by human macrophages. J Immunol. 1998;160:3513-3521.

[44] Ziolkowska M, Koc A, Luszczykiewicz G, Ksiezopolska-Pietrzak K, Klimczak E, Chwalinska-Sadowska H, Maslinski W. High levels of IL-17 in rheumatoid arthritis patients: IL-15 triggers in vitro IL-17 production via cyclosporin A-sensitive mechanism. J Immunol. 2000;164:2832-2838. DOI: 10.4049/jimmunol.164.5.2832.

[45] Taub DD, Oppenheim JJ. Review of the chemokine meeting the Third International Symposium of Chemotactic Cytokines. Cytokine. 1993;5:175-179. DOI: 10.1016/1043-4666(93)90001-l.

[46] Koch AE, Kunkel SL, Harlow LA, Johnson B, Evanoff HL, Haines GK, Burdick MD, Pope RM, Strieter RM. Enhanced production of monocyte chemoattractant protein-1 in rheumatoid arthritis. J Clin Invest. 1992;90:772-779. DOI: 10.1172/JCI115950.

[47] Kasama T, Strieter RM, Lukacs NW, Lincoln PM, Burdick MD, Kunkel SL. Interleukin-10 expression and chemokine regulation during the evolution of murine type II collagen-induced arthritis. J Clin Invest. 1995;95:2868-2876. DOI: 10.1172/JCI117993.

[48] Tchetverikov I, Lard LR, DeGroot J, Verzijl N, TeKoppele JM, Breedveld FC, Huizinga TW, Hanemaaijer R. Matrix metalloproteinases-3, −8, −9 as markers of disease activity and joint damage progression in early rheumatoid arthritis. Ann Rheum Dis. 2003;62: 1094-1099. DOI: 10.1136/ard.62.11.1094.

[49] Xue M, March L, Sambrook PN, Jackson CJ. Differential regulation of matrix metalloproteinase 2 and matrix metalloproteinase 9 by activated protein C: relevance to inflammation in rheumatoid arthritis. Arthritis Rheum. 2007;56:2864-74.

[50] Nagase H, Visse R, Murphy G. Structure and function of matrix metalloproteinases and TIMPs. Cardiovasc Res. 2006;562-73. DOI: 10.1016/j.cardiores.2005.12.002.

[51] van den Steen PE, Grillet B, Opdenakker G. Gelatinase B participates in collagen II degradation and releases glycosylated remnant epitopes in rheumatoid arthritis, Adv Exp Med Biol. 2005;564:45-55.

[52] Brew K, Dinakarpandian D, Nagase H. Tissue inhibitors of metalloproteinases: evolution, structure and function. Biochim Biophys Acta. 2000;1477:267-283. DOI: 10.1016/s0167-4838(99)00279-4.

[53] Lohi J, Harvima I, Keski-Oja J. Pericellular substrates of human mast cell tryptase: 72,000 dalton gelatinase and fibronectin. J Cell Biochem. 1992;50:337-349. DOI: 10.1002/jcb.240500402.

[54] Fang KC, Raymond WW, Lazarus SC, Caughey GH. Dog mastocytoma cells secrete a 92-kD gelatinase activated extracellularly by mast cell chymase. J Clin Invest. 1996;97:1589-1596. DOI: 10.1172/JCI118583.

[55] Ries C, Petrides PE. Cytokine regulation of matrix metalloproteinase activity and its regulatory dysfunction

in disease. Biol Chem Hoppe Seyler. 1995;376:345-355.

[56] Vaday GG, Schor H, Rahat MA, Lahat N, Lider O. Transforming growth factor-beta suppresses tumor necrosis factor alpha-induced matrix metalloproteinase-9 expression in monocytes. J Leukoc Biol. 2001;69: 613-621.

[57] Sopata I, Dancewicz AM. Presence of a gelatin-specific proteinase and its latent form in human leucocytes. Biochim Biophys Acta. 1974;370:510-523. DOI: 10.1016/0005-2744(74) 90112-0.

[58] Okada S, Kita H, George TJ, Gleich GJ, Leiferman KM. Migration of eosinophils through basement membrane components in vitro: role of matrix metalloproteinase-9. Am J Respir Cell Mol Biol. 1997;17:519-528. DOI: 10.1165/ajrcmb.17.4.2877.

[59] Yu Q, Stamenkovic I. Cell surface-localized matrix metalloproteinase-9 proteolytically activates TGF-beta and promotes tumor invasion and angiogenesis. Genes Dev. 2000;14:163-176.

[60] Tanaka, A., K. Aria, Y. Kitamura, H. Matsuda. Matrix metalloproteinase-9 production, a newly identified function of mast cell progenitors, is downregulated by c-kit receptor activation. Blood.1999;94:2390-2395.

[61] Baram D, Vaday GG, Salamon P, Drucker I, Hershkoviz R, Mekori YA. Human mast cells release metalloproteinase-9 on contact with activated T cells: juxtacrine regulation by TNF-α. J. Immunol. 2001;167: 4008-4016.

[62] Kanbe N, Tanaka A, Kanbe M, Itakura A, Kurosawa M, Matsuda H. Human mast cells produce matrix metalloproteinase 9. Eur J Immunol. 1999;29:2645-2649. DOI: 10.1002/(SICI)1521-4141(199908)29:08 <2645::AID-IMMU2645>3.0.CO;2-1.

[63] Di Girolamo N, Indoh I, Jackson N, Wakefield D, McNeil HP, Yan W, Geczy C, Arm JP, Tedla N. Human mast cell-derived gelatinase B (matrix metalloproteinase-9) is regulated by inflammatory cytokines: role in cell migration. J Immunol. 2006;177:2638-2650. DOI: 10.4049/jimmunol.177.4. 2638.

[64] Kim KS, Choi HM, Lee YA, Choi IA, Lee SH, Hong SJ, Yang HI, Yoo MC. Expression levels and association of gelatinases MMP-2 and MMP-9 and collagenases MMP-1 and MMP-13 with VEGF in synovial fluid of patients with arthritis. Rheumatol Int. 2011;31:543-547. DOI: 10.1007/s00296-010-1592-1.

[65] Itoh T, Matsuda H, Tanioka M, Kuwabara K, Itohara S, Suzuki R. The role of matrix metalloproteinase-2 and matrix metalloproteinase-9 in antibody-induced arthritis. J Immunol. 2002;169:2643-2647. DOI: 10.4049/ jimmunol.169.5.2643.

[66] Koenders MI, van den Berg WB. Novel therapeutic targets in rheumatoid arthritis. Trends Pharmacol Sci. 2015;36:189-195. DOI: 10.1016/j. tips.2015.02.001.

[67] Laporte JR, Ibáñez L, Vidal X, Vendrell L, Leone R. Upper gastrointestinal bleeding associated with the use of NSAIDs: newer versus older agents. Drug Saf. 2004;27:411-420. DOI: 10.2165/00002018-2004270 60-00005.

[68] Satyanarayanasetty D, Pawar K, Nadig P, Haran A. Multiple Adverse Effects of Systemic Corticosteroids: A Case Report. J Clin Diagn Res. 2015;9:FD01-2. DOI: 10.7860/ JCDR/2015/12110.5939.

[69] Gilani ST, Khan DA, Khan FA, Ahmed M. Adverse effects of low dose

methotrexate in rheumatoid arthritis patients. J Coll Physicians Surg Pak. 2012;22:101-104.

[70] Shire MG, Muller GW. TNF-α inhibitors and rheumatoid arthritis. Expert Opin. Ther. Patents. 2005;8:531-544.

[71] Lekander I, Borgström F, Lysholm J, van Vollenhoven RF, Lindblad S, Geborek P, Kobelt G. The cost-effectiveness of TNF-inhibitors for the treatment of rheumatoid arthritis in Swedish clinical practice. Eur J Health Econ. 2013;14:863-873. DOI: 10.1007/s10198-012-0431-6.

[72] Gautam R, Jachak SM. Recent developments in anti-inflammatory natural products. Med Res Rev. 2009;29:767-820. DOI: 10.1002/med.20156.

[73] Shinde CG, Venkatesh MP, Kumar TM, Shivakumar HG. Methotrexate: a gold standard for treatment of rheumatoid arthritis. J Pain Palliat Care Pharmacother. 2014;28:351-358.

[74] Salliot C, van der Heijde D. Long-term safety of methotrexate monotherapy in patients with rheumatoid arthritis: a systematic literature research. Ann Rheum Dis. 2009;68:1100-1104. DOI: 10.1136/ard.2008.093690.

[75] Cronstein BN, Aune TM. Methotrexate and its mechanisms of action in inflammatory arthritis. Nat Rev Rheumatol. 2020;16:145-154. DOI: 10.1038/s41584-020-0373-9.

[76] Olsen NJ, Spurlock CF 3rd, Aune TM. Methotrexate induces production of IL-1 and IL-6 in the monocytic cell line U937. Arthritis Res Ther. 2014;16:R17. DOI: 10.1186/ar4444.

[77] Merrill JT, Shen C, Schreibman D, Coffey D, Zakharenko O, Fisher R, Lahita RG, Salmon J, Cronstein BN. Adenosine A1 receptor promotion of multinucleated giant cell formation by human monocytes: a mechanism for methotrexate-induced nodulosis in rheumatoid arthritis. Arthritis Rheum. 1997;40:1308-1315. DOI: 10.1002/1529-0131(199707)40:7<1308::AID-ART16>3.0.CO;2-M.

[78] Williams AJ, Cronstein BN. The effect of A(2A) adenosine receptor activation on C-C chemokine receptor 7 expression in human THP1 macrophages during inflammation. Inflammation. 2012;35:614-622. DOI: 10.1007/s10753-011-9353-1.

[79] Leibovich SJ, Chen JF, Pinhal-Enfield G, Belem PC, Elson G, Rosania A, Ramanathan M, Montesinos C, Jacobson M, Schwarzschild MA, Fink JS, Cronstein B. Synergistic up-regulation of vascular endothelial growth factor expression in murine macrophages by adenosine A(2A) receptor agonists and endotoxin. Am J Pathol. 2002;160:2231-2244. DOI: 10.1016/S0002-9440(10)61170-4.

[80] Murphy EP, Crean D. Molecular Interactions between NR4A Orphan Nuclear Receptors and NF-κB Are Required for Appropriate Inflammatory Responses and Immune Cell Homeostasis. Biomolecules. 2015;5:1302-1318. DOI: 10.3390/biom5031302.

[81] Koscsó B, Csóka B, Kókai E, Németh ZH, Pacher P, Virág L, Leibovich SJ, Haskó G. Adenosine augments IL-10-induced STAT3 signaling in M2c macrophages. J Leukoc Biol. 2013;94:1309-1315. DOI: 10.1189/jlb.0113043.

[82] Miranda-Carús ME, Balsa A, Benito-Miguel M, Pérez de Ayala C, Martín-Mola *E. IL*-15 and the initiation of cell contact-dependent synovial fibroblast-T lymphocyte cross-talk in

rheumatoid arthritis: effect of methotrexate. J Immunol. 2004;173: 1463-1476. DOI: 10.4049/jimmunol.173.2.1463.

[83] Linde H. Ein neues Diterpen aus *Salvia officinalis* L. und eine Notiz zur Konstitution von Pikrosalvin. HCA. 1964;47: 1234-1239. https://DOI.org/10.1002/hlca.19640470517.

[84] Hill RA, Connolly JD. Triterpenoids. Nat Prod Rep. 2013;30:1028-1065. DOI: 10.1039/c3np70032a.

[85] Visanji JM, Thompson DG, Padfield PJ. Induction of G2/M phase cell cycle arrest by carnosol and carnosic acid is associated with alteration of cyclin A and cyclin B1 levels.Cancer Lett. 2006;231:130-136.

[86] Chen JH, Ou HP, Lin CY, Lin FJ, Wu CR, Chang SW, Tsai CW. Carnosic acid prevents 6-hydroxydopamine-induced cell death in SH-SY5Y cells via mediation of glutathione synthesis. Chem Res Toxicol. 2012;25:1893-1901. DOI: 10.1021/tx300171u.

[87] Bauer J, Kuehnl S, Rollinger JM, Scherer O, Northoff H, Stuppner H, Werz O, Koeberle A. Carnosol and carnosic acids from *Salvia officinalis* inhibit microsomal prostaglandin E2 synthase-1. J Pharmacol Exp Ther. 2012; 342:169-176.

[88] Oh J, Yu T, Choi SJ, Yang Y, Baek HS, An SA, Kwon LK, Kim J, Rho HS, Shin SS, Choi WS, Hong S, Cho JY. Syk/Src pathway-targeted inhibition of skin inflammatory responses by carnosic acid. Mediators Inflamm. 2012;2012:781375.

[89] Lian KC, Chuang JJ, Hsieh CW, Wung BS, Huang GD, Jian TY, Sun YW. Dual mechanisms of NF-kappaB inhibition in carnosol-treated endothelial cells.Toxicol Appl Pharmacol. 2010; 245:21-35. DOI: 10.1016/j.taap.2010.01.003.

[90] Poeckel D, Greiner C, Verhoff M, Rau O, Tausch L, Hörnig C, Steinhilber D, Schubert-Zsilavecz M, Werz O. Carnosic acid and carnosol potently inhibit human 5-lipoxygenase and suppress pro-inflammatory responses of stimulated human polymorphonuclear leukocytes. Biochem Pharmacol. 2008;76:91-97. DOI: 10.1016/j.bcp.2008.04.013.

[91] Hall ED, Wang JA, Miller DM, Cebak JE, Hill RL. Newer pharmacological approaches for antioxidant neuroprotection in traumatic brain injury. Neuro pharmacology. 2019;145(Pt B):247-258. DOI: 10.1016/j.neuropharm.2018.08.005.

[92] Takada T, Miyaki S, Ishitobi H, Hirai Y, Nakasa T, Igarashi K, Lotz MK, Ochi M. Bach1 deficiency reduces severity of osteoarthritis through upregulation of heme oxygenase-1. Arthritis Res Ther. 2015;17:285. DOI: 10.1186/s13075-015-0792-1.

[93] Wang LC, Wei WH, Zhang XW, Liu D, Zeng KW, Tu PF. An Integrated Proteomics and Bioinformatics Approach Reveals the Anti-inflammatory Mechanism of Carnosic Acid. Front Pharmacol. 2018;9:370.

[94] de Oliveira MR, de Souza ICC, Fürstenau CR. Carnosic Acid Induces Anti-Inflammatory Effects in Paraquat-Treated SH-SY5Y Cells Through a Mechanism Involving a Crosstalk Between the Nrf2/HO-1 Axis and NF-κB. Mol Neurobiol. 2018;55:890-897. DOI: 10.1007/s12035-017-0389-6.

[95] Chae IG, Yu MH, Im NK, Jung YT, Lee J, Chun KS, Lee IS. Effect of Rosemarinus officinalis L. on MMP-9, MCP-1 levels, and cell migration in RAW 264.7 and smooth muscle cells. J Med Food. 2012;15:879-886. DOI: 10.1089/jmf.2012.2162.

[96] Liu M, Zhou X, Zhou L, Liu Z, Yuan J, Cheng J, Zhao J, Wu L, Li H,

Qiu H, Xu J. Carnosic acid inhibits inflammation response and joint destruction on osteoclasts, fibroblast-like synoviocytes, and collagen-induced arthritis rats. J Cell Physiol. 2018; 233:6291-6303. DOI: 10.1002/jcp.26517.

[97] Pu WL, Zhang MY, Bai RY, Sun LK, Li WH, Yu YL, Zhang Y, Song L, Wang ZX, Peng YF, Shi H, Zhou K, Li TX. Anti-inflammatory effects of *Rhodiola rosea* L.: A review. Biomed Pharmacother. 2020;121:109552. DOI: 10.1016/j.biopha.2019.109552.

[98] Guan S, Feng H, Song B, Guo W, Xiong Y, Huang G, Zhong W, Huo M, Chen N, Lu J, Deng X. Salidroside attenuates LPS-induced pro-inflammatory cytokine responses and improves survival in murine endotoxemia. Int Immunopharmacol. 2011;11:2194-2209. DOI: 10.1016/j.intimp.2011.09.018.

[99] Qi Z, Qi S, Ling L, Lv J, Feng Z. Salidroside attenuates inflammatory response via suppressing JAK2-STAT3 pathway activation and preventing STAT3 transfer into nucleus. Int Immunopharmacol. 2016;35:265-271. DOI: 10.1016/j.intimp.2016.04.004.

[100] Wang J, Jin RG, Xiao L, Wang QJ, Yan TH. Anti-asthma effects of synthetic salidroside through regulation of Th1/Th2 balance. Chin J Nat Med. 2014;12:500-4. DOI: 10.1016/S1875-5364(14)60078-9.

[101] Chang X, Luo F, Jiang W, Zhu L, Gao J, He H, Wei T, Gong S, Yan T. Protective activity of salidroside against ethanol-induced gastric ulcer via the MAPK/NF-κB pathway in vivo and in vitro. Int Immunopharmacol. 2015;28:604-615. DOI: 10.1016/j.intimp.2015.07.031.

[102] Lee Y, Jung JC, Jang S, Kim J, Ali Z, Khan IA, Oh S. Anti-Inflammatory and Neuroprotective Effects of Constituents Isolated from *Rhodiola rosea*. Evid Based Complement Alternat Med. 2013;2013:514049. DOI: 10.1155/2013/514049.

[103] Huang Q, Hu XL. [Effects of salidroside on the secretion of inflammatory mediators induced by lipopolysaccharide in murine macrophage cell line J774.1]. Sheng Li Xue Bao. 2017;69:41-46.

[104] Hillmer EJ, Zhang H, Li HS, Watowich SS. STAT3 signaling in immunity. Cytokine Growth Factor Rev. 2016;31:1-15. DOI: 10.1016/j.cytogfr.2016.05.001.

[105] Gao H, Peng L, Li C, Ji Q, Li P. Salidroside Alleviates Cartilage Degeneration Through NF-κB Pathway in Osteoarthritis Rats. Drug Des Devel Ther. 2020;14:1445-1454. DOI: 10.2147/DDDT.S242862

[106] Wu M, Hu R, Wang J, An Y, Lu L, Long C, Yan L. Salidroside Suppresses IL-1β-Induced Apoptosis in Chondrocytes via Phosphatidylinositol 3-Kinases (PI3K)/Akt Signaling Inhibition. Med Sci Monit. 2019;25:5833-5840.

Chapter 13

Antiphospholipid Syndrome and Pregnancy-Diagnosis, Complications and Management: An Overview

Panagiotis Tsikouras, Christina Tsiggalou, Anastasia Bothou, Aggeliki Gerede, Ifigenia Apostolou, Fotini Gaitatzi, Anna Chalkidou, Xanthoula Anthoulaki, Spyridon Michalopoulos, Georgios Dragoutsos, Ioannis Tsirkas, Irini Babageorgaka, Theopi Nalbanti, Natalia Sachnova, Alexios Alexiou, Konstantinos Nikolettos, Christos Tsalikidis, Stefanos Zervoudis, Panagiotis Peitsidis and Nikolaos Nikolettos

Abstract

Antiphospholipid syndrome which is also known as APS is an autoimmune disease which represents an acquired form of thrombophilia. The etiology of APS remains unknown. This disorder occurs when the immune system mistakenly attacks some of the normal human proteins and manifests itself as recurrent arterial or venous thrombosis and it could emerge after abortions or in recurrent pregnancy loss. In APS, the body produces the wrong antibodies against phospholipid-binding proteins, that is present in the blood and plays an important role in coagulation. Antibodies are specific proteins that usually target and neutralize the body's invaders, such as viruses and bacteria. When antibodies attack phospholipid-binding proteins, blood clots abnormally. Specifically, it could cause blood clots in veins or arteries leading to stroke and various pregnancy complications such as: endometrial death, miscarriage, preeclampsia, intrauterine growth restriction and prematurity. APS is divided into primary and secondary, which is associated with autoimmune diseases and more often with systemic lupus erythematosus (SLE), while antibodies against cardiolipin are detected in many other conditions (infections, malignancies, drugs, etc.). The symptoms of APS, in addition to arterial and/or venous thrombosis and pregnancy complications, are multisystemic and the differential diagnosis of the primary APS from the secondary, in the context of SLE, is of particular clinical interest and is subject of this literature review.

Keywords: antiphospholipid syndrome, pregnancy, management neonatal outcome

1. Introduction

APS characterized by thrombosis of the arteries, veins and microvessels and/or with pregnancy morbidity, with persistently elevated antiphospholipid antibody (aPLs) titers. The syndrome was first described in 1983 by Professor G. Hughes, at Hammersmith Hospital (Hughes Syndrome) [1, 2]. APS is a prothrombotic condition (with related complications such as deep vein thrombosis, pulmonary embolism, etc.), belonging to autoimmune diseases of unknown cause, and is strongly associated with pregnancy [1–3]. Generally, autoimmune diseases namely Sjorgen's syndrome, Spondylanthritis, rheumatoid arthtritis RA have an incidence of 5–8% in the general population organoid or systemic, and represent the 2nd cause of hospitalization in Internal Medicine Departments and the 3rd cause of morbidity/mortality [1–4]. APS occurs as primary in the absence of findings of other autoimmune diseases or as secondary in 36% of cases in the context of another autoimmune disease (SEL, Sjogren's disease, inflammatory bowel disease, etc.), while it is present in about 5% of patients with subclinical SEL or coexists with another underlying systemic autoimmune disease in 6% of cases [5, 6].

2. Epidemiology

The incidence of the syndrome is increased with age. During pregnancy, aPLs detection ranges from 0 to 11%, with an average incidence of about 2%. On the contrary, the syndrome is detected in up to 37% of the patients with systemic erythematosus lupus (SEL). In the nonpregnancy setting, venous thromboses are more common than arterial ones and can be diagnosed by imaging techniques and/or histologic evidence [5–7].

3. Frequency

According to literature APS is the cause for 1 out of 5 Deep Vein Thrombosis ('DVTs'), 1 out of 5 cases of SLE (arterial stroke) in young patients (age <45 years) and 1 out of 5 miscarriages. Especially for Obstetrics Hughes Syndrome is currently recognized as the leading cause for the miscarriages [5–7]. In addition, APS is diagnosed as the underlying diagnosis in a still unknown percentage of cases previously misdiagnosed as migraine, Alzheimer's disease, and Multiple MS. It is estimated that the true incidence of the syndrome can be up to 1–2% or more in the general population [5–7]. Correlations-Percentages The mean age of APS onset is >30 years, with a female to male ratio of 5:1 and relapses usually take place at the same or similar area of the body. There is no apparent racial preference, but an increased incidence of SEL is reported in African Americans and Spaniards. Patients with SEL have positive aPLs in a percentage of 15–35%, but only about 50% of these patients will develop APS symptoms [5–7].

4. Clinical subtypes

Special categories of APS are described usually correlated to the target-organ or the severity of the manifestations. The following are included: Generalized APS, Arterial APS, APS and heart, APS and kidneys, Cerebral APS, Pediatric APS, Neonatal APS, Catastrophic CAPS and Obstetric APS [5–7].

5. Catastrophic APS

The 0.8% of the cases is characterized as Catastrophic Antiphospholipid Syndrome (CAPS). It is a very rare and severe form of APS. There are diffuse clots in the small vessels throughout the body. Sometimes it can appear as the first manifestation of APS and even without clinical or serological confirmation of SEL. Early diagnosis is necessary and immediate start of an aggressive treatment is inevitable [5, 7–9]. CAPS is caused when at least 3 different systems are affected at intervals of days or weeks, with multiple thrombosis in large and small vessels. The organs that are usually affected are: a) kidneys, b) lungs, c) heart, d) small-large vessels with consequences as peripheral limb ischemia, stroke, myocardial infarction, thrombosis of blood vessels of abdominal organs with a mortality rate of 50% [5, 7–9]. The observed thrombocytopenia is usually mild between 100-150x10^9/L but severe thrombocytopenia can be also observed. The prevalence of the syndrome in the general population ranges between 2% and 4% meaning 40–50 patients in 100,000 based on the criteria (mean age of diagnosis 34 years) and 7: 1 in the SEL/APS combination [5, 7–9].

6. Therapeutic interventions for catastrophic APS

Anticoagulant therapy + corticosteroids.
Anticoagulant therapy + corticosteroids + plasmapheresis.
Anticoagulant therapy + corticosteroids + IV γ-globin.
Anticoagulant therapy + corticosteroids + plasmapheresis + IV γ-globulin.

Diffuse intravascular coagulation is not usually seen in primary or secondary APS but it occurs in about 25% of patients with catastrophic APS. It is estimated that more than 53% of cases are related to the primary syndrome. It is estimated that approximately 10% of patients with primary APS will be diagnosed with another autoimmune, disorder, such as SEL, at some point in their lives which is estimated to coexist in up to 37% of patients with APS. Patients with primary APS and a female/male ratio incidence of 3.5: 1 should not be classified as SEL patients, as they are two different disease entities [5, 7–9]. Also, aPLs found in a variety of rheumatic and autoimmune diseases should not be confused with APS. The latter includes autoimmune hemolytic anemia, idiopathic thrombocytopenic purpura, rheumatoid arthritis and cutaneous manifestations such as edema. Also, the same antiphospholipid antibodies are detected either temporarily or permanently after various infections, such as hepatitis A, hepatitis B, acquired immune deficiency (AIDS), mumps, toxoplasmosis, erythema etc. The use of certain medicines, such as hydralazine, procainamide, and amoxicillin, phenothiazines may cause a serious differential diagnosis with APS, which requires immediate diagnostic and therapeutic treatment to reduce the increased maternal risk, and in particular perinatal morbidity and mortality due to placental infarction [5, 7–9].

7. Pathophysiology

Dysfunction of the vascular epithelium as well as oxidative damage and modifications of phospholipid-bound proteins that interfere with the regulation of coagulation are possible. It occurs when the immune system mistakenly attacks some of the normal proteins in the blood. The mechanism by which aPLs causes thrombosis is not fully understood. APLs consist of a heterogeneous group of autoantibodies that react primarily with plasma proteins associated with negatively charged phospholipids (epitope formation). Moreover, also react directly with both phospholipid-binding proteins and phospholipids [10–12].

However, aPLs have been shown to target not only cell membrane phospholipids, but also plasma proteins. Initially aPLs are directed directly against negative cell membrane phospholipids and autoantibodies are directed against plasma proteins with high affinity for these anionic phospholipids [10–14]. Phospholipids are like building blocks of cell membranes and the appearance of aPLs is due to the "projection" of their anions to the extracellular space [10–14]. This phenomenon is usually happening due to various causes, such as trauma, ischemia, inflammation, infections, or drug interactions. They were first observed in 1906 in 1–5% of the normal population.

The prevailing theory is that APS initially causes a disorder in cell apoptosis procedure resulting in the exposure of cell membrane phospholipids and their subsequent binding to various plasma proteins, such as β2-glycoprotein I. This binding leads, through activation, to generation of intracellular mediators (such as nuclear factor kappa B and mammalian target of rapamycin), and the formation of a phospholipid-protein complex resulting in the discovery of a new epitope, which then becomes target of autoantibodies [10–14].

Recent studies suggest that oxidized β2-glycoprotein I is capable of binding to and subsequently activating dendritic cells in a similar pathway to the one induced by activation via the Toll-like receptor 4 (TLR-4), resulting in its induction and the production of autoantibodies.

A total of 4 types of aPLs have been isolated [14–18].

1. Antibodies that give a false positive serological test for syphilis.

2. Lupus anticoagulants, which are antibodies to plasma proteins that bind to anionic phospholipids and cause prolonged results in laboratory methods of coagulation control, such as activated partial thromboplastin time (aPTT), kaolin clotting time (Kaoline Clotting)-KCT) and dilute Russell Viper Venom Time (dRVVT). These proteins are prothrombin or annexin V [14–18].

3. Antibodies to cardiolipin and phosphatidylserine. These antibodies may be IgA, IgG or IgM and may cross-react with lupus anticoagulants.

4. Antibodies to β2-glycoprotein-I, which are detected in a significant percentage of patients with primary or secondary antiphospholipid syndrome, while in 11% of patients it is the only laboratory finding [14–18]. This association results in either the discovery of "hidden" antigenic epitopes or the creation of new or simply increasing the concentration of weak antigenic sites in such quantities as to elicit an immune response.

Types of anti-b2 GPI antibodies [14–18]. There are several types of anti-β2 glycoprotein I antibodies, but not all of them are harmful. Those that target specific β-2 glycoprotein epitopes, such as the epitope in the N-terminal I domain of the molecule, are associated with the onset of clinical manifestations of the syndrome [14–18].

8. Correlation between APS clinical events and the type of anti-β2GPI antibodies

Patients with triple positivity in aPLs: have higher anti-β2GPI – domain I antibody titles, compared to patients with single or double positivity. Almost all anti-β2GPI – domain I IgG antibodies tested positive after 12 weeks, in contrast to innocent transient aPLs, which appear to be immune to infections. Although anti-β2GPI-Domain 1 (β2GPI-D1) IgG antibodies have been associated with thrombosis and pregnancy morbidity in APS patients, these antibodies are found in only one third of the patients [14–18].

9. Cell β2GPI/anti-β2GPI antibody receptors

Annexin A2 and Toll-like receptor (TLR) 4 are receptors for the entire β2GPI molecule. However, the absence of both of these receptors does not lead to the complete inhibition of the binding of the anti-β2GPI antibody, a finding that supports the view that there are additional surface adhesion molecules that play a role. TLR1, TLR2 and TLR6 are potential cell receptors [14–18].

10. Association of APS with pathogenic intestinal bacteria

B2GPI binds to LPS via domain V. Presence of a large amount of LPS probably increases the vascular distribution of APLs, by increasing the expression of TLR2 and especially TLR4. Because the main source of LPS in healthy people is the gut, it is possible that the presence of gut microbes in the gut increases them. Administration of intestinal flora-specific antimicrobial therapy to experimental animals showed a reduction in the thrombotic manifestations of APS [14–18].

11. The role of the complement in the pathogenesis of APS

Immediate evidence: In experimental models with C6-deficient rats and C5-depleted mice, it was shown that the addition of monoclonal anti-domain I MBB2 did not induce thrombosis or miscarriage. C4d and C3b sections have also been found in deposits on the placenta of women with APS [14–18].

Indirect evidence: In-vivo studies of the efficacy of drugs with C5 action. The non-complement-fixing anti-domain I monoclonal MBB2 [DELTA] Ch2 and the complement inhibitor C5-inhibitor rEV576 prevented the thrombotic complications of APS in vivo in experimental animals.

12. APL action mechanisms

APLs activate endothelial cells resulting in the expression of adhesion molecules (such as intercellular cell adhesion molecule-1 ICAM-1, vascular cell adhesion molecule-1 VCAM-1, E-selectin), and ultimately the overproduction of tissue factor TF.

APLs activate monocytes and cause increased tissue factor expression.

APLs activate platelets resulting in increased glycoprotein 2b-3a expression and thromboxane A2 synthesis. It has also recently been shown that aPLs induce the release of NETs from endothelial cells and these in turn further activate platelets. Their presence is enhanced by other conditions such as neoplasms, myelodysplastic syndromes, paraproteinemias, etc. [14–18].

These proteins (aPLs) normally bind to the phospholipid components of membranes and protect against activation of coagulation mechanisms. Autoantibodies displace these “protective” proteins and promote the formation of clots in the cells of the vascular endothelium resulting in arterial and venous thrombosis.

In particular, aPLs antibodies include antibodies to Lupus Anticoagulant (LA), antibodies to cardiolipin (aCL), antibodies to β2GPI (αβ2GPI) and antibodies to other phospholipid-binding proteins and other phospholipids. LA, aCL and αβ2GPI antibodies are important in the diagnosis of antiphospholipid syndrome [12–18].

13. The most likely explanation for the pathogenesis of APS

They occur in people with a genetic predisposition after accidental exposure to infectious agents or in a rheumatic disease environment such as SEL. It is the "second hit" theory required for the full development of the syndrome. Of course, not all people with antiphospholipid antibodies have thrombosis or obstetric complications.

The "two-hit theory" has been proposed, i.e. that in the manifestation of the disease only the presence of antiphospholipid antibodies is not sufficient but a second thrombotic risk factor must coexist (e.g. age, hypertension, infection, inflammation, diabetes mellitus, obesity, smoking, pregnancy and obstetrics, surgery, etc.) [14–18].

Regarding the pathophysiology of obstetric complications, trophoblast and perishable blood vessel thrombosis is at the heart of this process. Various mechanisms have been proposed that lead to this result:

1. aPLs bind to Annexin V molecules and reduce the active levels of the protein in the blood. Annexin V is a protein that covers the negatively charged phospholipids of the cell membrane when exposed to the extracellular space, thus making it impossible to activate the thrombosis mechanism, which would occur under other conditions. The reduction of the levels of this protein activates the thrombosis of the small vessels of the trophoblastic villi and consequently the abnormal penetration of the trophoblast into the myometrium.

2. aPLs may reduce the levels of endogenous anticoagulant proteins C and S.

3. aPLs can bind to and activate endothelial cells. This results in the production of cellular inflammatory agents (VCAM-1, ICAMP1, E-selectin), which eventually attract monocytes to the area, which contribute to the production of clots and the apoptosis of endothelial cells.

4. Binding of aPLs to the cell membrane β2-glycoprotein-1 complex and phospholipids reduces the efficacy of this complex, as an anticoagulant.

5. Binding of aPLs to platelet cell membrane components, such as phosphatidylserine, results in their injury, which promotes their adhesion and activation of the prothrombotic chain. Finally, the activation of the complement seems to play an important role in the pathophysiological chain of events, which may be necessary in those processes that lead to fetal death or intrauterine growth retardation [14–18].

14. Diagnostic criteria

"APL profile" includes: the type of autoantibodies and the presence of 2–3 types of autoantibodies. The title of aPLs is mid-high instead of low and their persistent positivity is certified by multiple tests. APS is characterized by the following lab test results [19–22].

Persistent presence of antiphospholipid antibodies (at least 2 positive results during a period of >12 weeks) including lupus anticoagulant, anticardiolipin antibodies and b2-glycoprotein 1^{α} antibodies [19–22].

Risk factors: pregnancy, labour, contraceptives, malignancy, infection (E-coli, Shigella, Salmonella, Streptococcus, Staphylococcus etc), injury, surgical procedures, operations, fractures, drugs, no compliance to the anticoagulant therapy and many other factors [19–22].

15. Laboratory findings

Usually there is severe thrombocytopenia, positive direct Coombs, microangiopathic hemolytic anemia, DIC findings in some patients and the presence of a heterogeneous group of antiphospholipid antibodies.

Laboratory confirmation is done with clotting assays for the detection of lupus anticoagulant and with solid phase assays-Elisa for the detection of anti-cardiolipin and anti-β2 glycoprotein antibodies [19–24].

1. The positive ACA IgG, Wolf Anticoagulant, ANA, ds-DNA, ENA (Ro, La) etc. are a heterogeneous group of IgG/IgM antibodies directed against plasma proteins involved in coagulation cataract activation. They are attached to PLs of the outer membrane of cells. While these antibodies cause thrombosis in vivo, in vitro prolong phospholipid-dependent coagulation tests. Detection of lupus anticoagulant (coagulation tests – 3-step procedure) prolongs the phospholipid-dependent coagulation time. Lupus anticoagulant is considered positive when it is detected in at least one of the two methods with the following diagnostic criteria – steps:

15.1 The screening test

a. Screening procedure when prolongation is observed in at least one of the phospholipid-dependent coagulation methods

    - Activated partial thromboplastin time (aPTT),

    - Russel snake venom dilution time (dRVVT)

b. Mixing patient plasma 50:50 with normal plasma fails to correct prolonged screening test time

    - Confirmation of the presence of coagulation inhibitor and not the absence of coagulation factor mixing test: Proof that the prolongation is due to the presence of coagulation inhibitor.

c. The addition of extra phospholipids corrects the prolonged clotting time. Confirmation test: Evidence that this inhibitor is directed against phospholipids [19–24].

15.2 Anti-cardiolipin antibodies (aCL) (IgG-IgM)

Presence of antibodies against cardiolipin (aCL) – IgG moderately to strongly positive (>15–20GPL) – IgM(> 15 – 20MPL) moderate to strongly positive, but with the simultaneous presence of LA [19–24].

They are directed against epitopes resulting from modulatory changes in the β2GPI (domains-V) molecule after binding to cardiolipin. They are directed directly against cardiolipin (CL). They are associated with infections, syphilis, in healthy individuals and are not related to APS [19–24].

15.3 Antiβ2 GPI antibodies (IgG-IgM)

Antibodies against β2GPI (anti-β2GPI), β2-glycoproteinI (β2 GPI) natural anticoagulant plasma protein associated with negatively charged molecules: phospholipids, heparin, lipoproteins (oxLDL), activated PLTs/Ecs, apoptotic cell membranes.

They turn directly against β2-GPI and are a heterogeneous population that recognizes epitopes in different regions (I-V) of the protein.

Antigen: purified human β2GPI with tight adhesion to plates for low avidity binding of antibodies and detection of domain I in situ.

Anti-LA/β2GPIs are positively associated with a particularly increased risk of thromboembolic complications and detection with new methods offers new opportunities for risk assessment [19–22].

ELISA: αCL/β2GPI detects various antibody specificity es with relatively low clinical utility – their exclusion from the criteria has been widely discussed, they are still a diagnostic criterion but current screening guidelines should be followed faithfully [19–22].

aβ2GPI antibodies: correlate very well with the clinical manifestations of APS – They are positive in patients with thrombosis who have negative LA and aCLs.

If aPL title > 40 GPL or IU at least 2 times in 12 week interval then APS is diagnosed. The most important are Abs against β2GPI and against prothrombin which show LA activity. Lupus anticoagulant is part of the APS antibody spectrum, reacting in the liquid phase. In contrast, other aPLs such as anti-CL and anti-β2-glycoprotein (β2-GPI-1) antibodies are detected by solid-phase immunoassay. For the APS diagnosis it is necessary to use both solid phase methods and coagulation tests for LA [19–24].

16. Other aPLs

Prothrombin antibodies: They have good association with LA, use in seronegative APS.

Antibodies to Annexin V, II Associated with thrombosis in APS.

Proteins against protein C and S: Lower sensitivity and specificity than aCLs/IgG.

Antibodies against vimentin (anti-Vim/CL: Positive (55%) in seronegative SN-APS, their use needs documentation.

The diagnosis of the syndrome should be avoided when a period of <12 weeks or > 5 years separates the clinical from the laboratory characteristics (regardless of the most presented first) [24–26].

17. Secondary antibodies in APS

- IgA anticardiolipin antibodies

- anti-β2 glycoprotein I IgA antibodies

- antiphosphatidylserine antibodies
- anti-phosphatidylethanolamine antibodies
- anti-prothrombin antibodies
- antibodies against the phosphatidylserine-prothrombin complex

APLs are a very heterogeneous family of antibodies and more than 30 different antibodies have been reported in patients with APS called 'antibody burst'. Their positivity does not offer much in the absence of clinical findings although confirmation is necessary for the duration of the symptoms. Ultimately the history and clinical picture determine the treatment [24–28].

- Presence of positive lupus anticoagulant (LA) in plasma, in at least two tests with an interval of at least 12 weeks between them offers reliable criteria for diagnosis.
- Moderate presence of high title of anticardiolipin antibodies (aCL) IgG or IgM in serum or plasma (eg> 40 IgG phospholipid units-GPL/mL or IgM phospholipid units-MPL/mL or> 99th percentile) in at least two intervals between them for at least 12 weeks.
- Moderate presence of high titer anti-beta-2 glycoprotein I IgG or IgM antibodies in plasma or serum (> 99th percentile) in at least two tests with an interval of at least 12 weeks [19–26].
- Extension Activated partial thromboplastin time (aPTT)
- Falsely positive test for syphilis
- Low levels of total protein S
- Hemolytic anemia. It occurs quite frequently and is particularly associated with the presence of anticardiolipin IgM antibodies
- Thrombopenia. It is quite common in patients with APS (22% at diagnosis, 30% overall) and is associated with paradoxical thrombosis even with low platelet counts. It is of course possible that when their number is <50,000/μL there is a coexistence risk of bleeding, making the treatment of these patients particularly difficult and urgent.

Positive antinuclear antibodies are often found at low titers, without necessarily being associated with the presence of SLE [19–26].

Coagulation methods for detecting anticoagulant lupus are affected by oral anticoagulant therapy (coumarin, newer anticoagulants), but also by therapeutic doses of standard heparin. For this reason, testing should be done before starting or after cessation of these drugs. In contrast, administration of low molecular weight heparin in prophylactic doses of aspirin or clopidogrel does not appear to significantly affect the detection of anticoagulant lupus.

18. APS-pregnancy

18.1 Clinical findings

APS is diagnosed in up to 40% of women with a history of miscarriage, intrauterine fetal death (> 18th week of gestation) or placental vascular disease, ie preeclampsia, intrauterine fetal growth retardation, placental abruption. However, in a percentage of 50–60% the causes remain unclear [26–34].

18.2 Manifested clinically with

- recurrent vascular thrombosis (venous and/or arterial, and/or capillary), and/or with
- obstetric vascular complications:
- abortions <10th week of pregnancy
- delayed miscarriages
- endometrial death
- preeclampsia and/or eclampsia, or HELLP syndrome
- intrauterine growth restriction (IUGR) [26–38]

18.3 Obstetric antiphospholipid syndrome triggered in pregnancy

The findings of some studies raise the suspicion of a subtype triggered by gestational APS, with a transient increase in antiphospholipid antibodies only during pregnancy.

18.4 Pregnancy morbidity

The morbidity of pregnancy is certified by the following parameters:

1. ≥1 unexplained fetal death > 10th week (morphologically healthy fetus)
2. ≥1 preterm birth <34th week (preeclampsia or severe placental insufficiency)
3. ≥3 consecutive miscarriages <10th week after exclusion of other pathologies such as anatomical, hormonal, chromosomal abnormalities, history of thromboembolic episodes

   - at least 1 unexplained fetal death in the 2nd or 3rd quarter (> 10 W)
   - at least 1 birth at gestational age <34 W, due to preeclampsia or placental insufficiency

According to the International Consensus Criteria of 2006, any of these antibodies, if tested positive in at least two laboratory tests at least 12 weeks apart, in combination with a clinical thrombosis or obstetric complication, leads to the diagnosis of APS.

There must be at least one laboratory and one clinical criterion for the diagnosis of primary APS. Antiphospholipid antibodies are detected by the enzyme-linked immunosorbent assay (ELISA) in which the phospholipid cardiolipin is used as the antigen. It is actually a complex of cardiolipin with a serum protein called β2-glycoprotein I (β2-GPI). The above protein plays an inhibitory role in blood clotting, and when the complex binds to antiphospholipid antibodies, its effectiveness as an anticoagulant decreases [26–42].

Laboratory findings usually show high titers of IgG or IgM antibodies against cardiolipin or lupus anticoagulant, which must be detected in the same patient in two different samples taken at least 6 weeks apart. The above mechanism is due to the frequent recurrent thrombi that affect both the large and small vessels of the arterial or venous limb. In addition, mild cytopenia occurs quite often, which usually subsides with the end of pregnancy.

18.5 The diagnosis of the syndrome can be suspected in

Arterial or venous thrombosis.

Presence of anticardiolipin antibodies, IgG, IgM, Anti-beta2-GPI and Lupus anticoagulant [26–42].

Adverse outcomes of pregnancy.

APS can be diagnosed, if one or more of the clinical criteria and one or more of the laboratory criteria are met.

Although a causal association between obstetric complications and antibody detection is difficult to identified, however the lupus anticoagulant is the major predictor of labor adverse events including both mother and fetus. Although spontaneous abortions before the 10th week are relatively common in the general population, it seems that this risk is higher in patients with the syndrome. Fetal demise due to insufficient blood flow is most probably caused by placental insufficiency triggered by placental infarctions [26–42].

This placental insufficiency is likely to be associated with delayed intrauterine fetal development, severe preeclampsia, premature rupture of the membranes, premature placental abruption, and preterm fetal death (preterm and preterm death) in the 20th week of pregnancy, which usually has the worst outcome, as well as the increased risk of premature ejaculation [26–42].

Regarding the relationship of aPLs with preeclampsia, their detection seems valuable only in cases of severe preeclampsia before the 34th week of pregnancy. For cases of severe intrauterine fetal growth retardation, there are studies that report its relationship to the presence of antibodies, while other studies do not seem to reach this conclusion.

19. Discussion

The risk of miscarriage in women with antiphospholipid antibodies is higher from the 10th week of pregnancy onwards. But also in women with a history of six miscarriages before the 10th week of pregnancy, antiphospholipid antibodies are detected in rates of 10 to 20% without the presence of other clinical manifestations [42–44].

Pregnancy complications in women with APS are due to decreased placental perfusion based on local thrombosis, which is probably caused by the interaction of aPL with annexin V of the trophoblast resulting in inhibition of its anticoagulant activity. Other manifestations of aPL include thrombocytopenia (40–50%), hemolytic anemia (14–23%), renal disease that has only recently been recognized as a consequence of APS, and Liveto redicularis [42–48]. Female patients with APS and kidney disease from antiphospholipid antibodies typically have high blood pressure, which is an additional serious risk to their pregnancy and can lead to the complications mentioned above [42–48].

20. When will we check a patient for aPLs

1. Spontaneous venous thrombosis at age <45 years (deep vein thrombosis, pulmonary embolism)

2. Arterial thrombosis in a person <45 years of age (myocardial infarction), without risk factors

3. Recurrent pregnancy loss

4. Thrombosis and vascular diseases associated with SLE

5. Recurrent thrombocytopenia of unknown etiology

6. Neurological manifestations

7. Acquired heart valve disease

8. Liveto redicularis

9. Patients with a false positive RPR test

10. Prolongation of any coagulation test [42–54].

Finally, for the presence of antiphospholipid syndrome, women of reproductive age who have any of the following characteristics should be screened (other than those mentioned above): False positive test for syphilis, stroke and venous thrombosis without other predisposing prolongation of aPTT, SLE and autoimmune hemolytic anemia [48–58].

Of course, from the medical history of the pregnant woman should always be sought the episodes of venous thrombosis that are usually observed in the veins of the lower extremities, which are not necessarily accompanied by episodes of pulmonary embolism, but also in rarer localizations, such as the sphenoid sinuses of the skull and the small visceral vessels. Autoantibodies and microthrombotic mechanisms could affect the normal implantation, the trophoblasts' expansion and the development of effective fetoplacental circulation leading to abortions of the first trimester [48–58].

At older gestational ages endometrial death is attributed to massive placental thrombosis while the mechanisms associated with other complications (preeclampsia) are unknown. In terms of laboratory findings, moderate to high IgG or IgM antibodies to cardiolipin (20–50 GPL, 20–80 MPL respectively) or lupus anticoagulant should be detected [48–58].

Patients who present with clinical manifestations of APS could be permanently negative for the three main autoantibodies. Women with positive aPLs are more likely to have thromboembolic events, miscarriage or fetal death, intrauterine growth retardation, severe preeclampsia, and placental abruption. However, the presence of these antibodies cannot exclude the possibility of a successful pregnancy and/or estimate the risk of potential complications. The existence of a burdensome obstetric or pathological history seems to play a more important role, since the reporting of thrombotic episodes, SLE or fetal death is associated with a 40% chance of premature birth and a greater than 30% chance of intrauterine growth retardation. From the beginning of pregnancy until the 20th week, visits should be made every 15 days and then every week until delivery [52–60].

Ultrasound examination of fetal development, but also the evaluation of the amount of amniotic fluid, should begin in the 16th week and be repeated every month unless there is a pathological finding. There is evidence that bilateral presence of notches in the uterine arteries, on Doppler screening at 24 weeks, can detect with satisfactory sensitivity those patients who develop preeclampsia and IUGR if they have a positive lupus anticoagulant. The umbilical artery test with Doppler from the 26th week until childbirth offers great help, while for the same period of time a weekly cardiotocographic test (non-stress test) should be performed, as well as an ultrasound control of the amount of amniotic fluid. The most commonly used regimen involves the administration of aspirin (80 mg daily) and heparin, either crystalline or low molecular weight, in prophylactic doses [60–64].

The patient's health condition before pregnancy will determine the resumption of therapy after childbirth. Thus, two to three days after delivery, women taking coumarin derivatives before pregnancy (due to a history of a thromboembolic event) should discontinue heparin (after an INR of 2–2.5) and resume taking these drugs. To decrease the possibility of a new thromboembolic event, women with a thrombotic history during the late pregnancy should be treated with prophylactic doses of heparin or coumarin derivatives for 6 weeks postpartum. For women without a thrombotic history, the anticoagulant therapy could be continued for the first five postpartum days at most. Compared to conventional heparin, less complications were related to low molecular weight heparins. Regarding the duration of the treatment, some recommend the prophylactic administration until the completion of the 37th week, then proposing induction of labor and others the administration until the automatic onset of labor with the simultaneous administration of vitamin K antagonists.

Hyperimmune γ-globin is no longer recommended because there is no clear evidence of improved perinatal outcome. Coumarin is not administered particularly in the 1st and 3rd trimesters as potential teratogens and due to easy passage through the placenta coagulation disorders in the fetus and because they are associated with greater maternal morbidity. Their administration is indicated only in rare cases of contraindication to heparin or aspirin [60–68].

Complications of anticoagulant therapy in pregnancy include embryopathy (nasal hypoplasia, spotted epiphyses), CNS abnormalities (Dandy-Walker syndrome, visual atrophy), fetal bleeding, hemorrhagic manifestations, skin allergies, thrombocytopenia and osteoporosis [60–72].

The basic principles of APS treatment include the systematic monitoring of the pregnant woman, the continuous assessment of the condition of the fetus, the administration of medication and the selection of the most appropriate time and manner of delivery. Despite the lack of large cross investigations, the usual therapeutic directions includes the corticosteroids, the aspirin, heparin, hyperimmune gamma globulin and coumarins.

Treatment should be applied only when the risk of complications is considered to be higher and after a thorough discussion with the pregnant woman. The prognostic factors of poor outcome are the title of anticardiolipin antibodies and the obstetric history [60–72].

Aspirin significantly reduces the risk of thrombosis by blocking platelet aggregation. It is considered safe during pregnancy. Until now, there are no final conclusions regarding the efficacy of the above therapy as monotherapy. Hydroxychloroquine inhibits aPL-B2GPI complexes on phospholipid surfaces, annexin A5, TF tissue factor, TLPs *Toll-like receptors*, statins such as pravastatin inhibition of *Nuclear factor kappa B* (*NF-κB*) is protein transcription factor, *Anti-CD20* monoclonal antibodies (mAbs) resistant APS and aspirin are recommended to prevent and treat preeclampsia [60–72].

The choice of time and method of delivery depends mainly on the presence or absence of complications of the disease during pregnancy. In any case of intra-uterine suffocation of the fetus, induction of labor is required with all the possible harmful consequences of prematurity. In asymptomatic forms of the disease and when there are no signs of fetal difficulty, childbirth is preferred as much as possible at the end of pregnancy.

Worldwide, the route of delivery has been the subject of intense controversy and it is not clear if vaginal delivery or cesarean (c-)section is safer for the mother. Thus, prelabour c-section or vaginal delivery should be guided by obstetric criteria [60–72].

APS (primary or secondary) is a chronic systemic autoimmune disorder that mainly affects young women of childbearing age. APL can impair trophoblast function and can cause implantation failure by not allowing fusion of the cytotrophoblast and can also developing small thrombophilia increase abortion rate. Natural killer cells attach to the cytotrophoblast of the embryo. However, the mechanisms by which such cells may or may not affect the embryo is not proven. Moreover, after the implantation, there is a slight inflammatory response. Patient with recurrent miscarriages and infertility develop less prominent reaction that may prevent the fetus from implantation [72–74].

21. Conclusion

The effect of the syndrome on pregnancy is accompanied by a multitude of serious complications that significantly increase the rates of maternal and especially perinatal morbidity and mortality.

There is an urgent need to create a new laboratory method, which will detect with great sensitivity and specificity all antiphospholipid antibodies and for this purpose large multicenter studies are already being done, the results of which are awaited.

Acknowledgements

I would like to warmly thank Ms. Dr. Lefkou Eleftheria and Associate Professor Panagiotis Skendros, who with their vast experience and valuable help and guidance on resolving various problems related to antiphospholipidemic syndrome contributed significantly to complete the background of the chapter.

Author details

Panagiotis Tsikouras[1*], Christina Tsiggalou[2], Anastasia Bothou[1], Aggeliki Gerede[1], Ifigenia Apostolou[3], Fotini Gaitatzi[1], Anna Chalkidou[1], Xanthoula Anthoulaki[1], Spyridon Michalopoulos[1], Georgios Dragoutsos[1], Ioannis Tsirkas[1], Irini Babageorgaka[1], Theopi Nalbanti[1], Natalia Sachnova[1], Alexios Alexiou[1], Konstantinos Nikolettos[1], Christos Tsalikidis[4], Stefanos Zervoudis[4], Panagiotis Peitsidis[1,5] and Nikolaos Nikolettos[1]

1 Department of Obstetrics and Gynecology, Democritus University of Thrace Medical School, Alexandroupolis, Greece

2 Department of Laboratory, Democritus University of Thrace Medical School, Alexandroupolis, Greece

3 Neonatal Intensive Unit Care, University Hospital of Thrace Medical School, Alexandroupolis, Greece

4 Second Department of Surgery University Hospital of Thrace Medical School, Alexandroupolis, Greece

5 Technological Educational Institute of Athens and Rea Maternity Hospital, Athens, Greece

*Address all correspondence to: tsikouraspanagiotis@gmail.com

References

[1] S Miyakis, M D Lockshin, T Atsumi, D W Branch, R L Brey, R Cervera, et al. International consensus statement on an update of the classification criteria for definite antiphospholipid syndrome (APS) J Thromb Haemost Feb;4(2):295-306. 2006 PMID: 16420554. DOI:10. 1111/j.1538-7836.2006.01753.x

[2] Kaul M, Erkan D, Sammaritano L, Lockshin MD. Assessment of the 2006 revised antiphospholipid syndrome classification criteria. Ann Rheum Dis. 2007 Jul;66(7):927-30. DOI:10.1136/ ard.2006.067314. Epub 2007 Mar 2. PMID: 17337473 Free PMC article

[3] Cervera R, Tektonidou MG, Espinosa G, Cabral AR, González EB, Erkan D, et al. Task force on catastrophic Antiphospholipid syndrome (APS) and non-criteria APS manifestations (II): Thrombocytopenia and skin manifestations. Lupus. 2011 Feb;20(2):174-181. DOI:10.1177/ 0961203310395052. PMID: 21303834

[4] Pourrat O, Jollit C, Gombert JM, Boinot C, Pierre F clinical relevance of the recent update of the classification criteria for definite antiphospholipid syndrome: An obstetric medicine clinic series of 107 patients. J Thromb Haemost. 2006 Oct;4(10):2276-2277. DOI:10.1111/j.1538-7836.2006.02142.x. Epub 2006 Jul 26. PMID: 16869832

[5] Gómez-Puerta JA, Cervera R. Diagnosis and classification of the antiphospholipid syndrome. J Autoimmun. 2014 Feb-Mar;48-49:20-5. DOI:10.1016/j.jaut.2014.01.006. Epub 2014 Jan 24. PMID: 24461539 Review.

[6] Bart PA When should consider antiphospholipid syndrome?. Rev Med Suisse. 2008 Jan 16;4(140):97-9. PMID: 18309870 Review

[7] Cohen H, Cuadrado MJ, Erkan D, Duarte-Garcia A, Isenberg DA, Knight JS, et al. 16th international congress on Antiphospholipid antibodies task force report on Antiphospholipid syndrome treatment trends. Lupus. 2020 Oct;29(12):1571-1593. DOI:10.1177/0961203320950461. PMID: 33100166

[8] Maria G Tektonidou, Laura Andreoli, Marteen limper, Zahir Amoura, Ricard Cervera, Nathalie Costedoat-chalumeau, et al. EULAR recommendations for the management of antiphospholipid syndrome in adults PMID: 31092409, DOI:10.1136/ annrheumdis-2019-215213 Ann Rheum Dis 2019 Oct;78(10):1296-1304.

[9] Cervera R, Bucciarelli S, Espinosa G, Gómez-Puerta JA, Ramos-Casals M, Shoenfeld Y, et al. Catastrophic antiphospholipid syndrome: lessons from the "CAPS Registry"--a tribute to the late Josep Font. Ann N Y Acad Sci. 2007 Jun;1108:448-56. DOI:10.1196/ annals.1422.047. PMID: 17894009 Review

[10] Grenn RC, Yalavarthi S, Gandhi AA, Kazzaz NM, Núñez-Álvarez C, Hernández-Ramírez D, et al. Endothelial progenitor dysfunction associates with a type I interferon signature in primary antiphospholipid syndrome. Ann Rheum Dis. 2017 Feb;76(2):450-457. DOI:10.1136/ annrheumdis-2016-209442. Epub 2016 Jul 18. PMID: 27432357

[11] E Svenungsson, A Antovic the antiphospholipid syndrome – Often overlooked cause of vascular occlusions? J Intern Med. 2020 Apr;287(4):349-372. DOI:10.1111/joim.13022. Epub 2020 Feb 11.

[12] Pier Luigi Meroni, Cecilia Beatrice Chighizola, Francesca Rovelli, Maria Gerosa Antiphospholipid syndrome in 2014: more clinical manifestations, novel pathogenic players and emerging

biomarkers Arthritis Res Ther 2014;16(2):209. DOI:10.1186/ar4549. PMID: 25166960 PMCID: PMC4060447 DOI:10.1186/ar4549

[13] Amelia Ruffatti, Marta Tonello, Teresa Del Ross, Anna Cavazzana, Chiara Grava, Franco Noventa, et al. Antibody profile and clinical course in primary antiphospholipid syndrome with pregnancy morbidity Thromb Haemost. 2006 Sep;96(3):337-341. DOI:10.1160/TH06-05-0287. PMID: 16953276 DOI:10.1160/TH06-05-0287

[14] Skjeflo EW, Christiansen D, Fure H, Ludviksen JK, Woodruff TM, Espevik T, et al. TE Staphylococcus aureus-induced complement activation promotes tissue factor-mediated coagulation. J Thromb Haemost. 2018 May;16(5):905-918. DOI:10.1111/jth.13979. Epub 2018 Mar 23. PMID: 29437288

[15] Stevens MG, Van Poucke M, Peelman LJ, Rainard P, De Spiegeleer B, Rogiers C, et al. Anaphylatoxin C5a-induced toll-like receptor 4 signaling in bovine neutrophils. J Dairy Sci. 2011 Jan;94(1):152-164. DOI:10.3168/jds.2010-3358. PMID: 21183027

[16] Redecha P, Tilley R, Tencati M, Salmon JE, Kirchhofer D, Mackman N, et al. Tissue factor: a link between C5a and neutrophil activation in antiphospholipid antibody induced fetal injury. Blood. 2007 Oct 1;110(7):2423-31. DOI:10.1182/blood-2007-01-070631. Epub 2007 May 29. PMID: 17536017 Free PMC article.

[17] Samarkos M, Mylona E, Kapsimali V.The role of complement in the antiphospholipid syndrome: A novel mechanism for pregnancy morbidity. Semin Arthritis Rheum. 2012 Aug;42(1):66-69. DOI:10.1016/j.semarthrit.2012.01.001. Epub 2012 Mar 8. PMID: 22405029

[18] Guo RF, Riedemann NC, Ward PA Role of C5a-C5aR interaction in sepsis. Shock. 2004 Jan;21(1):1-7. DOI:10.1097/01.shk.0000105502.75189.5e. PMID: 14676676 Review.

[19] Pengo V, Bison E, Denas G, Jose SP, Zoppellaro G, Banzato A. Semin Laboratory Diagnostics of Antiphospholipid Syndrome. Thromb Hemost. 2018 Jul;44(5):439-444. DOI:10.1055/s-0037-1601331. Epub 2017 May 3. PMID: 28470652 Review

[20] Pengo V, Denas G. Diagnostics and treatment of thrombotic antiphospholipid syndrome (APS): A personal perspective. Thromb Res. 2018 Sep;169:35-40. DOI:10.1016/j.thromres.2018.07.011. Epub 2018 Jul 7. PMID: 30007134 Review

[21] Pengo V, Denas G, Zoppellaro G, Jose SP, Hoxha A, Ruffatti A, et al. Rivaroxaban vs warfarin in high-risk patients with antiphospholipid syndrome. Blood. 2018 Sep 27;132(13):1365-1371. DOI:10.1182/blood-2018-04-848333. Epub 2018 Jul 12. PMID: 30002145 Clinical Trial

[22] Pengo V, Del Ross T, Ruffatti A, Bison E, Cattini MG, Pontara E, et al. G. Lupus anticoagulant identifies two distinct groups of patients with different antibody patterns. Thromb Res. 2018 Dec;172:172-178. DOI:10.1016/j.thromres.2018.11.003. Epub 2018 Nov 9. PMID: 30466070

[23] Roberta Misasi, Antonella Capozzi, Agostina Longo, Serena Recalchi, Emanuela Lococo1, Cristiano Alessandri, et al. "New" antigenic targets and methodological approaches for refining laboratory diagnosis of antiphospholipid syndrome J Immunol Research 2015 2015:858542. DOI:10.1155/2015/858542. Epub 2015 Mar 19. PMID: 25874238 PMCID: PMC4383493 DOI:10.1155/2015/858542

[24] Elena Ortona, Antonella Capozzi, Tania Colasanti, Fabrizio Conti,

Cristiano Alessandri, Agostina Longo, et al. Vimentin/cardiolipin complex as a new antigenic target of the antiphospholipid syndrome Blood 2010 Oct 21;116(16):2960-7. DOI:10.1182/blood-2010-04-279208. Epub 2010 Jul 15. PMID: 20634382 DOI:10.1182/blood-2010-04-279208

[25] Silvia S Pierangeli, Emmanuel J Favaloro, Gabriella Lakos, Pier Luigi Meroni, Angela Tincani, Richard C W Wong et al. Standards and reference materials for the anticardiolipin and anti-β2glycoprotein I assays: a report of recommendations from the APL Task Force at the 13th International Congress on Antiphospholipid Antibodies Clin Chim Acta 2012 Jan 18;413(1-2):358-60.DOI:10.1016/j.cca.2011.09.048. Epub 2011 Oct 15,PMID: 22019907 DOI:10.1016/j.cca.2011.09.048

[26] Pier Luigi Meroni, Martina Biggioggero, Silvia S Pierangeli, Joanna Sheldon, Ingrid Zegers, Maria Orietta Borghi Standardization of autoantibody testing: a paradigm for serology in rheumatic diseases Nat Rev Rheumatol 2014 Jan;10(1):35-43. DOI:10.1038/nrrheum.2013.180. Epub 2013 Nov 26. PMID: 24275965 DOI

[27] Thomas Sailer, Claudia Zoghlami, Christine Kurz, Helmut Rumpold, Peter Quehenberger, Simon Panzer, et al. Anti-beta2-glycoprotein I antibodies are associated with pregnancy loss in women with the lupus anticoagulant Thromb Haemost 2006 May;95(5):796-801. PMID: 16676070

[28] Yu CK, Papageorghiou AT, Parra M, Palma Dias R, Nicolaides KH; Fetal Medicine Foundation second trimester screening group. Randomized controlled trial using low-dose aspirin in the prevention of pre-eclampsia in women with abnormal uterine artery Doppler at 23 weeks' gestation. PMID: 12942493 Ultrasound Obstet Gynecol 2003;22:233-9.

[29] Rolnik DL, Wright D, Poon LC, O'Gorman N, Syngelaki A, de Paco Matallana C, et al. Aspirin versus Placebo in Pregnancies at High Risk for Preterm Preeclampsia. N Engl J Med. 2017 Jun 28 PMID: 28657417 DOI:10.1056/NEJMoa1704559

[30] Trapani A Jr, Gonçalves LF, Pires MM. Transdermal nitroglycerin in patients with severe pre-eclampsia with placental insufficiency: Effect on uterine, umbilical and fetal middle cerebral artery resistance indices. Ultrasound in Obstetrics & Gynecology. 2011;38(4):389-394 PMID: 21374750 DOI:10.1002/uog.8983

[31] Groten T, Fitzgerald n T, Schneider U, Kähler C, et al. OS013. Reduction of preeclampsia related complications with the NO-donor penterythriltetranitrat (petn) in risk pregnancies—A prospective randomized double-blind placebo pilot study. Pregnancy Hypertension. 2012;2: 181 PMID: 26105227

[32] E E Camarena Pulido, L García Benavides, J G Panduro Barón, S Pascoe Gonzalez, A J Madrigal Saray, F E García Padilla, S E Totsuka Sutto Efficacy of L-arginine for preventing preeclampsia in high-risk pregnancies: A double-blind, randomized, clinical trial Hypertens Pregnancy 2016 May;35(2):217-25. DOI:10.3109/10641955.2015.1137586. Epub 2016 Mar 22. PMID: 27003763

[33] Belinda Jim1, S Ananth Karumanchi 2 Preeclampsia: Pathogenesis, Prevention, and Long-Term Complications PMID: 28711078 DOI:10.1016/j.semnephrol.2017.05.011

[34] Thadhani R, Kisner T, Hagmann H, Bossung V, Noack S, Schaarschmidt W, Jank A, et al. Pilot study of extracorporeal removal of soluble fms-like tyrosine kinase 1 in preeclampsia. Circulation. 2011 Aug 23;124(8):940-950. DOI:10.1161/

CIRCULATIONAHA.111.034793. Epub 2011 Aug 1. PMID: 21810665

[35] Collaboration to Understand Complex Diseases: Preeclampsia and Adverse Pregnancy Outcomes. Roberts JM, Mascalzoni D, Ness RB, Poston L; Global Pregnancy Collaboration. Hypertension. 2016 Apr;67(4):681-7. DOI:10.1161/HYPERTENSIONAHA.115.06133. Epub 2016 Feb 16. PMID: 26883267 Review.

[36] Nariaki Kokuho1, Yasuhiro Terasaki2, Shinobu Kunugi3, Naomi Onda4, Hirokazu Urushiyama3, Mika Terasaki3, et al. Localized pulmonary crystal-storing histiocytosis complicating pulmonary mucosa-associated lymphoid tissue lymphoma presenting with multiple mass lesions Hum Pathol 2017 Jul;65:180-186. DOI:10.1016/j.humpath.2016.10.028. Epub 2017 Feb 21. PMID: 28232159

[37] Alessia Leone 1, Massimo Radin 2, Ahlam M Almarzooqi 3, Jamal Al-Saleh 3, Dario Roccatello 4, Savino Sciascia 5, Munther Khamashta 6 Autologous hematopoietic stem cell transplantation in Systemic Lupus Erythematosus and antiphospholipid syndrome: A systematic review Autoimmun Rev 2017 May;16(5):469-477. DOI:10.1016/j.autrev.2017.03.008. Epub 2017 Mar 7. PMID: 28279836

[38] Spradley FT Metabolic abnormalities and obesity's impact on the risk for developing preeclampsia. Am J Physiol Regul Integr Comp Physiol. 2017 Jan 1;312(1):R5-R12. DOI:10.1152/ajpregu.00440.2016. Epub 2016 Nov 30. PMID: 27903516

[39] Patricia Redecha 1, Claus-Werner Franzke, Wolfram Ruf, Nigel Mackman, Guillermina Girardi Neutrophil activation by the tissue factor/Factor VIIa/PAR2 axis mediates fetal death in a mouse model of antiphospholipid syndrome J Clin Invest 2008 Oct;118(10):3453-61. PMID: 18802482 PMCID: PMC2542852 DOI:10.1172/JCI36089

[40] Abdulwahab Ahmed 1, Jameel Singh, Ysodra Khan, Surya V Seshan, Guillermina Girardi A new mouse model to explore therapies for preeclampsia PLoS One 2010 Oct 27;5(10):e13663. PMID: 21048973 PMCID: PMC2965104 DOI:10.1371/journal.pone.0013663

[41] Bauer AJ, Banek CT, Needham K, Gillham H, Capoccia S, Regal JF, Gilbert JS. Pravastatin attenuates hypertension, oxidative stress, and angiogenic imbalance in rat model of placental ischemia-induced hypertension. Hypertension. 2013 May;61(5):1103-1110. DOI:10.1161/HYPERTENSIONAHA.111.00226. Epub 2013 Mar 4. PMID: 23460290

[42] Eleftheria Lefkou, Apostolos Mamopoulos, Themistoklis Dagklis, Christos Vosnakis, David Rousso, Guillermina Girardi Pravastatin improves pregnancy outcomes in obstetric antiphospholipid syndrome refractory to antithrombotic therapy J Clin Invest 2016 Aug 1;126(8):2933-40. DOI:10.1172/JCI86957. Epub 2016 Jul 25. PMID: 27454295 PMCID: PMC4966313

[43] Brian T Bateman, Sonia Hernandez-Diaz, Michael A Fischer, Ellen W Seely, Jeffrey L Ecker, Jessica M Franklin, et al. Statins and congenital malformations: cohort study BMJ 2015 Mar 17;350:h1035. DOI:10.1136/bmj.h1035. PMID: 25784688 PMCID: PMC4362473

[44] Maged M Costantine, Kirsten Cleary, Mary F Hebert, Mahmoud S Ahmed, Linda M Brown, National Institute of Child Health and Human Development Obstetric-Fetal Pharmacology Research Units Network Safety and pharmacokinetics of pravastatin used for the prevention of preeclampsia in high-risk pregnant women: a pilot randomized controlled trial Am J Obstet Gynecol 2016

Jun;214(6):720.e1-720.e17. DOI:10.1016/j.ajog.2015.12.038. Epub 2015 Dec 23. PMID: 26723196,PMCID: PMC4884459, DOI:10.1016/j.ajog.2015.12.038

[45] Alissa R Carver, Esther Tamayo, J Regino Perez-polo, George R Saade, Gary D V Hankins, Maged M Costantine the effect of maternal pravastatin therapy on adverse sensorimotor outcomes of the offspring in a murine model of preeclampsia Int J Dev Neurosci 2014 Apr;33:33-40. DOI:10.1016/j.ijdevneu.2013.11.004. Epub 2013 Nov 25. PMID: 24287098

[46] Garcia D, Erkan D. Diagnosis and Management of the Antiphospholipid Syndrome. N Engl J Med. 2018 May 24;378(21):2010-2021. DOI:10.1056/NEJMra1705454. PMID: 29791828 Review.

[47] Garcia D, Erkan D. Diagnosis and Management of the Antiphospholipid Syndrome. N Engl J Med. 2018 Sep 27;379(13):1290. DOI:10.1056/NEJMc1808253. PMID: 30257161

[48] Ricarte IF, Dutra LA, Abrantes FF, Toso FF, Barsottini OGP, Silva GS, de Souza AWS, Andrade D. Neurologic manifestations of antiphospholipid syndrome. Lupus. 2018 Aug;27(9):1404-1414. DOI:10.1177/0961203318776110. Epub 2018 May 17. PMID: 29768970

[49] Boura P, Tselios K, Skendros P, Kountouras J. Antiphospholipid syndrome in Greece: Clinical and immunological study and review of the literature. Angiology. 2004 Jul-Aug;55(4):421-430. DOI:10.1177/000331970405500409. PMID: 15258688

[50] Pasquale Pignatelli, Evaristo Ettorre, Danilo Menichelli, Arianna Pani, Francesco Violi, Daniele Pastori Seronegative antiphospholipid syndrome: refining the value of "non-criteria" antibodies for diagnosis and clinical management Haematologica 2020 Mar;105(3):562-572. DOI:10.3324/haematol.2019.221945. Epub 2020 Jan 30. PMID: 32001534 PMCID: PMC7049333

[51] Matsuura E, Shen L, Matsunami Y, Quan N, Makarova M, Geske FJ, et al. Pathophysiology of beta2-glycoprotein I in antiphospholipid syndrome. Lupus. 2010 Apr;19(4):379-84. DOI:10.1177/0961203310361352. PMID: 20353973 Review.

[52] Gioulia Romanidou, Theocharis G Konstantinidis, Odysseas Koutsogiannis, Anastasia Grapsa, Christina Tsigalou Study of Antiphospholipid Antibodies in Patients with Arterial Hypertension Med Sci (Basel) 2018 Nov 13;6(4):102. DOI:10.3390/medsci6040102. PMID: 30428599 PMCID: PMC6313595

[53] Boura P, Papadopoulos S, Tselios K, Skendros P, Dioritou O, Malamis G, Makris P, Lefkos N. Intracerebral hemorrhage in a patient with SLE and catastrophic antiphospholipid syndrome (CAPS): Report of a case. Clin Rheumatol. 2005 Aug;24(4):420-424. DOI:10.1007/s10067-004-1062-9. Epub 2005 May 24. PMID: 15912267

[54] Alijotas-Reig J, Esteve-Valverde E, Ferrer-Oliveras R, Sáez-Comet L, Lefkou E, A, Farran-Codina I; EUROAPS study GroupThe European registry on obstetric Antiphospholipid syndrome (EUROAPS): A survey of 1000 consecutive cases. Autoimmun Rev. 2019 Apr;18(4):406-414. DOI:10.1016/j.autrev.2018.12.006. PMID: 30772493

[55] Alijotas-Reig J, Esteve-Valverde E, Ferrer-Oliveras R, LLurba E, Lefkou E, EUROAPS Study Group. Comparative study between obstetric antiphospholipid syndrome and obstetric morbidity related with antiphospholipid antibodies. Med Clin (Barc). 2018 Sep 21;151(6):215-222.

DOI:10.1016/j.medcli.2017.11.017. Epub 2017 Dec 20. PMID: 29274674 English, Spanish.

[56] Cyprian F, Lefkou E, Varoudi K, Girardi G. Immunomodulatory effects of vitamin D in pregnancy and beyond. Front Immunol. 2019 Nov 22;10:2739. DOI:10.3389/fimmu.2019.02739. PMID: 31824513

[57] Alijotas-Reig J, Esteve-Valverde E, Ferrer-Oliveras R, Sáez-Comet L, Lefkou E, Farran-Codina I; Comparative study of obstetric antiphospholipid syndrome (OAPS) and non-criteria obstetric APS (NC-OAPS): Report of 1640 cases from the EUROAPS registry. EUROAPS study group. Rheumatology (Oxford). 2020 Jun 1;59(6):1306-1314. DOI:10.1093/rheumatology/kez419. PMID: 31580459

[58] Alijotas-Reig J, Ferrer-Oliveras R, Ruffatti A, Tincani A, Lefkou E, Farran-Codina I; The European Registry on Obstetric Antiphospholipid Syndrome (EUROAPS): A survey of 247 consecutive cases. (EUROAPS Study Group Collaborators). Autoimmun Rev. 2015 May;14(5):387-95. DOI:10.1016/j.autrev.2014.12.010. Epub 2014 Dec 31. PMID: 25555817 Review.

[59] Alijotas-Reig J, Ferrer-Oliveras R, Esteve-Valverde E, Ruffatti A, Lefkou E, EUROAPS study group. Inherited thrombophilia in women with poor aPL-related obstetric history: Prevalence and outcomes. Survey of 208 cases from the European registry on obstetric Antiphospholipid syndrome cohort. Am J Reprod Immunol. 2016 Aug;76(2):164-171. DOI:10.1111/aji.12534. PMID: 27401589

[60] Alijotas-Reig J, Ferrer-Oliveras R; EUROAPS Study Group. The European registry on obstetric Antiphospholipid syndrome (EUROAPS): A preliminary first year report. Lupus. 2012 Jun;21(7):766-768. DOI:10.1177/0961203312440058. PMID: 22635227

[61] Lefkou E, Mamopoulos A, Fragakis N, Dagklis T, Vosnakis C, Nounopoulos E, Rousso D, Girardi G. Clinical improvement and successful pregnancy in a preeclamptic patient with antiphospholipid syndrome treated with pravastatin. Hypertension. 2014 May;63(5):e118-e119. DOI:10.1161/HYPERTENSIONAHA.114.03115. PMID: 24591337

[62] Lefkou E, Varoudi K, Pombo J, Jurisic A, Jurisic Z, Contento G, Girardi G.Triple therapy with pravastatin, low molecular weight heparin and low dose aspirin improves placental haemodynamics and pregnancy outcomes in obstetric antiphospholipid syndrome in mice and women through a nitric oxide-dependent mechanism. Biochem Pharmacol. 2020 Dec;182:114217. DOI:10.1016/j.bcp.2020.114217. Epub 2020 Sep 12. PMID: 32926874

[63] Sircar M, Thadhani R, Karumanchi SA. Pathogenesis of preeclampsia.Curr Opin Nephrol Hypertens. 2015 Mar;24(2):131-8. DOI:10.1097/MNH.0000000000000105. PMID: 25636145 Review

[64] Astrid Bergmann, Shakil Ahmad, Melissa Cudmore, Achim D Gruber, Petra Wittschen, Werner Lindenmaier, et al. Reduction of circulating soluble Flt-1 alleviates preeclampsia-like symptoms in a mouse model J Cell Mol Med.2010 Jun;14(6B):1857-1867. DOI:10.1111/j.1582-4934.2009.00820.x. Epub 2009 Jun 16. PMID: 19538465

[65] Kenji Onda, Stephen Tong, Sally Beard, Natalie Binder, Masanaga Muto, Sevvandi N Senadheera,et al. Proton Pump Inhibitors Decrease Soluble fms-Like Tyrosine Kinase-1 and Soluble Endoglin Secretion, Decrease Hypertension, and Rescue Endothelial Dysfunction Hypertension 2017 Mar;69(3):457-468. doi10.1161/HYPERTENSIONAHA.116.08408. Epub 2017 Jan 23.PMID: 28115513

[66] Saleh L, van den Meiracker AH, Geensen R, Kaya A, Roeters van Lennep JE, Duvekot JJ, et al. soluble fms-like tyrosine kinase-1 and placental growth factor kinetics during and after pregnancy in women with suspected or confirmed pre-eclampsia. Ultrasound Obstet Gynecol. 2018 Jun;51(6):751-757. DOI:10.1002/uog.17547. Epub 2018 May 6. PMID: 28600845

[67] Anton A Turanov, Agnes Lo, Matthew R Hassler, Angela Makris, Ami Ashar-Patel, Julia F Alterman,et al. RNAi modulation of placental sFLT1 for the treatment of preeclampsia Nat Biotechnol 2018 Nov 19;10.1038/nbt.4297.DOI:10.1038/nbt.4297. Online ahead of print. PMID: 30451990 PMCID: PMC6526074

[68] Zhihe Li, Ying Zhang, Jing Ying Ma, Ann M Kapoun, Qiming Shao, Irene Kerr,et al. Recombinant vascular endothelial growth factor 121 attenuates hypertension and improves kidney damage in a rat model of preeclampsia Hypertension 2007 Oct;50(4):686-692. DOI:10.1161/HYPERTENSIONAHA.107.092098. PMID: 17724276

[69] Rokosh RS, Ranganath N, Yau P, Rockman C, Sadek M, Berland T, et al. High prevalence and mortality associated with upper extremity deep venous thrombosis in hospitalized patients at a tertiary care Center. Ann Vasc Surg. 2020 May;65:55-65. DOI:10.1016/j.avsg.2019.10.055. Epub 2019 Oct 24. PMID: 31669473

[70] Ly S, Echeverria D, Sousa J, Khvorova A. Single-Stranded Phosphorothioated Regions Enhance Cellular Uptake of Cholesterol-Conjugated siRNA but Not Silencing Efficacy. Mol Ther Nucleic Acids. 2020 Sep 4;21:991-1005. DOI:10.1016/j.omtn.2020.07.029. Epub 2020 Jul 25. PMID: 32818923 Free PMC article.

[71] Albrecht ED, Pepe GJ. Regulation of Uterine Spiral Artery Remodeling: a Review. Reprod Sci. 2020 Oct;27(10):1932-1942. DOI:10.1007/s43032-020-00212-8. Epub 2020 Jun 16. PMID: 32548805 Free PMC article. Review.

[72] Li L, Yang H, Chen P, Xin T, Zhou Q, Wei D, et al. Trophoblast-Targeted Nanomedicine Modulates Placental sFLT1 for Preeclampsia Treatment. Front Bioeng Biotechnol. 2020 Feb 11;8:64. DOI:10.3389/fbioe.2020.00064. eCollection 2020. PMID: 32117942 Free PMC article.

[73] Ribeiro M, Furtado M, Martins S, Carvalho T, Carmo-Fonseca M • RNA Splicing Defects in Hypertrophic Cardiomyopathy: Implications for Diagnosis and Therapy. Int J Mol Sci. 2020 Feb 16;21(4):1329. DOI:10.3390/ijms21041329. PMID: 32079122 Free PMC article. Review.

[74] Chen Y, Ding H, Wei M, Zha W, Guan S, Liu N,et al. MSC-secreted Exosomal H19 promotes Trophoblast cell invasion and migration by Downregulating let-7b and Upregulating FOXO1. Mol Ther Nucleic Acids. 2020 Mar 6;19:1237-1249. DOI:10.1016/j.omtn.2019.11.031. Epub 2019 Dec 6. PMID: 32069774

Section 6

Miscellaneous Inflammatory Diseases

Chapter 14

Non-Allergic Rhinitis

Erkan Yildiz

Abstract

Non-allergic rhinitis is a term used for situations where no allergen can be detected as the cause of rhinitis. In non-allergic rhinitis; Skin test positivity or specific Ig E response cannot be detected. The pathophysiology of nonallergic rhinitis (NAR) is heterogeneous. The most common type is vasomotor rhinitis, also called idiopathic. In addition, there are many types such as hormonal, gustatory, occupational, atrophic, cold air-induced and systemic diseases. Patients; They present with symptoms such as nasal congestion, runny nose, sneezing, and itching in the nose, the symptoms of the patients do not show a seasonal pattern. There are family stories, but they are not as common as allergic rhinitis (AR). An underlying factor such as infection, sinusitis or polyps cannot be detected in patients. It was determined that the patients showed more neurogenic abnormalities in the pathophysiology. These patients have been shown to be hypersensitive to substances with ingredients such as cold air or capsaicin. The diagnosis is made clinically, the onset of the disease is in adolescence. Oral/nasal antihistamines, steroids, leukotriene antagonists are used in the treatment.

Keywords: non-allergic rhinitis, IgE, vasomotor rhinitis, eosinophilic nonallergic rhinitis, rhinitis medicomentosa

1. Introduction

1.1 Non-allergic rhinitis

Non-allergic rhinitis is a term used for situations where no allergen can be detected as the cause of rhinitis. Non-allergic rhinitis occurs in approximately one third of allergic rhinitis. Affects 22 million people (7% of the population) in the USA [1]. In non-allergic rhinitis; Skin test positivity or specific Ig E response cannot be detected. The pathophysiology of nonallergic rhinitis (NAR) is heterogeneous [2]. The most common type is vasomotor rhinitis, also called idiopathic. In addition, there are many types such as hormonal, gustatory, occupational, atrophic, cold air-induced and systemic diseases [3]. Patients; They present with symptoms such as nasal congestion, runny nose, sneezing, and itching in the nose, the symptoms of the patients do not show a seasonal pattern. There are family stories, but they are not as common as allergic rhinitis (AR). An underlying factor such as infection, sinusitis or polyps cannot be detected in patients. It was determined that the patients showed more neurogenic abnormalities in the pathophysiology. These patients have been shown to be hypersensitive to substances with ingredients such as cold air or capsaicin. The diagnosis is made clinically, the onset of the disease is in adolescence [4].

IntechOpen

2. Pathophysiology

Non-Allergic rhinitis occurs due to non-IgE mediated mechanisms. Prostaglandins, leukotrienes are found in both the upper and lower airways. These cause mast cell secretion, eosinophils, after exposure to the allergen in rhinitis. Prostaglandins and leukotrienes released from mast cells cause vasodilatation and hypersecretion from the gland, leading to rhinitis symptoms. Although this mechanism is not fully active in non-allergic rhinitis, symptoms occur with a similar effect [5].

3. Vasomotor rhinitis

Vasomotor rhinitis; It constitutes the most important part of rhinitis in the definition of non-allergic rhinitis. Its other name is known as non-allergic rhinopathy. It occurs as a result of impaired vasomotor balance in the nose. There is a loop in the form of sympathetic/parasympathetic innervation in the nose. This cycle is disrupted due to reasons such as exercise, cold, stress, insufficient thyroid functions, pregnancy, excessive or prolonged use of some blood pressure drugs, birth control pills and decongestant drugs. At the beginning of all these reasons, nasal congestion is temporary and reversible. So if the cause is removed, the disease will improve. In addition, if it lasts long enough, this time the blood vessels will lose their elasticity and the event turns into an irreversible situation. Metabolic (Acromegaly, Pregnancy, Hypothyroidism), Autoimmune (Sjogren's syndrome SLE Relapsing polychondritis Churg-Straus),Granulomatous diseases (Sarcoidosis and Wegener's granulomatosis), Other (Cystic fibrosis, Cilia dyskinesia syndromes, Immunodeficiency, Amyloidosis, Chronic fatigue syndrome) are the most common causes of NAR [6].

4. Gustatuar rhinitis

Typically, it starts after consuming hot or spicy food and alcohol. It starts with a food allergy or an unknown mechanism and continues with profuse rhinorrhea. Ipratropium bromide is used in the treatment [7].

5. Occupational rhinitis

Occupationally allergic and non-allergic can occur. There are four types. The first is an uncomfortable rhinitis without inflammation in the nose caused by smell. The second type is rhinitis that is caused by irritant and causes inflammation in the mucosa. The third type is corrosive rhinitis that occurs due to high concentration of chemicals in the nasal mucosa. Ammonia etc. occurs with inhalation of substances. The fourth type is rhinitis, which causes Ig E due to occupational exposure. Latex allergy in healthcare workers depends on this. Nasal saline irrigation solutions, nasal steroids and antihistamines are used in the treatment of this rhinitis [8] (**Table 1**).

6. Hormonal rhinitis

It is divided into two as gestational rhinitis induced by the menstrual cycle. Gestational rhinitis begins in the second trimester of pregnancy and continues until the second week of postpartum. It is related to pregnancy in another form of hormonal rhinitis. This can start in any week of pregnancy. Nasal saline irrigation is used in the treatment. In addition, they can benefit from the tapes used for the

Drugs	Usage areas	Side effects
Antihistaminics	Sneezing, runny nose, itchy nose	Anti-cholinergic side effects such as dryness of mucosal membranes, urinary retention, constipation, tachycardia, decreased visual acuity; Central side effects such as attention deficit and sleep
Steroids (Oral prednisolone, methylprednisolone, nasal mometasone, fluticasone)	Nasal discharge, itching, sneezing (Due to the systemic side effects of oral steroids, nasal steroids are in common use and are used as the first choice in treatment..	Besides growth retardation in children, metabolism disorders in all cases, glaucoma and cataract formation, immunosuppression, suppression of the growth axis, thinning of the skin, behavioral disorders, osteoporosis
Leukotriene antagocytes (Montelukast, zileuton etc.)	It is the gold standard in rhinitis that does not respond to antihistamines and nasal steroids.	Agitation aggression, anxiety, hallucination, depression, insomnia, irritability, restlessness, and suicidal thoughts.
Oral / Nasal decongestants 1. Pseudoephedrine and phenylephrine-oral 2. oxymetazoline, xylo-metazoline and naphazoline (intranasal)	Nasal congestion	When used orally, irritability, insomnia, irritability, headache, tachycardia, hypertension, increased intraocular pressure, urinary difficulty

Table 1.
Drugs used in treatment [15].

nose wings at night. The benefit of intranasal steroids in these patients has not been determined. The use of pseudoephedrine should be avoided during pregnancy, especially in the 1st trimester [9].

7. Rhinitis medicamentosa (drug-induced rhinitis)

It is a severe nasal congestion caused by the continuous use of agents such as oxymetazoline and phenylephrine, which are sympathomimetic agents. They use oral or topical steroids in treatment and sympathomimetic sprays are discontinued. Drugs such as ACE inhibitors, NSAIDs and Aspirin also have similar effects [10].

8. Atrophic rhinitis

Progressive nzal atrophy and Klebsiella ozaenae etc. It occurs due to mucosal colonization with microbial agents. There is a disturbing foul-smelling discharge on the jas. It can also develop after inferior turbinate surgery. Oral antibiotics, salty and oily washing solutions are used for malodorous discharge. Since the disease is very persistent, symptomatic patients should be followed up from time to time [11].

9. Non-allergic rhinitis with eosinophilia syndrome (NARES)

Known as non-allergic rhinitis with eosinophilic syndrome (NARES), the disease usually begins in adulthood; It is a type of non-allergic rhinitis characterized by negative skin test and normal IgE levels. Aspirin sensitivity, asthma and nasal polyps may develop in these patients. Eosinophilia is observed in patients. There is also an increased risk of obstructive sleep apnea syndrome. Another variant is Non-Allergic rhinitis disease with eosinophilia in the blood called BENARES. Although the clinic of the disease is the same as NARES; In this disease, there is eosinophilia in the blood instead of nasal eosinophilia. Intranasal corticosteroids are sufficient in both NARES and BENARES [12].

10. Infectious rhinitis

Infectious rhinitis is a type of rhinitis with acute or chronic runny nose, nasal congestion, frontal headache, smell disorders, post nasal discharge and cough. Most infectious rhinitis in children are viral and resolve with symptomatic treatment. If it is bacterial, antibiotics are used. In addition, nasal solutions, nasal steroids are also effective in treatment [13].

What are the risk factors?

- Exposure to smoke, exhaust fumes, or tobacco smoke
- Being over 20 years old. (Allergic rhinitis occurs before this age, non-allergic rhinitis occurs after the age of 20)
- Continuous use of decongestants: Nasal decongestants, which solve acute nasal congestion, cause congestion when used for a long time and increase congestion with rebaunt effect.
- Gender: Being a woman increases non-allergic rhinitis with hormonal effect.
- Occupation: Exposure to fumes from building materials, solvents or other chemicals
- Chronic diseases: such as hypothyroidism and chronic fatigue syndrome
- Stress. Emotional or physical stress increases susceptibility.

10.1 Complications

1. **Nasal polyposis**: Congestion and fluid increase in the sinuses trigger inflammation. As a result, benign masses form and cause chronic obstruction in the nose.
2. **Chronic Sinusitis:** Congestion and fluid increase in the nasal area disrupt the nasal drainage and cause inflammation.
3. **Middle ear infections**: Congestion and increased fluid in the nasal area can obstruct the eustachian tube, leading to middle ear infections.
4. **Disruption of daily activities:** It can cause disruption of daily activities. It can lead to school failure or business difficulties in school children.

10.2 Diagnosis

In non-allergic rhinitis, the diagnosis is made by exclusion. First of all, allergic rhinitis is ruled out. Sinus problems are then ruled out. So there are no definitive diagnostic criteria. To exclude, respectively.

1. Prick test: It is done to determine whether the symptoms are caused by an allergen. Allergens are applied to the skin and decided as positive or negative depending on the reaction.

2. Blood test: IgE levels are checked to measure immune response.

3. Nasal endoscopy: Pathologies such as nasal polyps and acute sinusitis are ruled out in endoscopy.

4. CT Imaging: Detailed imaging is performed for paranasal sinuses.

11. Treatment

Non-allergic rhinitis treatment is similar to allergic rhinitis. In treatment;

1. **Avoiding causative factors**: Cigarette smoke, perfume, spice or chemical odors should be avoided. Again, some drugs should be avoided. (Antihypertensives, antidepressants, birth control drugs etc.)

2. **Nasal irrigation**: The use of saline nasal solutions provides both opening and moistening of the nose. In addition, oil-containing solutions cause further moistening of the nose and ensure the success of the treatment.

3. **Pharmacotherapy**: First of all, drug therapy should be tried. Treatment can be used with oral or nasal antihistamines, oral or nasal steroids, leukotriene antagonists [14].

- Antihistamines

Antihistamines are molecules that bind competitively to H1 receptors. They help us treat sneezing, runny nose and itchy nose by reducing the sensation of vascular permeability, smooth muscle contraction and itching.

Although first generation antihistamines are cheap, we know that there is serious central nervous system penetration. For this reason, unfortunately, almost 10–40% of the patients cause severe distraction, sleepiness and concentration impairment. Anti-cholinergic side effects such as dryness in mucosal membranes, urinary retention, constipation, tachycardia, and decreased visual acuity limit the use of these drugs in elderly patients. In addition, the antagonistic effects of these drugs, which require long-term use, related to serotonin receptors, unfortunately, can cause weight gain. Trefenadine and astemizole are the first 2nd generation antihistamines and their central nervous system penetration is less than the old generation; However, they were removed from use in clinical practice due to arrhythmia caused by susceptible patients. Loratadine and cetirizine are generally less sedating new generation drugs. Levocetirizine is an enantiomer of the cetirizine molecule and unfortunately causes sedation at the effective doses. Fexofenadine, terfenadine; deslarotadine are also active metabolites of loratadine; these are sometimes referred to as 3rd generation antihistamines. It is reported that fexofenadine does not cross the blood brain barrier and therefore does not sedate. However, unfortunately, this is not the case in clinical use. Desloratadine is also reported to have more sedation and anti-cholinergic side effects [15].

Recently, anti-inflammatory effects of antihistamines have been mentioned. It is stated that mast cells and basophils stabilize the receptor independently by inhibiting the transmembrane passage of calcium and intracellular cAMP, thus reducing the release of inflammatory mediators such as histamine, tryptase and prostaglandin. However, many antihistamines are unfortunately unable to stabilize these cells at therapeutic doses. Ketotifen, olopatadine, azelastine, bepotastine and alkaftadine are mostly known as both H1 receptor antagonists and dual-acting antihistamines with mast cell stability. It is stated that some antihistamines inhibit NF-□B and GATA3 transcription via H1 receptor and thus achieve anti-inflammatory effect.

- Corticosteroids

Corticosteroids are the first-line anti-inflammatory drugs we know best for the treatment of many inflammatory diseases. Although corticosteroids have well-known side effects, we see that they are still one of the most important pharmacological agents. In addition to growth retardation in children, side effects such as metabolism disorders, glaucoma and cataract formation, immunosuppression, suppression of the HPA axis, thinning of the skin, behavioral disorders and osteoporosis are the most common ones in all cases. Due to these restrictions arising in systemic use, it is mostly used intranasally in AR. Among the intranasal preparations, they are currently the most used pharmacological products in primary care. Although the anti-inflammatory mechanisms of corticosteroids are not very clear, the most important effects are seen as cytokine and chemokine inhibition. They bind to glucocorticoid receptors (GR) in the cytoplasm, dimerize and pass into the nucleus; they then associate with the glucocorticoid response element (GRE) and consequently increase the transcription of the gene codes of anti-inflammatory proteins such as lipocortin-1, IL-10, IL-1 receptor antagonist and neutral endopeptidase.

Glucocorticoids also cause a considerable reduction in the number of inflammatory cells in nasal lavage fluid. Especially, they cause a significant decrease in eosinophil numbers. This is due to their inhibitory functions on both IL-5 and GM-CSF. Currently, beclamethasone monohydrate, budesonide, flunisolide, triamcinolone acetonide, fluticasone (propionate and furoate), mometasone furoate, and ciclesonide are commercially available nasal topical corticosteroids. There are no significant differences in clinical efficacy between these preparations.

Local burning and stinging sensation, irritation, dryness and sometimes nosebleeds can be encountered as topical side effects with these preparations [15].

- Leukotriene antagocytes

Leukotrienes are inflammatory lipid mediators synthesized from arachidonic acid that can be produced by mast cells, eosinophils, basophils and macrophages. The adventure of arachidonic acid cleavage that started with the posfolipase A2 enzyme from the nuclear membrane continues with leukotriene synthesis. Arachidonic acid is metabolized to LTA4 via the 5-lipoxygenase (5-LO) enzyme. LTC4, LTD4 and LTE4 are then formed through different convertases. We call these leukotrienes "cysteinyl leukotrienes (CsyLTs)". CsyLTs has serious bronchial smooth muscle contraction, mucus production, edema and vascular permeability enhancing effects. LTD4 enhances the P-selectin pathway, increasing leukocyte adhesion and leukocyte aggregation to the inflammation site. It also plays an important role in eosinophil adhesion by increasing β2-integrins. As a result of nasal provocation with LD4 in normal humans, it was observed that nasal mucosal blood flow accelerated and airway resistance increased.

Leukotrienes can be physiologically antagonized by blocking their synthesis or receptors. Zileuton is a 5-LO synthesis inhibitor and it is a pharmacological product that can block nasal congestion in patients with AR after allergen provocation. For now, only montelukast, which is a Cys LT1 receptor antagonist, has been approved for AR and is a commercial product. Montelukast is observed to improve congestion during the day and at night, nasal discharge, nasal itching and sneezing, difficulty falling asleep, and sleeping at night. It is thought to reduce the number of peripheral eosinophils and thus create an anti-inflammatory effect. However, despite all these, there are many publications showing that it is much less effective than intranasal corticosteroids in terms of these effects. Although it looks like a safe preparation in general; Some psychiatric side effects such as agitation, aggression, anxiety, hallucination, depression, insomnia, irritability, restlessness and suicidal thoughts are mentioned [15].

- Nasal decongestants

These drugs slow down nasal blood flow by antagonizing α1 and α2 adrenergic receptors in nasal capacitance vessel endothelium. In this way, they reduce nasal mucosal congestion and swelling. Better results can be obtained when combined with an antihistamine. Pseudoephedrine and phenylephrine, which are catecholamines, have oral forms. Although a runny nose can improve symptoms, it has no effect on itching, sneezing and eye symptoms in the nose. The imidazoline derivatives oxymetazoline, xylometazoline and naphazoline are suitable for intranasal use. Although they are fast intranasal decongestants and have fewer side effects, severe rebound congestion effects occur when the drug is discontinued. In some publications, it is mentioned that oxymetazoline inhibits T cells and cytokines such as IL-1β, TNF-α, IL-6 and IL-8. Some local nasal side related to these preparations.

11.1 Monoclonal anti-IgE antibodies

Omaluzimab is a humanized, recombinant, monoclonal antibody that blocks the binding of circulating IgE antibodies to the high affinity receptors in cells such as mast cells and basophil by complexing with the Ce3 region. There are many publications showing that patients with AR provide a very serious clinical benefit by significantly decreasing circulating IgE levels. In addition, it reduces FcR1 expressions on mast cells in both blood and tissue. It improves the nasal symptoms and increases the quality of life. It is an antibody that is well tolerated and has a very low risk of anaphylaxis (0.9/1000 applications). There are studies showing that SIT treatment applied together with omalizumab is more effective in single applications. The most important handicap is that it is currently an expensive treatment model [15].

11.2 Capsaicin treatment, complementary and alternative medicine, surgery

Capsaicin is bound to vanilloid resertors expressed in nasal C-fibers. It has been observed that repeated applications to the skin or intranasally cause desensitization in the peripheral nerve endings. It works well in vasomotor rhinitis in which neurotransmitters play an important role. It has been observed that it reduces symptoms such as nasal congestion, runny nose, and sneezing in AR. However, there are also publications showing that it has no clinical efficacy, especially in patients with house dust mite-sensitive PAR patients.

Nasal irrigation or irrigation with saline is a complementary treatment model in AR. In this form of treatment, it is ensured that the contact of the sinuses and pharynx with allergens and mucus is reduced. At the same time, edema in the nose is reduced. It has been shown that nasal saline application reduces the need for topical corticosteroids in children with AR.

It has been shown that exposure to microbes in children increases the expression of IL-10 and TGF-β inhibitory cytokines as well as the development of Th1-type immune response. There is evidence that beneficial microorganisms do this through toll-like respectors. Especially bifidobacteria and lactobacilli have such effects. There are studies showing that such probiotics can be effective in AR.

There is no sufficient and scientific evidence that acupuncture is effective in AR.

It has been stated that UV-A and UV-B are used, and that the patients are not able to use drugs or get sufficient response in a few small series. In only one study on AR, infrared radiation therapy (FIR) has been tried. It has been stated that the application of the oven affects the thermo-receptors due to the heat it emits and can be effective by increasing the microcirculation.

Surgical intervention may be beneficial for sinusitis, nasal polyps, enlarged turbinates, or nasal septal deviation, if any, that do not respond to medical treatment [15].

Author details

Erkan Yildiz
Department of Otorhinolaryngology, Afyonkarahisar Şuhut State Hospital, Şuhut, Afyonkarahisar, Turkey

*Address all correspondence to: dr.erkanyildiz@hotmail.com

References

[1] Settipane RA, Kaliner MA. Nonallergic Rhinitis. *American Journal of Rhinology & Allergy*. 2013;27(3_suppl):S48-S51. doi:10.2500/ajra.2013.27.3927

[2] Eifan AO, Durham SR. Pathogenesis of rhinitis. *Clin Exp Allergy*. 2016;46(9): 1139-1151. doi:10.1111/cea.12780

[3] Sur DKC, Plesa ML. Chronic Nonallergic Rhinitis. *Am Fam Physician*. 2018;98(3):171-176.

[4] Ellis AK, Keith PK. Nonallergic rhinitis with eosinophilia syndrome and related disorders. *Clin Allergy Immunol*. 2007;19:87-100.

[5] Shahab R, Phillips DE, Jones AS. Prostaglandins, leukotrienes and perennial rhinitis. J Laryngol Otol. 2004 Jul;118(7):500-7. doi: 10.1258/0022215041615155. PMID: 15318955.

[6] Leader P, Geiger Z. Vasomotor Rhinitis. 2020 Aug 16. In: StatPearls [Internet]. Treasure Island (FL): StatPearls Publishing; 2020 Jan–. PMID: 31613484.

[7] Hellings PW, Klimek L, Cingi C, et al. Non-allergic rhinitis: Position paper of the European Academy of Allergy and Clinical Immunology. *Allergy*. 2017;72(11):1657-1665. doi:10.1111/all.13200

[8] Shao Z, Bernstein JA. Occupational Rhinitis: Classification, Diagnosis, and Therapeutics. *Curr Allergy Asthma Rep*. 2019;19(12):54. Published 2019 Nov 27. doi:10.1007/s11882-019-0892-0

[9] Wei J, Gerlich J, Genuneit J, et al. Hormonal factors and incident asthma and allergic rhinitis during puberty in girls. *Ann Allergy Asthma Immunol*. 2015;115(1):21-27.e2. doi:10.1016/j.anai.2015.04.019

[10] Zucker SM, Barton BM, McCoul ED. Management of Rhinitis Medicamentosa: A Systematic Review. *Otolaryngol Head Neck Surg*. 2019;160(3):429-438. doi:10.1177/0194599818807891

[11] Balur MB, Koçak HE, Altınay S, Özdamar K, Taşkın Ü, Oktay MF. Is submucosal fat injection effective in atrophic rhinitis? An experimental animal study. *Eur Arch Otorhinolaryngol*. 2017;274(10):3637-3642. doi:10.1007/s00405-017-4670-0

[12] Becker S, Rasp J, Eder K, Berghaus A, Kramer MF, Gröger M. Non-allergic rhinitis with eosinophilia syndrome is not associated with local production of specific IgE in nasal mucosa. *Eur Arch Otorhinolaryngol*. 2016;273(6):1469-1475. doi:10.1007/s00405-015-3769-4

[13] Marti J, López F, Gascón I, Julve J. Propolis nasal spray effectively improves recovery from infectious acute rhinitis and common cold symptoms in children: a pilot study. *J Biol Regul Homeost Agents*. 2017;31(4):943-950.

[14] Lieberman PL, Smith P. Nonallergic Rhinitis: Treatment. *Immunol Allergy Clin North Am*. 2016;36(2):305-319. doi:10.1016/j.iac.2015.12.007

[15] Daramola OO, Kern RC. An update regarding the treatment of nonallergic rhinitis. *Curr Opin Otolaryngol Head Neck Surg*. 2016;24(1):10-14. doi:10.1097/MOO.0000000000000225

Chapter 15

Islet Inflammation: The Link between Type 2 Diabetes and Pancreatic Cancer

Alpana Mukhuty

Abstract

The role of islet inflammation in type 2 diabetes (T2DM) and pancreatic ductal adenocarcinoma (PDAC) is complex. About 80% of pancreatic cancer patients have glucose intolerance or T2D. Chronic type 2 diabetes increases risk for pancreatic cancer, but the mechanisms are unknown. In this context two hypotheses exist: (i) pancreatic cancer causes diabetes and (ii) diabetes promotes the development of pancreatic cancer. Pancreatic ductal adenocarcinoma is the most common and deadly form of pancreatic cancer that is associated with diabetes. There are many possibilities by which obesity links to pancreatic cancer. These possibilities include insulin resistance, hyperinsulinemia and inflammation. Adipose tissue deposition near pancreas (peri-pancreatic depot) increase proinflammatory response to a high fat or high calorie containing diet. Inflammatory processes in the islets act as main mediators during the development and progression of pancreatic cancer. Recently, studies have been carried out to investigate the underlying mechanisms that contribute to tumorigenesis induced by inflammation. Tumor-elicited inflammation, secretion of pro-inflammatory cytokines and migration of immune cells play the key roles in initiation, promotion and progression of malignant metastasis in pancreatic cancer. Initiation and progression of islet inflammation in diabetes and pancreatic cancer occurs as a result of various protein–protein interactions and genetic events. The increase in pancreatic cancer cases may be attributed to the obesity endemic and obesity mediated Type 2 diabetes. The existence of link between islet inflammation in chronic diabetes and pancreatic cancer cannot be ignored, although the details about the underlying mechanisms are not clear, and must be studied in detail.

Keywords: Islet inflammation, type 2 diabetes, pancreatic cancer, obesity, insulin resistance

1. Introduction

Type 2 diabetes (T2D) is characterized by hyperglycemia which occurs due to impaired insulin production and reduced pancreatic beta cell population during insulin resistance. Most diabetes patients are able to compensate increasing insulin resistance by increasing insulin production. Now the decrease in insulin secretion occurs due to increased beta cell apoptosis, and the reason behind apoptosis remains endoplasmic reticulum stress, mitochondrial dysfunction and inflammation. Since a long time T2D and pancreatic cancer have been associated and development of diabetes is related to occurrence of pancreatic cancer. The causes behind association of T2D with pancreatic cancer may be chronic inflammation and common progenitor cells for endocrine and exocrine pancreas, however still more research is needed in this field, and every detail about diabetes and pancreatic cancer must be studied [1].

Firstly, Type 2 diabetes is the third most possible risk factor for pancreatic cancer after obesity and cigarette smoking. Studies have shown that chronic type 2 diabetes increases risk of pancreatic cancer by 1.5- to 2.0-fold. Prediagnostic assessment of glucose and insulin levels may help in early diagnosis. The reasons behind development of diabetes-associated pancreatic cancer remain insulin resistance, hyperglycemia, hyperinsulinemia, and inflammation. On the other hand, people diagnosed with Type 2 diabetes may be part of a population of pancreatic cancer patients who have been detected earlier. There are several signaling pathways regulating metabolic processes which dictate cell proliferation and tumor growth. Better insight on the different mechanisms common in Type 2 diabetes and pancreatic cancer can be helpful in the development of new biomarkers and potent preventive or therapeutic strategies [1].

Ductal adenocarcinoma of pancreas is the fifth major cause of death in cancer in developed countries after lung, stomach, colorectal and breast cancer. 23% of the patients can live for 1 year after diagnosis and 6% of the patients have a 5-year survival rate due to advanced stage of cancer at the time of the diagnosis. Ductal adenocarcinoma of pancreas is also the thirteenth most common type of cancer and eight most common cause of cancer-related deaths. Here it must be mentioned that 80% of pancreatic cancer patients have been ailing with Type 2 diabetes or compromised glucose tolerance at the time of diagnosis [2–4].

Patients with ductal adenocarcinoma of pancreas and also Type 2 diabetes, have a record of diagnosis of diabetes less than 24 months before the diagnosis of ductal adenocarcinoma of pancreas in 74–88% of cases [5]. It means that Type 2 diabetes and ductal adenocarcinoma of pancreas show "dual causality," while chronic Type 2 diabetes remains a risk factor for the development of ductal adenocarcinoma of pancreas and, on the other hand, ductal adenocarcinoma of pancreas is also presumed to be a cause for Type 2 diabetes in many cases.

The Centre for Disease Control and Prevention recorded that ~29 million people in the U.S. suffered from Type 2 diabetes in 2014, while about 8 million of these patients have not yet been diagnosed. Also, ~86 million adults in the U.S. are known to be prediabetic, having a fasting plasma glucose level of 100–125 mg/dL, a 2-h plasma glucose level of 140–199 mg/dL, or a glycohemoglobin (HbA1c) level of 5.7–6.4% [6]. The global increase of ductal adenocarcinoma of pancreas further escalates the need to understand the pathophysiology of Type 2 diabetes. Chronic Type 2 diabetes is established to be a risk factor for ductal adenocarcinoma of pancreas [7]. Type 2 diabetes is also linked with obesity, and obesity also increases the risk for developing ductal adenocarcinoma of pancreas [8]. Type 2 diabetes is also associated with defective insulin function since insulin fails to suppress hepatic glucose release. As a result, peripheral glucose utilization mainly by skeletal muscle, is compromised, with initial increase in insulin levels since the beta cells try to overcome insulin resistance by producing more insulin [9]. With chronic Type 2 diabetes, beta cells undergo failure leading to apoptosis and decreased beta cell mass [10]. Patients with obesity and Type 2 diabetes are likely to suffer for long time periods with high intrapancreatic insulin levels due to beta cell compensation to overcome the increasing insulin demand and to maintain glucose homeostasis. Insulin is released into the circulation by beta cells through intrapancreatic portal circulation that also supplies blood to acinar and ductal cells near the islets. Acinar and ductal cells neighboring the islets may also get blood supply from intrapancreatic portal circulation [11]. This close association allows high levels of islet hormones to directly get supplied to acinar and ductal cells, resulting in proxicrine effects on insulin receptors present on acinar cells and also on insulin like growth factor-I receptors in any differentiated cells in the region, enhancing survival and proliferation of the cells. Hence, intrapancreatic hyperinsulinemia, arising due to obesity and insulin resistance in prediabetic patients or in early diabetic patients contribute to increased risk in ductal adenocarcinoma of pancreas.

Compromised glycemic control is also associated with increased levels of advanced glycation end products (AGE) which activate RAGE, a receptor for AGE [12]. RAGE receptor belongs to the immunoglobulin super family and can bind to several ligands apart from AGE, including some proinflammatory cytokines that have role in inflammation and ductal adenocarcinoma of pancreas [12]. Also, activation of RAGE contributes to obesity and inflammation [13]. Excess of activation of RAGE also contribute to the higher prognosis of ductal adenocarcinoma of pancreas in Type 2 diabetes.

2. Mechanisms between type 2 diabetes and pancreatic cancer

The mechanism behind the association of Type 2 diabetes and pancreatic cancer is elaborate and include metabolic, hormonal, and immunological modifications that regulate tumor growth (**Figure 1**). The most presumed mechanisms behind the association between Type 2 diabetes and pancreatic cancer are insulin resistance, compensatory hyperinsulinemia and increased levels of circulating insulin-like growth factors (IGFs). In-vivo studies showed that islet cell turnover, linked with insulin resistance, is important for pancreatic cancer. Like, in hamsters, islet cell proliferation increase pancreatic ductal cancer [14], while destruction of islet cells by streptozotocin or alloxan impede pancreatic cancer prevalence [15, 16]. Also, biguanide metformin treatment inhibit the creation of pancreatic tumors by N-nitrosobis-(2-oxopropyl) amine, a potent pancreatic carcinogen. High-fat containing diet in hamsters normalize the islet cell turnover rate [17].

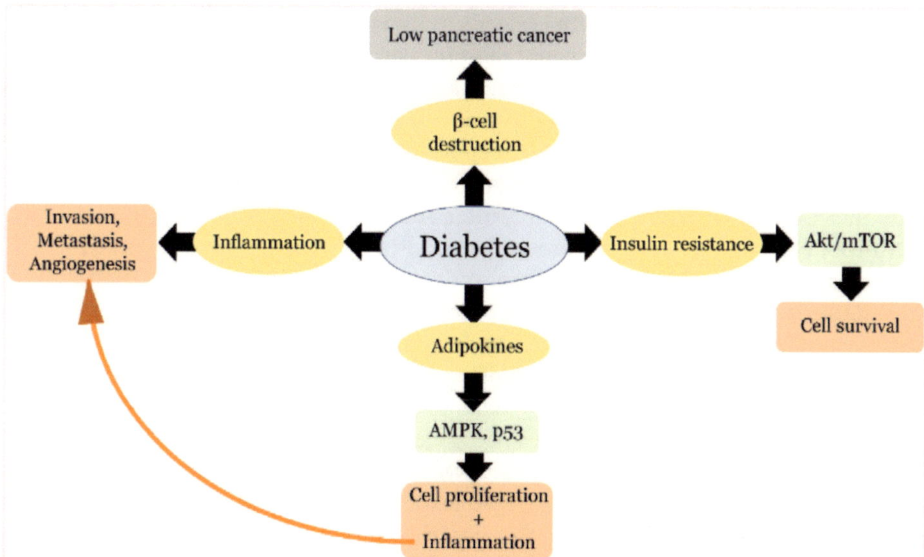

Figure 1.
Association between diabetes and pancreatic cancer [1].

Pancreatic β-cells become hyperactive, their mass increase which together led to insulin over secretion to combat insulin resistance. The exocrine part of pancreatic tissue is exposed to much higher level of local insulin concentrations than the amount of insulin in the circulation of hyperinsulinemic patients. Insulin also acts as a growth-promoting hormone which increases cell proliferation. Hence, insulin not only promotes cell proliferation but also increases uptake of glucose [18], and both of these processes are important for development and progression of tumor. Moreover, insulin increases the availability of insulin like growth factors by decreasing hepatic production of binding proteins for insulin like growth factors [19, 20]. The two main properties of insulin like growth factor-1 (IGF-1) are mitogenic and antiapoptotic activities which increase growth of cells expressing insulin as well as IGF-1 receptor (IGF1R). Here it must be noted that IGF-1 and IGF1R are overexpressed in pancreatic cancer cells [21]. Also, IGF-1 regulated signal transduction elevates proliferation, invasion, and expression of different mediators of angiogenesis and decrease apoptosis of pancreatic cancer cells as well [22–24]. IGF1R-induced signal transduction also activates several intracellular signal pathways, like Ras/Raf/mitogen-activated protein kinase and phosphoinositide-3 kinase/Akt/mammalian target of rapamycin (mTOR) pathways [25]. Decreased levels of IGF binding protein 1 can predict increased risk of pancreatic cancer [26]. Unusual glucose metabolism can also predict presence of tumor cells, since most tumors have upregulated insulin-independent glucose uptake mechanisms while, diabetic animals with β-cell destruction induced by alloxan show reduced tumor growth [27]. This suggests that hyperglycemia has no role in increasing neoplastic growth in insulin deficiency. High dietary glycemic index increases the risk of pancreatic cancer due to deleterious effects of high postprandial glucose and increasing insulin demands [28]. Type 2 diabetes and diabetes associated obesity increase the risk of pancreatic cancer due to increased oxidative stress and inflammation during type 2 diabetes and also due to the link between oxidative stress and insulin resistance [29–32]. Antioxidant supplementation with vitamin E or α-lipoic acid can be preventive or curative in insulin resistance [33, 34]. Moreover, postprandial hyperglycemia directly increases oxidative stress leading to overproduction of superoxide by the mitochondrial electron-transport chain [35]. Impairment of the cellular redox state reduces tyrosine phosphorylation and elevates serine phosphorylation of insulin receptor substrate 1, which leads to impaired insulin-signaling pathway [35]. Moreover, obesity and macronutrient intake activate inflammatory signaling pathways [36, 37], and glucose and fat intake stimulate inflammation by increasing oxidative stress and the activating transcriptional factors such as nuclear factor-κB, activating protein-1 and early growth response-1 [38–40]. Also, adipose tissues may act as an endocrine organs to regulate the release of fatty acids, hormones, and cytokines like tumor necrosis factor-α, interleukin-6, and resistin [41].

Adipocytokines, which are secreted from adipocytes, are mainly involved in apoptosis, development, metabolism, innate immunity and inflammation. Proinflammatory cytokines are known to stimulate angiogenesis, tumor progression, and metastasis. During obesity or Typ2 2 diabetes altered levels or dysfunctions of many molecules like leptin [42], IGF-1 [43], and peroxisome proliferator-activated receptor-γ [44], lead to development of pancreatic cancer by impeding immune system.

Several genome-wide studies have shown new genetic variants that increase the risk of diabetes, and some of the susceptible loci already established in Type 2 diabetes are known to be involved in differentiation and development [45]. NR5A2 (or LRH1) is one such pancreatic cancer susceptibility gene identified in genome-wide association studies [46]. NR5A2 is a direct target of pancreatic duodenal homeobox (PDX-1) gene in pancreatic development and differentiation [47]. It regulates the expression of developmental genes, like transcription factors hepatocyte nuclear factor (HNF)-3β, HNF-4α, and HNF-1β. On the other hand, NR5A2 expression is regulated by HNF-3β and HNF-1, so the case is regulated both ways. PDX-1 is necessary for pancreatic development and also for casual function of β-cell and secretion of insulin [48]. Mutations in HNF-1β gene is associated with maturity-onset diabetes in the young people [49]. Better insight about the function of NR5A2 gene in the progression and development of pancreatic cancer can be helpful in curbing the risk of diabetes-linked pancreatic cancer and also decipher the genetic mechanisms behind Type 2 diabetes and pancreatic cancer.

2.1 Genomic associations between type 2 diabetes, chronic pancreatitis and pancreatic ductal adenocarcinoma

Several clinical and epidemiological studies associate the risk of ductal adenocarcinoma of pancreas to chronic Type 2 diabetes and chronic pancreatitis (CP). The genetic reasons of susceptibility among all these three diseases are quite variant however, some reasons are common. The mechanism behind the function of these genes and how they influence susceptibility is not common because of the difference in methodology of identification of the genes. Interestingly, all three diseases share these characteristics: 1) all patients have a report of family history or familial clustering, which indicate shared genetic or environmental influence, 2) difference in age of patients at the time diagnosis is due to familial risk, and 3) analyzing Mendelian segregation prove that in some families there are some hereditary components which demonstrate the common features of the gene [11]. Apart from genetics factors, there are epidemiological factors like obesity in diabetes, alcohol intake in chronic pancreatitis, and smoking in ductal adenocarcinoma of pancreas that may work with genetic factors to increase the risk. Several approaches have been evolved to discover these susceptibility genes, from family-based case control studies and cohort studies, from where a list of candidate genes is identified, and large-scale genome-wide association studies (GWAS) are conducted to search for single nucleotide polymorphisms (SNPs) or next-generation sequencing. The genetic basis of Type 2 diabetes is characterized as polygenic, having implication of over 50 genes [50]. Any single major gene cannot explain the genetic risk of Type 2 diabetes except in some rare cases [51]. However, chronic pancreatitis and ductal adenocarcinoma of pancreas can be explained by mutations in some major genes. Genome-wide association studies (GWAS) have identified many low-penetrance common SNPs which are associated with risk of ductal adenocarcinoma of pancreas. Among all these three diseases, Type 2 diabetes has been studied in detail, which depict that Type 2 diabetes is a multifactorial disease and is genetically complex. Variants of more than 50 genes have been studied which increase genetic risk. These genes are divided into some having modest effect like PPARG and KDNJ11, and others having strong association like TCF7L2, WFS1, HDF1B, FTO, CDKN2A, and SLC20A8. New strategies have been developed which have characterized the genetic basis of the disease through subclinical or related phenotypes by predisposition of the genes [52]. Since Type 2 diabetes is a polygenic risk model, each genetic variant has a small effect. These genetic variants improve risk assessment from common risk factors like age, sex, family history and BMI (Body Mass Index) [53]. Family-based studies and data on pathophysiology of chronic pancreatitis facilitate success in explaining the genetic heterogeneity [54]. Most of the variations in susceptibility are due to acute and chronic pancreatitis being related to genetic variations among patients. Alcohol was considered to be the primary reason behind genetic contributions but after the discovery of PRSS1, CFTR, and SPINK1 variants which associated with pancreatitis the reasons have been resolved [55]. Hence, no single factor can cause pancreatitis, and majority of cases having acute and chronic pancreatitis have multiple variants of a gene, or multiple genes having epistatic interactions, or genetic factors coupled with environmental cues.

The genetic predisposition to ductal adenocarcinoma of pancreas is difficult due to the poor collection and analysis of biospecimens from patients owing to their low survival rate. Alike Type 2 diabetes and chronic pancreatitis, ductal adenocarcinoma of pancreas is also genetically heterogeneous. The identification of susceptibility genes has led to discovery of some rare gene mutations which are associated with cancer syndromes linked with common single nucleotide polymorphisms (SNPs). Study designs on family hierarchy and case-controls have led to discovery of mutations in known syndrome-associated genes, like BRCA1, BRCA2, CDKN2A, and CFTR. Moreover, next-generation sequencing has led to identification of additional mutations like PALB2 [56] and ATM [57]. Patients with sporadic ductal adenocarcinoma of pancreas carry germline mutations in major genes [58] and it changes the present knowledge for risk assessment. Large numbers of sporadic cases of ductal adenocarcinoma of pancreas and healthy subjects have exposed SNPs in chromosomal regions containing ABO, TERT, and CLPTM1L and other genes. Nevertheless, risk modeling using GWAS SNPs cannot provide sufficient genetic information that can improve prediction of pancreatic cancer [59].

2.2 Role of obesity and pancreatitis mediated inflammation in pancreatic ductal adenocarcinoma

Obesity is linked with an elevated risk of cancer, including pancreatic cancer [60]. The observed increase in pancreatic cancer epidemiology and deaths can be partially attributed to obesity taking the form of an endemic disease. Obesity can lead to pancreatic cancer, insulin resistance, hyperinsulinemia and inflammation by many possible ways [61]. Pancreatic cancer development can be attenuated in genetically engineered mouse model by using nonsteroidal anti-inflammatory drugs, which indicate that tissue inflammation plays an important role in this disease [62]. Tissue inflammation during obesity creates a perfect microenvironment for tumor initiation and promotion. Besides obesity, increase in BMI and visceral adiposity bears a strong link with metabolic diseases and gastrointestinal cancers, together with pancreatic cancer [63]. The accumulation of adipose tissue near the pancreas (peri-pancreatic depot) lead to an enhanced proinflammatory reaction in response to high-fat or high-calorie containing diet compared to peri-gonadal depot [64]. The association between adipose tissue depot-specific reactions to diet-induced obesity and the effect of these adipose tissue depots on cancer development is very crucial to understand the connection between body condition and risk of cancer. Moreover, high-fat or high-calorie containing diet increases the progression of pancreatic intraepithelial neoplasia, which is a known precursor of ductal adenocarcinoma of pancreas, and this accelerates the incidence of pancreatic cancer in an invasive and metastatic manner in conditional KrasG12D mouse model [65, 66].

2.3 Mechanisms behind type 2 diabetes in pancreatic ductal adenocarcinoma

To be specific, prevalence of Type 2 diabetes among ductal adenocarcinoma of pancreas patients is really very high. Type 2 diabetes is found in 47% of ductal adenocarcinoma of pancreas patients compared with only 7% of healthy subjects, and a normal fasting glucose occurs in 59% of healthy subjects, while it is found only in 14% of ductal adenocarcinoma of pancreas patients [5] (**Figure 2**). In 74% of ductal adenocarcinoma of pancreas patients with diabetes, diabetes is diagnosed within 24 months before the diagnosis of ductal adenocarcinoma of pancreas [67].

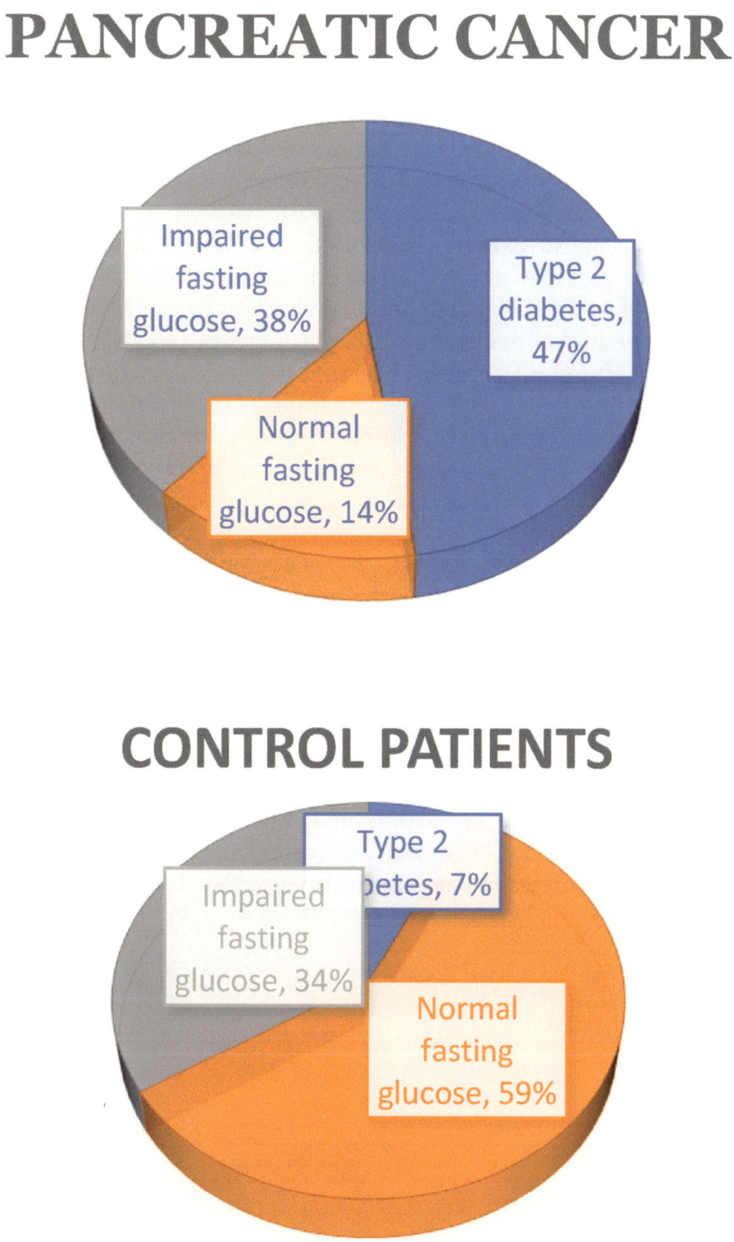

Figure 2.
Prevalence of type 2 diabetes in ductal pancreatic adenocarcinoma [5, 11].

This remarks that in most of the patients, new-onset diabetes is due to the tumor and this diagnosis of diabetes may be a useful "biomarker" for the diagnosis of ductal adenocarcinoma of pancreas. Although known risk factors for Type 2 diabetes like obesity, age and family history of diabetes are also the common risk factors in case of risk factors for ductal adenocarcinoma of pancreas, the occurrence of Type 2 diabetes in ductal adenocarcinoma of pancreas is pretty higher than the occurrence of Type 2 diabetes among all other common types of cancer. Type 2 diabetes is found in 68% of patients with ductal adenocarcinoma of pancreas while it occurs in 14.8–23.5% of patients with breast, colon, lung, and prostate cancers [68]. Also, insulin resistance is common in patients with both ductal adenocarcinoma of pancreas and Type 2 diabetes, while many patients with ductal adenocarcinoma of pancreas undergo weight loss. Deteriorating glycemic control along with weight loss occurs in ductal adenocarcinoma of pancreas along with its incidence in Type 2 diabetes. These common characteristics give alert to the clinicians for the possibility of ductal adenocarcinoma of pancreas -associated diabetes. New-onset diabetes associated with ductal adenocarcinoma of pancreas can be cured after tumor resection, if there are enough islets left in the pancreatic tissue. Several reports show that Type 2 diabetes improves after resection of pancreatic tumors [69]. 57% of the patients with new-onset diabetes get cured of diabetes post operation of pancreatic tumors, while all of ductal adenocarcinoma of pancreas patients with long-standing diabetes cannot be cured of diabetes even after pancreatic resection [5] (**Figure 3**). These data strongly support that new-onset diabetes is associated with ductal adenocarcinoma of pancreas and it can be a paraneoplastic phenomenon, where malignancy interferes with insulin secretion or insulin function, finally leading to Type 2 diabetes. Numerous studies have tried to identify the mechanisms behind Type 2 diabetes caused by ductal adenocarcinoma of pancreas or the genomic and protein markers of Type 2 diabetes caused by ductal adenocarcinoma of pancreas. Connexin 26, a gap junction protein, is highly overexpressed in islets of ductal adenocarcinoma of pancreas patients with Type 2 diabetes [70], and a pancreatic ductal adenocarcinoma -derived S-100A8 N-terminal peptide is a diabetogenic agent [71, 72] which is also upregulated patients with ductal adenocarcinoma of pancreas associated with new-onset diabetes. Vanin-1 and matrix metalloproteinase 9 can also act as predictors of ductal adenocarcinoma of pancreas associated diabetes [73]. Vanin-1, is also overexpressed during inflammation, which means that mediators of inflammation play an important role in damaged islet function and insulin function in ductal adenocarcinoma of pancreas. Pancreatic Polypeptide (PP) release increases in Type 2 diabetes, and a deficit in PP response due to nutrient ingestion can transform into new-onset diabetes caused by pancreatic exocrine

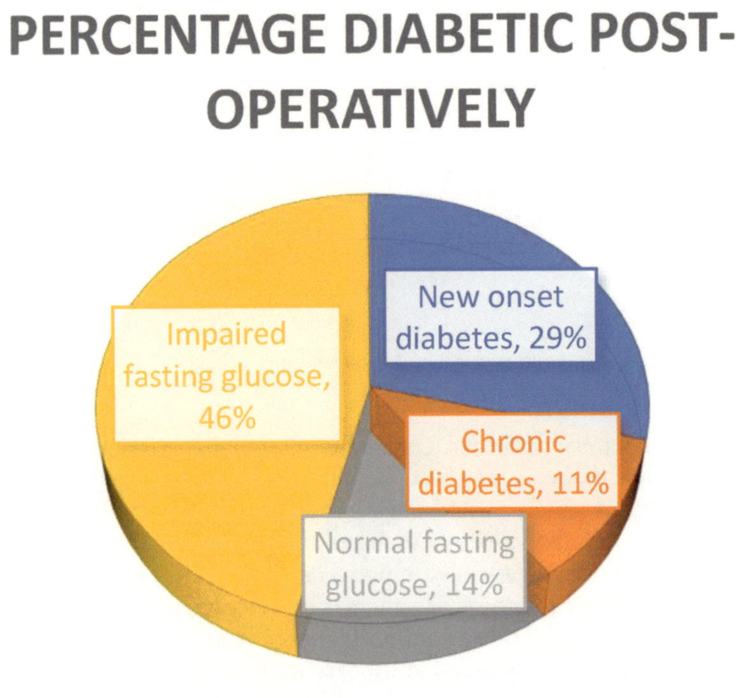

Figure 3.
Prevalence of type 2 diabetes after pancreaticoduodenectomy for ductal pancreatic adenocarcinoma [5, 11].

disease. Basal and meal-stimulated PP release significantly decreases in patients with diabetes associated with ductal adenocarcinoma of pancreas localized in the head of pancreas in comparison to patients with Type 2 diabetes [11].

2.4 Significance of type 2 diabetes in pancreatic ductal adenocarcinoma

Some researchers say that diabetes does not contribute to earlier diagnosis or clinical features or tumor size or prognosis of pancreatic cancer [74], although, previous studies had established that diabetes can predict pancreatic cancer [75]. A study compared diabetic and non-diabetic patients and observed a worse overall mortality and median survival in diabetic patients [76]. In another study, patients with diabetes had a better overall survival [77]. On the other hand, Type 2 diabetes is known to confer a poor survival in ductal adenocarcinoma of pancreas patients [78]. Actually, gender and mean age of the patients in these two studies regulated the number of comorbidities, time of diabetes and also time for development of complications in diabetes [75]. Use of preventive medicine, frequent clinical follow-up and earlier diagnosis of ductal pancreatic adenocarcinoma can generate a better median survival.

3. Future perspectives of dealing with pancreatic ductal adenocarcinoma

The explanation of hormonal [79], paracrine [21] and autocrine [22, 23] mediators of pancreatic cancer and its association with new-onset diabetes can be helpful in pathogenesis and showing new therapeutic targets. A better explanation of the epidemiology of pancreatic cancer, is poorly controlled diabetes or it can be an intrinsically genetic [8] or epigenetic [80–82] or immunologic [83, 84] or gastrointestinal microbiota [85, 86] or tissue microenvironment which are characteristic of Type 2 diabetes [87–89] patients progressing towards pancreatic cancer.

The various techniques like gene sequencing, lymphocyte flow cytometry, mRNA profiling, PCR studies and microbe identification microarray from Type 2 diabetes patients in different stages of progression can help in early diagnosis and prevent diabetic complications in pancreatic cancer and diabetes. Molecular biomarkers can be very crucial to diagnose patients with new-onset diabetes who should be tested with endoscopic ultrasound for identifying pancreatic cancer [75]. Hyperinsulinemia can negatively predict value development of new-onset diabetes associated with pancreatic cancer if all other hormonal, paracrine or autocrine factors play against development of insulin resistance [75].

Metformin, a well-known medication for Type 2 diabetes, improves survival in pancreatic cancer patients and has prognostic effects [90]. The knowledge available on the mechanism of action of metformin helps in the understanding of the ductal adenocarcinoma of the pancreas cancer pathways [75].

4. Altered intracellular metabolism in pancreatic ductal adenocarcinoma

Deregulated systemic physiology is the effect of disruption of energy homeostasis, and metabolic processes within the cells of a pancreatic tumor can also be knowledgeable [91]. Malignant cells of a pancreatic tumor, have alterations that are mediated by both oncogene-driven programs and also by the rare physiology of tumor. Pancreatic tumors have a dense, fibrotic stroma which inhibits vascular function and also disrupts delivery of nutrients and oxygen [92]. Mutant Kras expression regulates metabolic networks facilitating redox balance, bioenergetics, and anabolic metabolism for better survival and cell proliferation under these poor circumstances [93–95]. Nutrients recycled by autophagy fuel these pathways [96, 97] and also the nutrients scavenged by nonspecific bulk extracellular space engulfment or by micropinocytosis [98] as well as overexpressed nutrient importers help in regulating these pathways [93, 99]. Together, the regulation of metabolism of pancreatic cancer cells are controlled by oncogene-driven pathways, and they engage nutrient scavenging mechanisms as well as improve nutrient utilization to overcome the problems of insufficient vascularization [91].

Malignant cells constitute 10% of the total cellular content of a pancreatic tumor [92]. As a result, the non-malignant cells help in shaping the metabolic condition and facilitate tumor growth [91]. These processes can be divided into 2 types: First, the cooperative reactions between non-malignant cells and malignant cells support the metabolism in cancer cells, and second, the reaction between malignant and non-malignant cells is competitive and it happens between tumor cells and the antitumor immune reaction [100].

One main cooperative reaction is the nutrient exchange pathway that occurs between pancreatic cancer cells and activated pancreatic stellate cells (PSCs) [101]. Pancreatic cancer cells are known to induce autophagy in the PSCs. As a result, protein breakdown occurs through autophagy and nonessential amino acids are released. Now, the pancreatic cancer cells engulf alanine and utilize it to in mitochondrial metabolism and also in the biosynthesis of cellular building blocks. Here it must be mentioned that alanine can be used in metabolism in replacement of glucose and glutamine, and the biosynthetic substrates also aid in cancer cell metabolism. If this metabolic crosstalk pathway is blocked or inhibited by suppressing autophagy particularly in the PSCs then it can lead to a dramatic decrease in tumor growth. Interestingly, pancreatic tumors can suppress immune responses and are highly resistant to immunotherapies [102]. Local nutrient depletion and waste accumulation indeed play important roles in aiding tumor immune suppression [100]. Moreover, Cytotoxic T-cells, are intrinsically less apt at obtaining nutrients than oncogene-driven cells, and they are compelled to compete for the limited nutrients like carbohydrates and amino acids, in a tumor microenvironment, and later result in defective antitumor immune response. The compromised antitumor T-cell response in melanoma and sarcoma is directly connected with glucose deprivation [103, 104], while high titres of lactate aid in the polarization of anti-inflammatory macrophages [105]. Mutant Kras-expressing pancreatic cancer cells vigorously consume glucose and then release lactate (so-called, Warburg metabolism) [93], and all of these mechanisms result in suppressed immune function in pancreatic cancer. Moreover, M2 type anti-inflammatory macrophages and cancer cells can exhaust tumors of amino acids such as arginine and tryptophan [106]. These processes also restrict antitumor T-cell responses and aids the differentiation of T-cells into anti-inflammatory T-regulatory cells.

5. Role of bariatric surgery in obesity and pancreatic ductal adenocarcinoma

Premorbid obesity unpleasantly influences ductal adenocarcinoma of pancreas associated mortality in a dose-dependent manner [107, 108]. A high BMI is also linked with an increased risk of ductal adenocarcinoma of pancreas [107, 108]. The etiology of obesity-linked diseases starts with excess energy and deposition of triglyceride in the adipose tissue. This excess of triglyceride cannot be completely deposited in the adipose tissue, hence ectopic fat deposition occurs in various organs like liver and pancreas. Triglyceride deposition in the liver leads to oxidative stress and inflammation, resulting in cirrhosis, steatohepatitis and hepatocellular carcinoma. Similar mechanisms occur in the pancreas. Free fatty acids and inflammatory mediators remain in high amounts in the pancreas of obese high fat fed mice [109], and this accelerates tumor growth [110]. Fat depots in liver and pancreas increase in obese individuals. After bariatric surgery, weight loss occurs, and hepatic and pancreatic fats rapidly disappear [111]. After weight loss, insulin resistance and circulatory levels of inflammatory factors also rapidly normalize [112]. Weight loss occurring after bariatric surgery decreases cancer mortality by 40–60% [113, 114]. Also, the risk of ductal adenocarcinoma of pancreas is significantly lower among the patients who have undergone bariatric surgery [115]. Nevertheless, bariatric surgery is restricted to individuals with high obesity (mean BMI >40 kg/m2). Substantial weight loss (mean > 30% total body weight) occurs in these individuals after bariatric surgery. Moreover, intentional weight loss by bariatric surgery or changes in lifestyle or pharmacotherapy or less invasive surgical or endoscopic procedures also helps in reducing the risk of cancer in obese patients [115].

6. Role of visceral and Peripancreatic fat in pancreatic ductal adenocarcinoma

BMI is a well-known marker for adiposity, and can also be linked with insulin resistance, metabolic syndrome and gastrointestinal malignancies, like ductal adenocarcinoma of pancreas [116]. Highly inflamed visceral adipose tissue (VAT) in obese patients remains the main reason behind metabolic dysfunction and gastrointestinal cancer due to the close proximity of the visceral organs with the portal system. VAT has a high correlation with occurrence of ductal adenocarcinoma of pancreas. Interestingly, conditional KRasG12D (KC) mice fed high-fat and high calorie containing diet gained more weight than the standard diet fed mice and ended up developing hyperinsulinemia and hyperleptinemia with extensive VAT expansion and high inflammation [64, 65, 117]. These obese KC mice had highly inflamed pancreas and were more prone to develop ductal adenocarcinoma of pancreas than the control mice fed on standard diet and this occurred in the male mice, which meant that the sex hormones had a role in it [117]. Interestingly, the increased incidence of pancreatic ductal adenocarcinoma in obese KC mice was largely seen in male mice, suggesting a role for sex hormones in this process, since the female mice gained more adipose tissue subcutaneously [64, 65, 117].

7. Role of gut microbiome in pancreatic ductal adenocarcinoma

Human microbiome has gained a lot of popularity recently to tackle prevention, as well as early diagnosis, and treatment of ductal adenocarcinoma of pancreas, since many diseases have now started to be linked with composition of microbiome [118–120]. The composition of microbiome also interferes with development of ductal adenocarcinoma of pancreas and its relation with diabetes, obesity, and inflammation [121]. Ductal adenocarcinoma of pancreas is an inflammation-mediated cancer and gut microbiome can stimulate chronic inflammation via changes in molecular pattern recognition receptors. These pattern recognition receptors and their downstream signaling cascade leads to the incidence of inflammation-mediated cancers. These bacteria regulate the efficiency of calorie absorption in the intestines and hence lead to obesity. Many diseases like Type 2 diabetes, obesity, and chronic pancreatitis are linked with chronic inflammation, which also result in ductal adenocarcinoma of pancreas [122]. Moreover, alteration of oral microbiome increases risk of ductal adenocarcinoma of pancreas, and it can be a useful biomarker of the disease. Specific abundance in certain oral bacteria and gut microbiome in pancreatic secretions or fecal matter may be associated with risk of ductal adenocarcinoma of pancreas, hence these knowledges can help in preventing or in early diagnosis of ductal adenocarcinoma of pancreas [122].

8. Role of inflammation in pancreatic ductal adenocarcinoma

As already mentioned above, chronic inflammation in pancreas or chronic pancreatitis is a major reason behind ductal adenocarcinoma of pancreas. Activated PSCs play a key role in progression of chronic pancreatitis. Activation of PSCs is also increased by cytokines secreted from injured acinar and immune cells. The mechanisms underlying triggering of macrophages and survive the fibrotic processes by reacting with PSCs, if interfered end in suppression of inflammation and fibrosis in chronic pancreatitis [123]. Alcohol and smoking are also potent risk factors for chronic pancreatitis and ductal adenocarcinoma of pancreas. IL-22 signaling during inflammation and cross talk between immune cells and PSCs is one of the signaling involved in smoking-induced progression of chronic pancreatitis [124]. The other pathways that are behind progression of ductal adenocarcinoma of pancreas are IL-6 and histone deacetylases in immune and cancer cell interactions, which together mean that immune signals are key factors in promoting pancreatitis and pancreatic cancer progression [125]. However, most cases of ductal adenocarcinoma of pancreas are resistant to immunotherapies treatment with immune checkpoint antibodies because inflammatory processes are important in promoting the malignant transformation, growth, and metastasis of pancreatic cancer. For example, Kras mutations stimulate profuse cytokine and chemokine secretion in tumor epithelial cells and recruit immune cells like macrophages, dendritic cells (DCs), and myeloid-derived suppressive cells, all of which stimulate tumor growth and progression. So, all these cells need to be reprogrammed in ductal adenocarcinoma of pancreas to create a favorable immunostimulatory environment for efficient immunotherapy. Since, ductal adenocarcinoma of pancreas is often followed by metastatic relapse even after complete surgical pancreatic resection, the newly developed cancer cells fail in immunotherapy, which means that a better knowledge about the factors affecting metastasis is important for the development of more effective immunotherapies and treatments [126]. Early metastases are linked with dense networks of CD11b + CD11c + MHC-II + CD24 + CD64 and low F4/80 cells, and all of these cells develop from monocytes and aid in promoting metastasis by increasing regulatory T-cells and suppressing the development of cytotoxic T-cells. Phenotypically similar dendritic cells are seen to accumulate at primary and secondary sites in pancreatic portions of ductal adenocarcinoma of pancreas patients [127]. Dendritic cells can be reprogrammed into immunostimulatory antigen-presenting cells in tumor metastasis, which is one of the most popular immunotherapeutic strategies at present. Another strategy is based on the availability of tumor-binding immunoglobulin G antibodies along with some dendritic cell-stimulating molecules which help the enable tumor-associated dendritic cells to uptake, process, and present a variety of tumor antigens to T-cells. Then the T-cells proliferate and attack the tumors throughout the host. This technique can eradicate metastases, and also primary tumors in many types of cancers, including ductal adenocarcinoma of pancreas by overcoming tumor-mediated immunosuppression [128]. But the tumor cells tend to enter into the circulation and metastasize and end up colonizing distant organs [129]. Metastatic ductal adenocarcinoma of pancreas has many epigenetic modifications in the primary tumor. While the cancer cells circulate in clusters and colonize different organs, the establishment of a new premetastatic niche in a new organ includes proinflammatory processes, exosomes and immune cells [130]. All of this information can help in developing new therapeutic approaches targeting different agents for primary ductal adenocarcinoma of pancreas and also in its metastasis.

9. Conclusion

Ductal adenocarcinoma of pancreas is a very challenging malignancy with a high incidence and high lethality. Moreover, the disease has intricate relationships with diabetes and obesity. Type 2 diabetes has its own risks and can be both a risk factor for ductal adenocarcinoma of pancreas as well as an early manifestation of the disease. Obesity is also strongly associated with increasing risk of ductal adenocarcinoma of pancreas. However, every detail about all these diseases and their association is not fully understood, particularly the specific mechanisms that contribute to ductal adenocarcinoma of pancreas are not clear, which makes the diagnosis and treatment of ductal adenocarcinoma of pancreas very difficult. Hence present research is targeted in bringing out all the minute details and the mechanisms to tame this malignancy and preferably find a cure or a preventive mechanism or at least a better biomarker in near future.

Acknowledgements

AM is thankful to the Science & Engineering Research Board (SERB), Department of Science & Technology, Govt. of India, for her JRF fellowship (Grant No. ECR/2017/001028/LS). The author is thankful to Dr. Rakesh Kundu, Chandrani Fouzder, Snehasis Das and Dipanjan Chattopadhyay for technical assistance and constant encouragement.

Conflict of interest

The author declares no conflict of interest.

Notes/thanks/other declarations

The author thanks to the Head of the Department of Zoology, for providing the assistance in the research work.

Author details

Alpana Mukhuty
Cell Signaling Laboratory, Department of Zoology, Visva-Bharati University, Santiniketan, India

*Address all correspondence to: alpanamukhuty@yahoo.com

References

[1] Li D. Diabetes and pancreatic cancer. Mol Carcinog. 2012 Jan;51(1):64-74.

[2] Karnevi E, Said K, Andersson R, Rosendahl AH. Metformin-mediated growth inhibition involves suppression of the IGF-I receptor signalling pathway in human pancreatic cancer cells. BMC Cancer. 2013 May;13:235.

[3] Parkin DM, Bray F, Ferlay J, Pisani P. Global cancer statistics, 2002. CA Cancer J Clin. 2005;55(2):74-108.

[4] Jemal A, Siegel R, Ward E, Hao Y, Xu J, Thun MJ. Cancer statistics, 2009. CA Cancer J Clin [Internet]. 2009;59(4):225-249. Available from: http://europepmc.org/abstract/MED/19474385

[5] Pannala R, Leirness JB, Bamlet WR, Basu A, Petersen GM, Chari ST. Prevalence and clinical profile of pancreatic cancer-associated diabetes mellitus. Gastroenterology. 2008 Apr;134(4):981-987.

[6] Menke A, Casagrande S, Geiss L, Cowie CC. Prevalence of and Trends in Diabetes Among Adults in the United States, 1988-2012. JAMA. 2015 Sep;314(10):1021-1029.

[7] Wolpin BM, Bao Y, Qian ZR, Wu C, Kraft P, Ogino S, et al. Hyperglycemia, insulin resistance, impaired pancreatic β-cell function, and risk of pancreatic cancer. J Natl Cancer Inst. 2013 Jul;105(14):1027-1035.

[8] Tang H, Dong X, Hassan M, Abbruzzese JL, Li D. Body mass index and obesity- and diabetes-associated genotypes and risk for pancreatic cancer. Cancer Epidemiol biomarkers Prev a Publ Am Assoc Cancer Res cosponsored by Am Soc Prev Oncol. 2011 May;20(5):779-792.

[9] Kahn SE. The relative contributions of insulin resistance and beta-cell dysfunction to the pathophysiology of Type 2 diabetes. Diabetologia. 2003 Jan;46(1):3-19.

[10] Dooley J, Tian L, Schonefeldt S, Delghingaro-Augusto V, Garcia-Perez JE, Pasciuto E, et al. Genetic predisposition for beta cell fragility underlies type 1 and type 2 diabetes. Nat Genet. 2016 May;48(5):519-527.

[11] Andersen DK, Korc M, Petersen GM, Eibl G, Li D, Rickels MR, et al. Diabetes, Pancreatogenic Diabetes, and Pancreatic Cancer. Diabetes. 2017 May;66(5):1103-1110.

[12] Leclerc E, Vetter SW. The role of S100 proteins and their receptor RAGE in pancreatic cancer. Biochim Biophys Acta. 2015 Dec;1852(12):2706-2711.

[13] Song F, Hurtado del Pozo C, Rosario R, Zou YS, Ananthakrishnan R, Xu X, et al. RAGE regulates the metabolic and inflammatory response to high-fat feeding in mice. Diabetes. 2014 Jun;63(6):1948-1965.

[14] Pour PM, Kazakoff K. Stimulation of islet cell proliferation enhances pancreatic ductal carcinogenesis in the hamster model. Am J Pathol. 1996 Sep;149(3):1017-1025.

[15] Pour PM, Donnelly K, Stepan K. Modification of pancreatic carcinogenesis in the hamster model. 3. Inhibitory effect of alloxan. Am J Pathol. 1983 Mar;110(3):310-314.

[16] Pour PM, Patil K. Modification of pancreatic carcinogenesis in the hamster model. X. Effect of streptozotocin. J Natl Cancer Inst. 1983 Nov;71(5):1059-1065.

[17] Schneider MB, Matsuzaki H, Haorah J, Ulrich A, Standop J, Ding XZ, et al. Prevention of pancreatic cancer

induction in hamsters by metformin. Gastroenterology. 2001 Apr;120(5): 1263-1270.

[18] Ding XZ, Fehsenfeld DM, Murphy LO, Permert J, Adrian TE. Physiological concentrations of insulin augment pancreatic cancer cell proliferation and glucose utilization by activating MAP kinase, PI3 kinase and enhancing GLUT-1 expression. Pancreas. 2000 Oct;21(3):310-320.

[19] Ooi GT, Tseng LY, Tran MQ, Rechler MM. Insulin rapidly decreases insulin-like growth factor-binding protein-1 gene transcription in streptozotocin-diabetic rats. Mol Endocrinol. 1992 Dec;6(12): 2219-2228.

[20] Powell DR, Suwanichkul A, Cubbage ML, DePaolis LA, Snuggs MB, Lee PD. Insulin inhibits transcription of the human gene for insulin-like growth factor-binding protein-1. J Biol Chem. 1991 Oct;266(28):18868-18876.

[21] Bergmann U, Funatomi H, Yokoyama M, Beger HG, Korc M. Insulin-like growth factor I overexpression in human pancreatic cancer: evidence for autocrine and paracrine roles. Cancer Res. 1995 May;55(10):2007-2011.

[22] Ohmura E, Okada M, Onoda N, Kamiya Y, Murakami H, Tsushima T, et al. Insulin-like growth factor I and transforming growth factor alpha as autocrine growth factors in human pancreatic cancer cell growth. Cancer Res. 1990 Jan;50(1):103-107.

[23] Stoeltzing O, Liu W, Reinmuth N, Fan F, Parikh AA, Bucana CD, et al. Regulation of hypoxia-inducible factor-1alpha, vascular endothelial growth factor, and angiogenesis by an insulin-like growth factor-I receptor autocrine loop in human pancreatic cancer. Am J Pathol. 2003 Sep;163(3): 1001-1011.

[24] Zeng H, Datta K, Neid M, Li J, Parangi S, Mukhopadhyay D. Requirement of different signaling pathways mediated by insulin-like growth factor-I receptor for proliferation, invasion, and VPF/VEGF expression in a pancreatic carcinoma cell line. Biochem Biophys Res Commun. 2003 Feb;302(1):46-55.

[25] Pollak M. Insulin and insulin-like growth factor signalling in neoplasia. Nat Rev Cancer. 2008 Dec;8(12): 915-928.

[26] Wolpin BM, Michaud DS, Giovannucci EL, Schernhammer ES, Stampfer MJ, Manson JE, et al. Circulating insulin-like growth factor binding protein-1 and the risk of pancreatic cancer. Cancer Res. 2007 Aug;67(16):7923-7928.

[27] Heuson JC, Legros N. Influence of insulin deprivation on growth of the 7,12-dimethylbenz(a)anthracene-induced mammary carcinoma in rats subjected to alloxan diabetes and food restriction. Cancer Res. 1972 Feb;32(2):226-232.

[28] Hine RJ, Srivastava S, Milner JA, Ross SA. Nutritional links to plausible mechanisms underlying pancreatic cancer: a conference report. Vol. 27, Pancreas. United States; 2003. p. 356-366.

[29] Ogihara T, Asano T, Katagiri H, Sakoda H, Anai M, Shojima N, et al. Oxidative stress induces insulin resistance by activating the nuclear factor-kappa B pathway and disrupting normal subcellular distribution of phosphatidylinositol 3-kinase. Diabetologia. 2004 May;47(5):794-805.

[30] Bastard J-P, Maachi M, Lagathu C, Kim MJ, Caron M, Vidal H, et al. Recent advances in the relationship between obesity, inflammation, and insulin resistance. Eur Cytokine Netw. 2006 Mar;17(1):4-12.

[31] Gopaul NK, Manraj MD, Hébé A, Lee Kwai Yan S, Johnston A, Carrier MJ, et al. Oxidative stress could precede endothelial dysfunction and insulin resistance in Indian Mauritians with impaired glucose metabolism. Diabetologia. 2001 Jun;44(6):706-712.

[32] Manning PJ, Sutherland WHF, Walker RJ, Williams SM, De Jong SA, Ryalls AR, et al. Effect of high-dose vitamin E on insulin resistance and associated parameters in overweight subjects. Diabetes Care. 2004 Sep;27(9):2166-2171.

[33] Midaoui AEL, Elimadi A, Wu L, Haddad PS, de Champlain J. Lipoic acid prevents hypertension, hyperglycemia, and the increase in heart mitochondrial superoxide production. Am J Hypertens. 2003 Mar;16(3):173-179.

[34] Blendea MC, Jacobs D, Stump CS, McFarlane SI, Ogrin C, Bahtyiar G, et al. Abrogation of oxidative stress improves insulin sensitivity in the Ren-2 rat model of tissue angiotensin II overexpression. Am J Physiol Endocrinol Metab. 2005 Feb;288(2):E353-E359.

[35] Tirosh A, Potashnik R, Bashan N, Rudich A. Oxidative stress disrupts insulin-induced cellular redistribution of insulin receptor substrate-1 and phosphatidylinositol 3-kinase in 3T3-L1 adipocytes. A putative cellular mechanism for impaired protein kinase B activation and GLUT4 translocation. J Biol Chem. 1999 Apr;274(15): 10595-10602.

[36] Shoelson SE, Herrero L, Naaz A. Obesity, inflammation, and insulin resistance. Gastroenterology. 2007 May;132(6):2169-2180.

[37] Gallagher EJ, LeRoith D. Insulin, insulin resistance, obesity, and cancer. Curr Diab Rep. 2010 Apr;10(2):93-100.

[38] Aljada A, Ghanim H, Mohanty P, Syed T, Bandyopadhyay A, Dandona P. Glucose intake induces an increase in activator protein 1 and early growth response 1 binding activities, in the expression of tissue factor and matrix metalloproteinase in mononuclear cells, and in plasma tissue factor and matrix metalloproteinase conce. Am J Clin Nutr. 2004 Jul;80(1):51-57.

[39] Dhindsa S, Tripathy D, Mohanty P, Ghanim H, Syed T, Aljada A, et al. Differential effects of glucose and alcohol on reactive oxygen species generation and intranuclear nuclear factor-kappaB in mononuclear cells. Metabolism. 2004 Mar;53(3):330-334.

[40] Mohanty P, Ghanim H, Hamouda W, Aljada A, Garg R, Dandona P. Both lipid and protein intakes stimulate increased generation of reactive oxygen species by polymorphonuclear leukocytes and mononuclear cells. Am J Clin Nutr. 2002 Apr;75(4):767-772.

[41] van Kruijsdijk RCM, van der Wall E, Visseren FLJ. Obesity and cancer: the role of dysfunctional adipose tissue. Cancer Epidemiol biomarkers Prev a Publ Am Assoc Cancer Res cosponsored by Am Soc Prev Oncol. 2009 Oct;18(10):2569-2578.

[42] Lago R, Gómez R, Lago F, Gómez-Reino J, Gualillo O. Leptin beyond body weight regulation--current concepts concerning its role in immune function and inflammation. Cell Immunol. 2008;252(1-2):139-145.

[43] Smith TJ. Insulin-like growth factor-I regulation of immune function: a potential therapeutic target in autoimmune diseases? Pharmacol Rev. 2010 Jun;62(2):199-236.

[44] Wohlfert EA, Nichols FC, Nevius E, Clark RB. Peroxisome proliferator-activated receptor gamma (PPARgamma) and immunoregulation: enhancement of regulatory T cells through PPARgamma-dependent

and -independent mechanisms. J Immunol. 2007 Apr;178(7):4129-4135.

[45] Duffy DL. Genetic determinants of diabetes are similarly associated with other immune-mediated diseases. Curr Opin Allergy Clin Immunol. 2007 Dec;7(6):468-474.

[46] Petersen GM, Amundadottir L, Fuchs CS, Kraft P, Stolzenberg-Solomon RZ, Jacobs KB, et al. A genome-wide association study identifies pancreatic cancer susceptibility loci on chromosomes 13q22.1, 1q32.1 and 5p15.33. Nat Genet. 2010 Mar;42(3):224-8.

[47] Annicotte J-S, Fayard E, Swift GH, Selander L, Edlund H, Tanaka T, et al. Pancreatic-duodenal homeobox 1 regulates expression of liver receptor homolog 1 during pancreas development. Mol Cell Biol. 2003 Oct;23(19):6713-6724.

[48] Brissova M, Shiota M, Nicholson WE, Gannon M, Knobel SM, Piston DW, et al. Reduction in pancreatic transcription factor PDX-1 impairs glucose-stimulated insulin secretion. J Biol Chem. 2002 Mar;277(13):11225-11232.

[49] Glucksmann MA, Lehto M, Tayber O, Scotti S, Berkemeier L, Pulido JC, et al. Novel mutations and a mutational hotspot in the MODY3 gene. Diabetes. 1997 Jun;46(6):1081-1086.

[50] Herder C, Roden M. Genetics of type 2 diabetes: pathophysiologic and clinical relevance. Eur J Clin Invest. 2011 Jun;41(6):679-692.

[51] Fuchsberger C, Flannick J, Teslovich TM, Mahajan A, Agarwala V, Gaulton KJ, et al. The genetic architecture of type 2 diabetes. Nature. 2016 Aug;536(7614):41-47.

[52] Zeggini E, Scott LJ, Saxena R, Voight BF, Marchini JL, Hu T, et al. Meta-analysis of genome-wide association data and large-scale replication identifies additional susceptibility loci for type 2 diabetes. Nat Genet. 2008 May;40(5):638-645.

[53] Meigs JB, Shrader P, Sullivan LM, McAteer JB, Fox CS, Dupuis J, et al. Genotype score in addition to common risk factors for prediction of type 2 diabetes. N Engl J Med. 2008 Nov;359(21):2208-2219.

[54] Whitcomb DC. Genetic aspects of pancreatitis. Annu Rev Med. 2010;61:413-424.

[55] Whitcomb DC, LaRusch J, Krasinskas AM, Klei L, Smith JP, Brand RE, et al. Common genetic variants in the CLDN2 and PRSS1-PRSS2 loci alter risk for alcohol-related and sporadic pancreatitis. Nat Genet. 2012 Dec;44(12):1349-1354.

[56] Jones S, Hruban RH, Kamiyama M, Borges M, Zhang X, Parsons DW, et al. Exomic sequencing identifies PALB2 as a pancreatic cancer susceptibility gene. Science. 2009 Apr;324(5924):217.

[57] Roberts NJ, Jiao Y, Yu J, Kopelovich L, Petersen GM, Bondy ML, et al. ATM mutations in patients with hereditary pancreatic cancer. Cancer Discov. 2012 Jan;2(1):41-46.

[58] Hu C, Hart SN, Bamlet WR, Moore RM, Nandakumar K, Eckloff BW, et al. Prevalence of Pathogenic Mutations in Cancer Predisposition Genes among Pancreatic Cancer Patients. Cancer Epidemiol biomarkers Prev a Publ Am Assoc Cancer Res cosponsored by Am Soc Prev Oncol. 2016 Jan;25(1):207-211.

[59] Klein AP, Lindström S, Mendelsohn JB, Steplowski E, Arslan AA, Bueno-de-Mesquita HB, et al. An absolute risk model to identify individuals at elevated risk for pancreatic cancer in the general population. PLoS One. 2013;8(9):e72311.

[60] Renehan AG, Zwahlen M, Egger M. Adiposity and cancer risk: new mechanistic insights from epidemiology. Nat Rev Cancer. 2015 Aug;15(8):484-498.

[61] Park J, Morley TS, Kim M, Clegg DJ, Scherer PE. Obesity and cancer--mechanisms underlying tumour progression and recurrence. Nat Rev Endocrinol. 2014 Aug;10(8):455-465.

[62] Funahashi H, Satake M, Dawson D, Huynh N-A, Reber HA, Hines OJ, et al. Delayed progression of pancreatic intraepithelial neoplasia in a conditional Kras(G12D) mouse model by a selective cyclooxygenase-2 inhibitor. Cancer Res. 2007 Aug;67(15):7068-7071.

[63] Vongsuvanh R, George J, Qiao L, van der Poorten D. Visceral adiposity in gastrointestinal and hepatic carcinogenesis. Cancer Lett. 2013 Mar;330(1):1-10.

[64] Hertzer KM, Xu M, Moro A, Dawson DW, Du L, Li G, et al. Robust Early Inflammation of the Peripancreatic Visceral Adipose Tissue During Diet-Induced Obesity in the KrasG12D Model of Pancreatic Cancer. Pancreas. 2016 Mar;45(3):458-465.

[65] Dawson DW, Hertzer K, Moro A, Donald G, Chang H-H, Go VL, et al. High-fat, high-calorie diet promotes early pancreatic neoplasia in the conditional KrasG12D mouse model. Cancer Prev Res (Phila). 2013 Oct;6(10):1064-1073.

[66] Philip B, Roland CL, Daniluk J, Liu Y, Chatterjee D, Gomez SB, et al. A high-fat diet activates oncogenic Kras and COX2 to induce development of pancreatic ductal adenocarcinoma in mice. Gastroenterology. 2013 Dec;145(6):1449-1458.

[67] Pelaez-Luna M, Takahashi N, Fletcher JG, Chari ST. Resectability of presymptomatic pancreatic cancer and its relationship to onset of diabetes: a retrospective review of CT scans and fasting glucose values prior to diagnosis. Am J Gastroenterol. 2007 Oct;102(10):2157-2163.

[68] Aggarwal G, Kamada P, Chari ST. Prevalence of diabetes mellitus in pancreatic cancer compared to common cancers. Pancreas. 2013 Mar;42(2): 198-201.

[69] Permert J, Ihse I, Jorfeldt L, von Schenck H, Arnquist HJ, Larsson J. Improved glucose metabolism after subtotal pancreatectomy for pancreatic cancer. Br J Surg. 1993 Aug;80(8): 1047-1050.

[70] Pfeffer F, Koczan D, Adam U, Benz S, von Dobschuetz E, Prall F, et al. Expression of connexin26 in islets of Langerhans is associated with impaired glucose tolerance in patients with pancreatic adenocarcinoma. Pancreas. 2004 Nov;29(4):284-290.

[71] Basso D, Greco E, Fogar P, Pucci P, Flagiello A, Baldo G, et al. Pancreatic cancer-derived S-100A8 N-terminal peptide: a diabetes cause? Clin Chim Acta. 2006 Oct;372(1-2):120-128.

[72] Huang H, Dong X, Kang MX, Xu B, Chen Y, Zhang B, et al. Novel blood biomarkers of pancreatic cancer-associated diabetes mellitus identified by peripheral blood-based gene expression profiles. Am J Gastroenterol. 2010 Jul;105(7):1661-1669.

[73] He X-Y, Yuan Y-Z. Advances in pancreatic cancer research: moving towards early detection. World J Gastroenterol. 2014 Aug;20(32):11241-11248.

[74] Dehayem YM, Phelip J-M, Kengne A-P, Choukem S-P, Benhamou P-Y, Halimi S. Impact of diabetes mellitus on clinical presentation and prognosis of pancreatic cancer. Ann Endocrinol (Paris). 2011 Feb;72(1):24-29.

[75] De Souza A, Irfan K, Masud F, Saif MW. Diabetes Type 2 and Pancreatic Cancer: A History Unfolding. JOP. 2016 Mar;17(2):144-148.

[76] Busaidy NL, Yazbeck CF, Shah P, Evans DB, Li D, Geraci JM, et al. Survival of resectable pancreatic cancer patients with diabetes. J Clin Oncol [Internet]. 2006 Jun 20;24(18_suppl):4098. Available from: https://doi.org/10.1200/jco.2006.24.18_suppl.4098

[77] Olowokure OO, Beg MS, Ali S, Tandra A, Safa MM, Havlin K, et al. Is diabetes mellitus (DM) associated with worse outcomes in pancreatic cancer (PC)? J Clin Oncol [Internet]. 2010 May 20;28(15_suppl):4114. Available from: https://doi.org/10.1200/jco.2010.28.15_suppl.4114

[78] Sahin IH, Shama MA, Tanaka M, Abbruzzese JL, Curley SA, Hassan M, et al. Association of diabetes and perineural invasion in pancreatic cancer. Cancer Med. 2012 Dec;1(3):357-362.

[79] Chang M-C, Chang Y-T, Su T-C, Yang W-S, Chen C-L, Tien Y-W, et al. Adiponectin as a Potential Differential Marker to Distinguish Pancreatic Cancer and Chronic Pancreatitis. Pancreas [Internet]. 2007;35(1). Available from: https://journals.lww.com/pancreasjournal/Fulltext/2007/07000/Adiponectin_as_a_Potential_Differential_Marker_to.2.aspx

[80] van Kampen JGM, Marijnissen-van Zanten MAJ, Simmer F, van der Graaf WTA, Ligtenberg MJL, Nagtegaal ID. Epigenetic targeting in pancreatic cancer. Cancer Treat Rev. 2014 Jun;40(5):656-664.

[81] Hidalgo B, Irvin MR, Sha J, Zhi D, Aslibekyan S, Absher D, et al. Epigenome-wide association study of fasting measures of glucose, insulin, and HOMA-IR in the Genetics of Lipid Lowering Drugs and Diet Network study. Diabetes. 2014 Feb;63(2):801-807.

[82] Gilbert ER, Liu D. Epigenetics: the missing link to understanding β-cell dysfunction in the pathogenesis of type 2 diabetes. Epigenetics. 2012 Aug;7(8):841-852.

[83] Salman B, Zhou D, Jaffee EM, Edil BH, Zheng L. Vaccine therapy for pancreatic cancer. Vol. 2, Oncoimmunology. 2013. p. e26662.

[84] Musilli C, Paccosi S, Pala L, Gerlini G, Ledda F, Mugelli A, et al. Characterization of circulating and monocyte-derived dendritic cells in obese and diabetic patients. Mol Immunol [Internet]. 2011;49(1-2):234-238. Available from: http://europepmc.org/abstract/MED/21940050

[85] Farrell JJ, Zhang L, Zhou H, Chia D, Elashoff D, Akin D, et al. Variations of oral microbiota are associated with pancreatic diseases including pancreatic cancer. Gut. 2012 Apr;61(4):582-588.

[86] Tsukumo DML, Carvalho-Filho MA, Carvalheira JBC, Prada PO, Hirabara SM, Schenka AA, et al. Loss-of-function mutation in Toll-like receptor 4 prevents diet-induced obesity and insulin resistance. Diabetes. 2007 Aug;56(8):1986-1998.

[87] Truty MJ, Urrutia R. Basics of TGF-beta and pancreatic cancer. Pancreatol Off J Int Assoc Pancreatol . [et al]. 2007;7(5-6):423-35.

[88] Lunardi S, Muschel RJ, Brunner TB. The stromal compartments in pancreatic cancer: are there any therapeutic targets? Cancer Lett. 2014 Feb;343(2):147-155.

[89] Dunmore SJ, Brown JEP. The role of adipokines in β-cell failure of type 2 diabetes. J Endocrinol. 2013;216(1).

[90] Stefanovski D, Richey JM, Woolcott O, Lottati M, Zheng D, Harrison LN, et al. Consistency of the disposition index in the face of diet

induced insulin resistance: potential role of FFA. PLoS One [Internet]. 2011 Mar 30;6(3):e18134–e18134. Available from: https://pubmed.ncbi.nlm.nih.gov/21479217

[91] Halbrook CJ, Lyssiotis CA. Employing Metabolism to Improve the Diagnosis and Treatment of Pancreatic Cancer. Cancer Cell. 2017 Jan;31(1):5-19.

[92] Ying H, Dey P, Yao W, Kimmelman AC, Draetta GF, Maitra A, et al. Genetics and biology of pancreatic ductal adenocarcinoma. Genes Dev. 2016 Feb;30(4):355-385.

[93] Ying H, Kimmelman AC, Lyssiotis CA, Hua S, Chu GC, Fletcher-Sananikone E, et al. Oncogenic kras maintains pancreatic tumors through regulation of anabolic glucose metabolism. Cell [Internet]. 2012;149(3):656-670. Available from: http://dx.doi.org/10.1016/j.cell.2012.01.058

[94] Son J, Lyssiotis CA, Ying H, Wang X, Hua S, Ligorio M, et al. Glutamine supports pancreatic cancer growth through a KRAS-regulated metabolic pathway. Nature. 2013 Apr;496(7443):101-105.

[95] DeNicola GM, Karreth FA, Humpton TJ, Gopinathan A, Wei C, Frese K, et al. Oncogene-induced Nrf2 transcription promotes ROS detoxification and tumorigenesis. Nature. 2011 Jul;475(7354):106-109.

[96] Yang S, Wang X, Contino G, Liesa M, Sahin E, Ying H, et al. Pancreatic cancers require autophagy for tumor growth. Genes Dev. 2011 Apr;25(7):717-729.

[97] Perera RM, Stoykova S, Nicolay BN, Ross KN, Fitamant J, Boukhali M, et al. Transcriptional control of autophagy-lysosome function drives pancreatic cancer metabolism. Nature. 2015 Aug;524(7565):361-365.

[98] Commisso C, Davidson SM, Soydaner-Azeloglu RG, Parker SJ, Kamphorst JJ, Hackett S, et al. Macropinocytosis of protein is an amino acid supply route in Ras-transformed cells. Nature [Internet]. 2013;497(7451):633-637. Available from: https://doi.org/10.1038/nature12138

[99] Kamphorst JJ, Nofal M, Commisso C, Hackett SR, Lu W, Grabocka E, et al. Human pancreatic cancer tumors are nutrient poor and tumor cells actively scavenge extracellular protein. Cancer Res. 2015 Feb;75(3):544-553.

[100] Lyssiotis CA, Kimmelman AC. Metabolic Interactions in the Tumor Microenvironment. Trends Cell Biol. 2017 Nov;27(11):863-875.

[101] Sousa CM, Biancur DE, Wang X, Halbrook CJ, Sherman MH, Zhang L, et al. Pancreatic stellate cells support tumour metabolism through autophagic alanine secretion. Nature [Internet]. 2016;536(7617):479-483. Available from: https://doi.org/10.1038/nature19084

[102] Zhang Y, Velez-Delgado A, Mathew E, Li D, Mendez FM, Flannagan K, et al. Myeloid cells are required for PD-1/PD-L1 checkpoint activation and the establishment of an immunosuppressive environment in pancreatic cancer. Gut. 2017 Jan;66(1):124-136.

[103] Chang C-H, Qiu J, O'Sullivan D, Buck MD, Noguchi T, Curtis JD, et al. Metabolic Competition in the Tumor Microenvironment Is a Driver of Cancer Progression. Cell. 2015 Sep;162(6):1229-1241.

[104] Ho P-C, Bihuniak JD, Macintyre AN, Staron M, Liu X, Amezquita R, et al. Phosphoenolpyruvate Is a Metabolic Checkpoint of Anti-tumor T Cell Responses. Cell. 2015 Sep;162(6):1217-1228.

[105] Colegio OR, Chu N-Q, Szabo AL, Chu T, Rhebergen AM, Jairam V, et al. Functional polarization of tumour-associated macrophages by tumour-derived lactic acid. Nature. 2014 Sep;513(7519):559-563.

[106] Murray PJ. Amino acid auxotrophy as a system of immunological control nodes. Nat Immunol. 2016 Feb;17(2):132-139.

[107] Calle EE, Rodriguez C, Walker-Thurmond K, Thun MJ. Overweight, obesity, and mortality from cancer in a prospectively studied cohort of U.S. adults. N Engl J Med. 2003 Apr;348(17):1625-1638.

[108] Eibl G, Cruz-Monserrate Z, Korc M, Petrov MS, Goodarzi MO, Fisher WE, et al. Diabetes Mellitus and Obesity as Risk Factors for Pancreatic Cancer. J Acad Nutr Diet. 2018 Apr;118(4):555-567.

[109] Mathur A, Zyromski NJ, Pitt HA, Al-Azzawi H, Walker JJ, Saxena R, et al. Pancreatic steatosis promotes dissemination and lethality of pancreatic cancer. J Am Coll Surg. 2009 May;208(5):986-989.

[110] Zyromski NJ, Mathur A, Pitt HA, Wade TE, Wang S, Nakshatri P, et al. Obesity potentiates the growth and dissemination of pancreatic cancer. Surgery. 2009 Aug;146(2):258-263.

[111] Gaborit B, Abdesselam I, Kober F, Jacquier A, Ronsin O, Emungania O, et al. Ectopic fat storage in the pancreas using 1H-MRS: importance of diabetic status and modulation with bariatric surgery-induced weight loss. Int J Obes (Lond). 2015 Mar;39(3):480-487.

[112] Purnell JQ, Selzer F, Wahed AS, Pender J, Pories W, Pomp A, et al. Type 2 Diabetes Remission Rates After Laparoscopic Gastric Bypass and Gastric Banding: Results of the Longitudinal Assessment of Bariatric Surgery Study. Diabetes Care. 2016 Jul;39(7):1101-1107.

[113] Adams TD, Gress RE, Smith SC, Halverson RC, Simper SC, Rosamond WD, et al. Long-term mortality after gastric bypass surgery. N Engl J Med. 2007 Aug;357(8):753-761.

[114] Sjöström L, Gummesson A, Sjöström CD, Narbro K, Peltonen M, Wedel H, et al. Effects of bariatric surgery on cancer incidence in obese patients in Sweden (Swedish Obese Subjects Study): a prospective, controlled intervention trial. Lancet Oncol. 2009 Jul;10(7):653-662.

[115] Schauer DP, Feigelson HS, Koebnick C, Caan B, Weinmann S, Leonard AC, et al. Bariatric Surgery and the Risk of Cancer in a Large Multisite Cohort. Ann Surg. 2019 Jan;269(1):95-101.

[116] Aune D, Greenwood DC, Chan DSM, Vieira R, Vieira AR, Navarro Rosenblatt DA, et al. Body mass index, abdominal fatness and pancreatic cancer risk: a systematic review and non-linear dose-response meta-analysis of prospective studies. Ann Oncol Off J Eur Soc Med Oncol. 2012 Apr;23(4):843-852.

[117] Chang H-H, Moro A, Takakura K, Su H-Y, Mo A, Nakanishi M, et al. Incidence of pancreatic cancer is dramatically increased by a high fat, high calorie diet in KrasG12D mice. PLoS One. 2017;12(9):e0184455.

[118] Memba R, Duggan SN, Ni Chonchubhair HM, Griffin OM, Bashir Y, O'Connor DB, et al. The potential role of gut microbiota in pancreatic disease: A systematic review. Pancreatol Off J Int Assoc Pancreatol . [et al]. 2017;17(6):867-74.

[119] Signoretti M, Roggiolani R, Stornello C, Delle Fave G, Capurso G.

Gut microbiota and pancreatic diseases. Minerva Gastroenterol Dietol. 2017 Dec;63(4):399-410.

[120] Ertz-Archambault N, Keim P, Von Hoff D. Microbiome and pancreatic cancer: A comprehensive topic review of literature. World J Gastroenterol. 2017 Mar;23(10):1899-1908.

[121] Boulangé CL, Neves AL, Chilloux J, Nicholson JK, Dumas M-E. Impact of the gut microbiota on inflammation, obesity, and metabolic disease. Genome Med [Internet]. 2016;8(1):42. Available from: https://doi.org/10.1186/s13073-016-0303-2

[122] Jandhyala SM, Madhulika A, Deepika G, Rao GV, Reddy DN, Subramanyam C, et al. Altered intestinal microbiota in patients with chronic pancreatitis: implications in diabetes and metabolic abnormalities. Sci Rep. 2017 Mar;7:43640.

[123] Xue J, Sharma V, Hsieh MH, Chawla A, Murali R, Pandol SJ, et al. Alternatively activated macrophages promote pancreatic fibrosis in chronic pancreatitis. Nat Commun. 2015 May;6:7158.

[124] Xue J, Zhao Q, Sharma V, Nguyen LP, Lee YN, Pham KL, et al. Aryl Hydrocarbon Receptor Ligands in Cigarette Smoke Induce Production of Interleukin-22 to Promote Pancreatic Fibrosis in Models of Chronic Pancreatitis. Gastroenterology. 2016 Dec;151(6):1206-1217.

[125] Edderkaoui M, Xu S, Chheda C, Morvaridi S, Hu RW, Grippo PJ, et al. HDAC3 mediates smoking-induced pancreatic cancer. Oncotarget. 2016 Feb;7(7):7747-7760.

[126] Tseng WW, Winer D, Kenkel JA, Choi O, Shain AH, Pollack JR, et al. Development of an Orthotopic Model of Invasive Pancreatic Cancer in an Immunocompetent Murine Host. Clin Cancer Res [Internet]. 2010 Jul 15;16(14):3684 LP – 3683695. Available from: http://clincancerres.aacrjournals.org/content/16/14/3684.abstract

[127] Kenkel JA, Tseng WW, Davidson MG, Tolentino LL, Choi O, Bhattacharya N, et al. An Immunosuppressive Dendritic Cell Subset Accumulates at Secondary Sites and Promotes Metastasis in Pancreatic Cancer. Cancer Res. 2017 Aug;77(15):4158-4170.

[128] Carmi Y, Spitzer MH, Linde IL, Burt BM, Prestwood TR, Perlman N, et al. Allogeneic IgG combined with dendritic cell stimuli induce antitumour T-cell immunity. Nature. 2015 May;521(7550):99-104.

[129] Makohon-Moore A, Iacobuzio-Donahue CA. Pancreatic cancer biology and genetics from an evolutionary perspective. Nat Rev Cancer. 2016 Sep;16(9):553-565.

[130] Giovannetti E, van der Borden CL, Frampton AE, Ali A, Firuzi O, Peters GJ. Never let it go: Stopping key mechanisms underlying metastasis to fight pancreatic cancer. Semin Cancer Biol. 2017 Jun;44:43-59.

Chapter 16

Hypomelanosis Secondary to Cutaneous Inflammation

Behzad Dalvand

Abstract

Hypomelanosis is a prevalent skin disorder in individuals with dark skin. Numerous inflammatory skin disorders cause hypomelanosis, even depigmentation. Its pathogenesis remains unknown, but it can be attributed to changes in melanin production in response to inflammation. The clinical manifestations, often including lesions with ill-defined borders limited to the site of inflammation, mostly appear in individuals with dark skin. The most important way to manage PIH is to effectively treat the underlying skin disorder that has led to it, however, medical therapy and phototherapy can be helpful, as well.

Keywords: PIH, hypomelanosis secondary to inflammation, depigmentation, pathogenesis, melanocytes

1. Introduction

Hypomelanosis is a prevalent skin disorder in dark-skinned Individuals. The numerous skin diseases that cause hypomelanosis include psoriasis, mycosis fungoides, sarcoidosis, pityriasis lichenoides chronica, lichen striatus, lupus erythematosus and lichen sclerosus. Different clinical pictures of lesions and multiple factors in developing post-inflammatory hypopigmentation (PIH) constitute a diagnostic challenge for dermatologists.

1.1 Pathogenesis

Although many studies have addressed PIH, its exact etiology remains unknown and needs the assistance of cytologists. PIH is actually caused by a disorder in melanocyte-keratinocyte interactions. The release of inflammatory agents can be involved in the synthesis of melanin or transfer of melanin to keratinocytes, especially by inhibiting the transfer of melanin from melanocytes to keratinocytes. Melanocytes can respond by changing melanin production in response to posttraumatic stress and inflammation.

Individuals inherit chromatic tendency in the predominantly autosomal dominant form. Hypopigmentation can develop as a result of damage to melanocytes, especially in patients with weak melanocytes. It is worth noting that melanocytes can be weak even in individuals with fair skin. Different factors control melanogenesis as a complex process that involves the synthesis, transfer and release of melanin. PIH is mostly caused by the inhibition rather than destruction of melanocytes.

Moreover, severe inflammatory responses of the skin can cause melanocyte loss or death and thus pigmentation changes.

1.2 Clinical manifestations

The clinical manifestations, often including lesions with ill-defined borders limited to the site of inflammation, mostly emerge in individuals with dark skin, especially in those prone to hypopigmentation or even depigmentation. They are associated with diagnostic challenges, especially in children, as they can be associated with minor or asymptomatic variations.

The clinical features normally vary based on the primary skin lesions and the lesion margins are often blurred.

The rate of hypopigmentation varies with the age and severity of the cutaneous lesions and severity of the inflammation. Identifying the underlying cause of hypopigmentation can be difficult upon the patient admission, as inflammation of advanced lesions may decrease in severity or even gradually disappear (**Figure 1**). A complex description and frequent examinations are therefore required in these cases. Biopsy and histological examinations are also required in the absence of inflammatory symptoms.

1.3 Treatment

The most important treatment is to effectively treat the underlying skin disorder that has led to PIH because PIH usually improves over time.

UVB phototherapy and epidermal melanocyte transplantation can help treat completely-destroyed or depigmented melanocytes. Photo protection, apply broad spectrum (UVAUVB) SPF 30 or 50 and reapply every 2–4 hours self-tanner (dihydroxyocetonc). Applying topical ironoxide (3%) can effectively protect the skin against blue visible light, especially in dark-skinned patients with PIH.

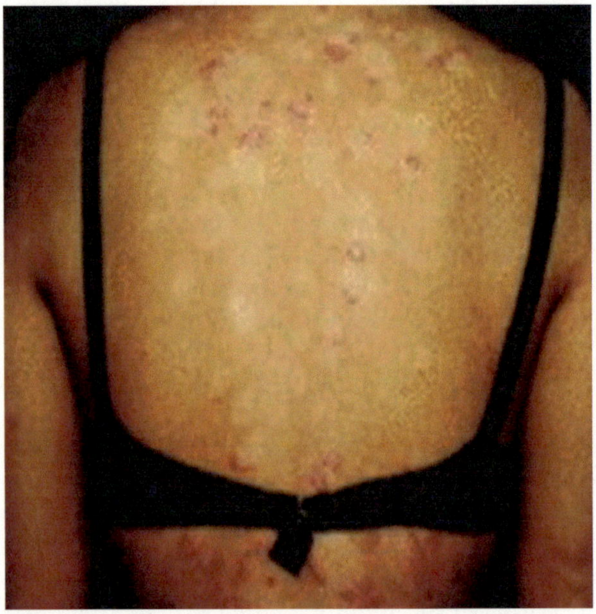

Figure 1.
Psoriasis, showing multiple-well dermarcated hypopigmented lesions.

2. Diseases of PIH

2.1 Pityriasis alba

2.1.1 Introduction

Pityriasis albais a prevalent benign but chronic and inflammatory dermatosis and a minor skin feature of atopic dermatitis that mostly emerges in 3 to 16-year-old individuals. Its prevalence is 1.9%–9.9% in children and up to 5%, especially when coupled with atopic dermatitis.

2.1.2 Pathogenesis

Different mechanisms can be considered for explaining the still-unknown etiology of pityriasis alba. A history of atopic dermatitis constitutes a pathogenic factor in pityriasis alba.

A Positive Relationship between health habits and pityriasis alba, frequent bathing and excessive washing may contribute to the lesion.

Nutritional factors and copper deficiency are also effective. Tyrosine in dermal cells involved in producing melanin is activated by copper. Pathological examinations with electron microscopy and light microscopy showed decreases in the number and size of melanosomes in the affected skin [1].

2.1.3 Clinical manifestations

The eruptions usually appear as round or oval macules or patches with an indistinct border with or without slight and often asymptomatic scales (**Figure 2**). The lesions normally become more visible in summer and may initially appear pink in

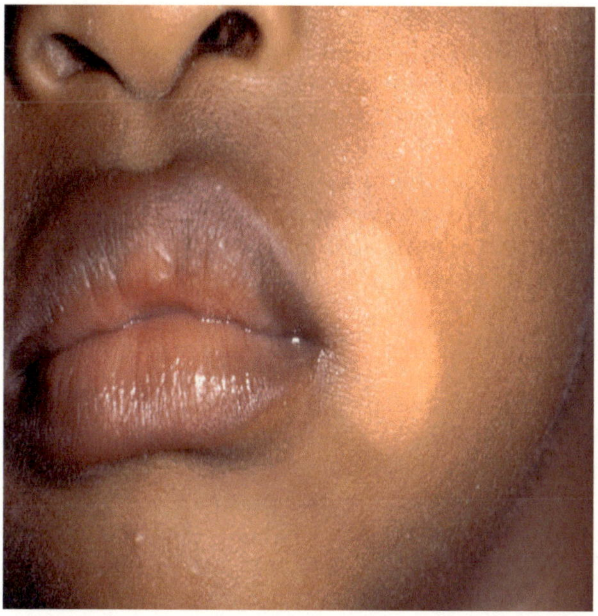

Figure 2.
Pityriasis alba: A common disfiguring hypomelanosis, which, as the name indicates, is a white area (alba) with very mild scaling (pityriasis). It is observed in a large number of children in the summer intemperate climates.

a way that the erythema subsides and turns white with powdery appearance and a pink border within a few weeks. With a size of 5–30 mm, the lesions mostly involve the face. Direct examination of scrapings with 10% KOH and slit-skin smear are respectively used to diagnose tinea versicolor and leprosy, and Wood's lamp examinations are performed for distinguishing vitiligo and the diseases associated with hypopigmentation.

It is mostly a cosmetic problem in persons with brown or black skin and commonly occurs on the face, as in this child. Among 200 patients with pityriasis alba, 90% ranged from 6–12 years of age. In young adults, PA quite often occurs on the arms and trunk [2].

2.1.4 Treatment

If pityriasis alba is left untreated, it can turn chronic and recurrent, although it self-heals in most cases after puberty. Topical steroids class V help reduce the lesion inflammation caused by pityriasis alba. Calcineurin inhibitors such as pimecrolimus cream1% and tacrolimus ointment 0.3% or 0.1% with anti-inflammatory properties can positively affect and activate tyrosinase and thus increase melanin synthesis [3]. Narrow-band UVB and excimer light or excimer laser treatment also yields proper responses through 5–10 treatments of 308 nm excimer laser.

2.2 Cutaneous lupus erythematosus

2.2.1 Introduction

Cutaneous lupus erythematosus is more prevalent in women with dark skin, especially in their fourth decade of life. One to five percent of the patients may progress to systemic lupus erythematosus.

2.2.2 Pathogenesis

Trauma and UVR may have been involved in the onset and exacerbation of symptoms in a person with a predisposed background. Photosensitivity is also observed in 50% of the patients. Histologic examinations can suggest lymphocytic interface dermatitis with basal layer degeneration (hydropic degeneration), keratinocyte apoptosis, basement membrane thickening (greatest in discoid lupus erythematosus), perivascular and periadnexal lymphohistiocytic infiltrate, follicular plugging, cutaneous mucinosis, epidermal atrophy, fibrosis, hypomelanosis and amelanosis, which are observed especially in the center of the lesions.

2.2.3 Clinical manifestations

As the most prevalent manifestations, sharply demarcated lesions in discoid lupus erythematosus (DLE) can be round, justifying the term "discoid". The face and scalp constitute the most commonly affected sites.

DLE lesions are usually asymmetric and asymptomatic with a well-defined and elevated margin, which explains their red to violaceous color. These lesions often appear atrophic and hypopigmented or depigmented, especially in black individuals with prominent follicular plugs (**Figure 3**). Their hypopigmented center is often surrounded by a hyperpigmented margin.

Systemic lupus erythematosus can be assessed by performing a complete blood count, an erythrocyte sedimentation rate and an antinuclear antibody test.

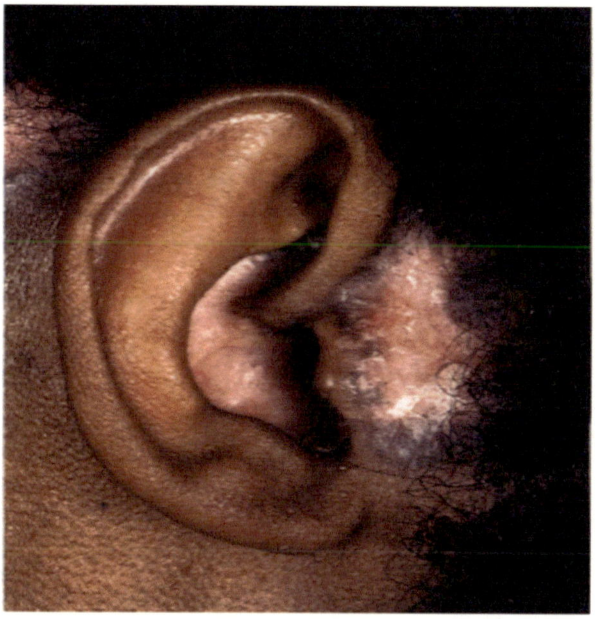

Figure 3.
Discoid lupus erythematosus; there are well-defined, erythematous, scaling lesions with a pigmented margin and central depigmention and behind the ear in this west Indian.

2.2.4 Treatment

Initial treatment options include topical steroids, intralesional steroids, antimalarial medications such as Hydroxychloroquine, and acitretin. High-potency corticosteroids are recommended for the facial lesions.

Intralesional triamcinolone, commonly at a concentration of 4 to 5 mg/ml, can be very effective especially in active discoid lesions.

Reports suggest the successful application of new topical immunomodulators such as tacrolimus to cutaneous lesions.

2.3 Systemic sclerosis (scleroderma)

2.3.1 Introduction

As a collagen vascular disease with cutaneous fibrosis as its skin manifestation, systemic sclerosis causes skin tightening and pigmentary changes. The incidence and prevalence of scleroderma are respectively below two per million and 25 per million [4, 5].

2.3.2 Pathogenesis

Abnormal immune responses, vascular dysfunction and activation of connective tissue cells have been reported in genetically-predisposed individuals. Different environmental and occupational factors such as silica and [6]. organic solvents can be involved.

Electron microscopy shows depigmentation, loss of melanocytes and degenerative changes.

2.3.3 Clinical manifestations

The clinical patterns of the disease include limited cutaneous systemic sclerosis, which is limited to distal limbs, reaches up to the knees and elbows and usually involves the face.

The patients may present only with fibrosis of the fingers. The other pattern, diffuse cutaneous systemic sclerosis, involves the trunk in its early stages and facial involvement is uncommon. This type is often associated with more systemic involvements and a worse prognosis.

Systemic sclerosis can cause diffuse hyperpigmentation that is exacerbated in sun-exposed areas, a specific manifestation of leukoderma. A combination of hypomelanosis and hypermelanosis can be present in the sclerotic and non-sclerotic skin areas of patients with systemic sclerosis, especially on their hands. Leukoderma emerging as complete depigmentation can be comorbid with supravenous hyper-pigmentation and perifollicular macules (**Figure 4**). This type of leukoderma can suggest suspected systemic scleroderma.

Histological examinations with an electron microscope shows complete or partial loss of melanocyte pigmentation coupled with degenerative changes.

It is actually a collagen vascular disease with some degree of cutaneous fibrosis that causes skin tightening.

2.3.4 Treatment

Topical and intralesional steroids are recommended for the inflammatory stages. Topical tacrolimus, calcipotriol and imiquimod have been also used. Combination therapies used in the absence of responses include calcipotriol and betamethasone or imiquimod or low dose PUVA alone or with calcipotriol.

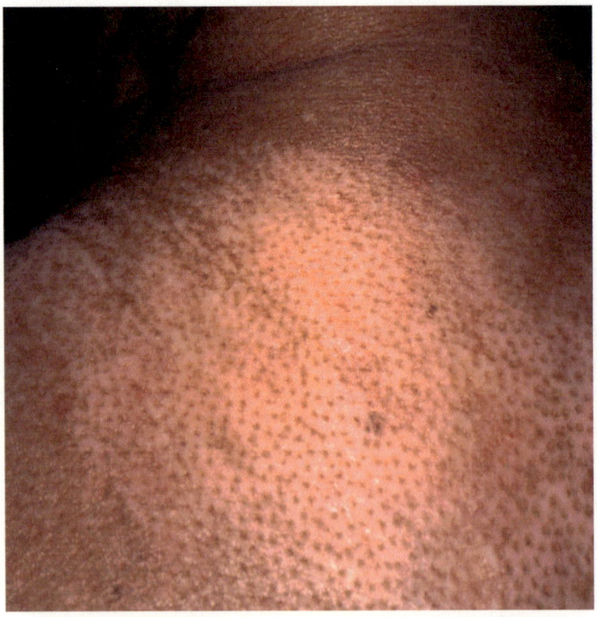

Figure 4.
"Salt and pepper" sign Leukoderma with the retention of perifollicular pigmentation in a patient with systemic sclerosis.

2.4 Hypopigmented mycosis fungoides (HMF)

2.4.1 Introduction

HMF is a variant of early MF, which is more prevalent in black individuals. HMF mostly affects ages of 30–40 years, although this type can involve 25–50% of children and adolescents. In fact, it is a prevalent type of MF in children. As a prevalent condition in the Middle East, HMF can be misdiagnosed as pityriasis alba or tinea versicolor in children. A study reported HMF in18 out of 34 subjects and 29 out of 50 adolescents and children [7].

2.4.2 Pathogenesis

Mycosis fungoides is a cutaneous T-cell lymphoma with a major phenotype of C8+T cells and a pathogenic similarity to vitiligo. Given the absence of clinically hypopigmented lesions in the majority of patients with mycosis fungoides and T cells, presence of cytotoxic T cell phenotypesis not adequate for inducing hypopigmentation. Although electron microscopy shows melanosome degradation in melanocytes and keratinocytes, the large number of normal melanosomes found in melanocytes suggests a defect in melanosome transfer.

2.4.3 Clinical manifestations

Patients with mycosis fungoides May present with hypopigmented patches and plaques, usually associated with mild erythema and pruritus (**Figure 5**). The lesions are distributed more in the trunk and proximal areas of the limbs, especially in the non-exposed areas. Closer examinations show erythematous lesions.

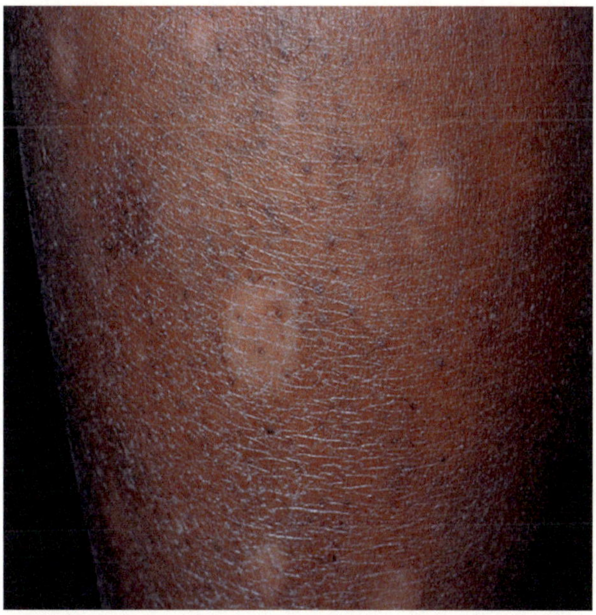

Figure 5.
Mycosis fungoides, hypopigmented patches.

2.4.4 Treatment

Repigmentation following treatments can be a sign of their effectiveness. Despite being the only manifestation of conventional mycosis fungoides, HMF is better in terms of its prognosis [8].

One year of treatment with a combination of steroids and tacrolimus, twice a week, was reported to significantly improve hypopigmented patches and cause no recurrence of lesions, and UVB phototherapy, 2–3 times a week, was found to yield proper responses [9].

2.5 Hypopigmented sarcoidosis

2.5.1 Introduction

Hypopigmented sarcoidosis is a multisystem granulomatous disease that affects organs such as the lungs, eyes and skin as well as lymph nodes. The exact cause of hypopigmentation in sarcoidosis is unknown. Cutaneous manifestations have been reported in one- quarter to one-third of patients with systemic sarcoidosis. The prevalence of the lesions with different morphologies has been reported as high as 60% in black individuals. The prevalence is also twice in females than in males.

2.5.2 Pathogenesis

Sarcoidosis can be caused by autoimmune reactions or genetic processes given the existing racial and ethnic differences. HLA haplotype diversity patterns can explain different manifestations between different races. This disorder is histopathologically categorized as a granulomatous disease given the non-caseating granulomas found in the dermis. Electron microscopy also shows vacuolated melanocytes and decreases in the number of melanosomes in keratinocytes. Granulomas mainly include epithelioid cells and occasionally giant cells, with lymphocytic infiltration around granulomasin the absence of caseous necrosis.

2.5.3 Clinical manifestations

The most prevalent skin manifestations of sarcoidosis include small erythematous-violaceous papules 3–5 mm. Sarcoidosis often initiates in an acute state and then becomes chronic. With a peripheral scaly marginand a hypopigmented center (**Figure 6**), the annular lesions are usually limited to the head and neck with a poor prognosis. A rare cutaneous form with patches or plaques usually appearing 1–10 mm in size mainly involves the trunk and face. Erythematous papules in the center of the patches resemble a fried egg [10].

The patients are often asymptomatic and usually diagnosed through radiological examinations. A skin biopsy and pathological examinations may also be ultimately required.

2.5.4 Treatment

Although acute sarcoidosis is a self-healing conditions, cutaneous sarcoidosis with systemic involvement can be treated with 1 mg/kg/day of prednisolone as an oral steroid to cleanse the skin lesions. The localized skin manifestations can be treated only with topical steroids or intralesional injections. Anti-TNF biologic medications can be used as alternatives to steroids, especially when steroids are

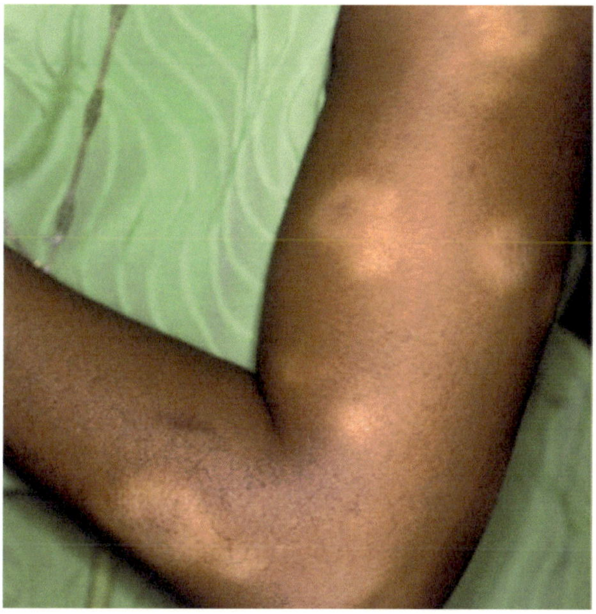

Figure 6.
Cutaneous sarcoidosis; clinical variants, the hypopigmented variant is more noticeable in individuals with a darkly-pigmented skin.

contraindicated. Hypopigmented cutaneous sarcoidosis is responsive to minocycline [11] and can be treated with 8-methoxypsoralen [12] and long-wave ultraviolet light.

2.6 Lichen Striatus

2.6.1 Introduction

Lichen striatus is a benign self-limiting dermatosis with an unknown etiology. It is more prevalent in children than in other age groups, it is acquired and unilaterally occurs along the lines of blaschko. Although the lesions are often transient, they may be of a prolonged form.

Lichen striatus is associated with vitiligo or atopic dermatitis. It mainly affects children at an age of 3.5 years, although it may occur in children of 4 months to 10 years of age.

2.6.2 Clinical manifestations

Lichen striatus usually manifests itself as smooth and scaly or hypopigmented flat-topped papules, which are 2-4 mm in size and initially inflammatory (**Figure 7**). The lesions appear as continuous or interrupted flat papules along the lines of blaschko within 2–3 weeks. The eruptions, being mainly distributed in the limbs, especially the lower limbs, normally leave a long-lasting hypopigmentation in 50% of the cases. According to recent studies in India, lichen striatus causes hypopigmentation in approximately 1.7% of the patients [13].

2.6.3 Treatment

No treatments are normally required given the benign and self-limiting nature of the disease. Tacrolimus ointment has been found to speed up the relief and cause complete healing without skin sequelae.

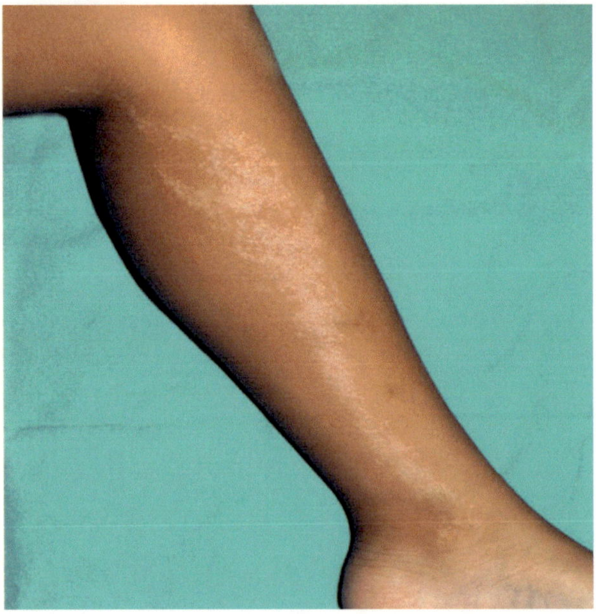

Figure 7.
Lichen striatus: Linear streaks on the leg alongthe lines of Blaschko, comparing numerous small, flat-topped tan (hypopigmented) papules.

3. Conclusion

Numerous inflammatory skin diseases can cause pigmentation disorders, which suggests that despite multiple inflammatory disease of skin, ultimately through the activation of inflammatory agents located in the skin, such as T cells, cytokines and other inflammatory cells that lead to disregulation of melanogenesis system.

However, the exact mechanism of PIH is not known and further studies are needed. Despite advance in treating the cause of the hypomelanosis, but PIH is still a challenge for dermatologists. Appropriate treatment for PIH is to identify the underlying cause and treat it, with applying symptomatic therapy.

Conflict of interest

The author declares no conflict of interest.

Author details

Behzad Dalvand
Artina Skin and Hair Clinic, Tehran, Iran

*Address all correspondence to: dalvandb@yahoo.com

References

[1] Bolognia J, Shaffer J, Cerroni L. Dermatology. 4th ed. Toronto: Elsevier; 2018. 2880 p. ISBN: 9780702062759.

[2] Dinalos J. Habif' clinical Dermatology. 7th ed. Toronto: Elesvier; 2020. 1086 p. E-ISBN: 9780323612708

[3] Hoeger P, Kinsler V, Yan A, Harper J, Oranje A, Bodemer C, et al. Harper's Textbook of pediatric Dermatology. 4th ed. Blackwell: Willy; 2020. 2413 p. DOI:10.1002/9781119142812

[4] Furst DE, Fernandes AVV, Lorga SR, Greth W, Bancroft T. Epidemiology of systemic sclerosis in a large US managed care population. J Rhematol. 2012;89:784-786. DOI: 10.3899/jrheum.111106

[5] Horimoto AMC, Matos ENN, da Costa MR, Takahashi F, Rezende MC, Kanomata LB, et al. Incidence and prevalence of systemic sclerosis in Compo Grorde, Sal, Brazil. Rev Bras Rheumafol. 2017;57:107-114. DOI: 10.1016/j.rbre.2016.09.005

[6] Callen J, Jorrizo J, Zone J, Piette W, Rosenbach M, Vleugels RA. Dermatological sign of systemic diseases. 5th ed. Toronto: Elsevier; 2017. 480 p. ISBN: 9780323358293

[7] Boulos S, Vaid R, Aladily TN, Ivan DS, Talpur R, Duvic M. Clinical presentation, immunopathology, and treatment of juvenile-onset mycosis fungoides; A case series of 34 patients. J Am Acad Dermatol. 2014;71(6):1117-1126. DOI:https://doi.org/10.1016/j.jaad.2014.07.049

[8] Cerroni L. Skin Lymphoma. The illustrated guide. 4th ed. Chichester. Wiley-Blackwell; 2020. 425 p. ISBN: 9781119485919

[9] Zaidi Z, Hussain K, Sudhakaran S. Treatment of skin disease: A practical guide. 1st ed. Switzerland: Springer; 2019. 551 p. DOI: 10.1007/978-3-319-89581-9

[10] Condrice RH, David J, Taylor SC. Sarcoidosis: Are there differences in your skin of color patients? J Am Acad Dermatol. 2012;66(1):121. DOI: 10.1016/j.jaad.2010.06.068

[11] Schmitt CE, Fabi SG, Kukreja T, Feinberg JS. Hypopigmented cutaneous sarcoidosis responsive to minocycline. J Drugs Dermatol. 2012;11(3):385-9. PMID: 22395590

[12] Patterson JW, Fitzwater JE. Treatment of hypopigmented sarcoidosis with 8-methoxypsoralen and long wave ultraviolet light. Int J Dermatol. 1982;21(8):476-80.DOI: 10.1111/j.1365-4362.1982.tb03187.x.

[13] Chong JH, Mermin D, Goussot JF, Taieb A. Vitiligo co existing with lichen striatus: more than a co incidence? J Eur Acad Dermatol Venereol. 2017;31(4):e200-e202. DOI: 10.1111/jdv.13954.

Section 7

Parasites as Immunomodulatory Approach in Chronic Inflammation

Chapter 17

Helminth Induced Immunomodulation against Metainflammation and Insulin Resistance

Vivekanandhan Aravindhan and Sibi Joy Manohar

Abstract

Filariasis mediated immunomodulation against metabolic diseases is a recently identified novel phenomenon. There seems to be an inverse relationship between filarial infections and type-2 diabetes. Rapid elimination of filarial diseases, due to mass drug administration has somehow fueled the sudden and rampant increase in type-2 diabetes, at least in certain tropical countries, like India and Indonesia. Filarial infections are in a way unique, since they bring about immunomodulation, in contrast to inflammation which is triggered by viral and bacterial infections. This dampens immunity and confers better survival for the pathogen. However, this also attenuates chronic inflammation and insulin resistance and thereby confers protection against type-2 diabetes. This chapter elucidates the various immune mechanisms involved in immunomodulation against insulin resistance and type-2 diabetes induced by helminth infection.

Keywords: Metainflammation, Insulin Resistance, Immunomodulation, Helminth infections, Metabolic diseases

1. Introduction

1.1 What is metainflammation?

Chronic inflammation has long been recognized as a major etiological factor for metabolic diseases [1]. The inflammation in metabolic diseases is chronic, low grade and non-antigen-specific but differs from one condition to other [2]. This is different from those seen in infectious diseases and has been named "Metainflammation". Meta inflammation leads to insulin resistance (IR) wherein the target organs of insulin become resistant to insulin action [2]. IR has now been identified as a major etiological factor for a variety of metabolic diseases, apart from obesity and Type-2 diabetes (T2DM) [2]. Meta inflammation typically starts as an organ-specific inflammation affecting the major target organs of insulin namely adipose tissue, skeletal muscles and liver [2]. With disease progression, it becomes more systemic and starts affecting the blood vessels leading to endothelial dysfunction called vasculopathy [2]. The exact cause of inflammation in IR is not clearly known even though dietary, genetic and environmental factors have been implicated [2].

1.2 Helminth infection as an immunomodulation strategy

Infections serve as an important source of inflammation especially in tropical countries and can serve as a link between infections and metabolic diseases [3]. The link between infections and metabolic diseases is less well explored and in recent years has gained tremendous interest [3]. Changes in the lifestyle of people living in industrialized countries have led to a decrease in the infectious burden and an increase in the prevalence of allergic and autoimmune diseases [4]. The leading idea is that some infectious agents – notably those that co-evolved with us – are able to protect us against a large spectrum of immune-related disorders [5]. The strongest evidence for a causal relationship between the decline of infectious diseases and the increase in immunological disorders originates from animal models and a number of clinical studies, suggesting the beneficial effect of infectious agents or their components known as immunomodulators [5]. Immunomodulators are drugs or molecules (Thalidomide. Macrolide antibiotics, and curcumin) that modify the dangerous immune response to prevent the inflammatory damage, while leaving the protective immune response intact [6]. It is speculated that infections as such are important in keeping the immunoregulatory network active and, in the absence of such infections, the immune system gets hyperactivated, resulting in allergies and autoimmunity [5]. In this regard, the helminth infections need a special mention since they were found to be alleviating numerous autoimmune disorders like atopic disorders, systemic lupus erythematosus, multiple sclerosis, sepsis, inflammatory bowel diseases [7].

Not all infections promote inflammation. While in general, viral and bacterial diseases induce inflammation, helminth infections are largely immunosuppressive in nature [3]. The link between fungal and protozoan diseases, with systemic inflammation, is not known. In general, infections which promote inflammation are thought to augment metabolic diseases while those which dampen inflammation by immunomodulation can confer protection against metabolic diseases [3]. Previously, we have shown a decreased prevalence of filarial infection (not disease) among both T1DM [8] and T2DM subjects [9]. Further, serum cytokine profiling revealed the downregulation of Interleukin-6 (IL-6), Tumour Necrosis Factor-alpha (TNF-α) and Granulocyte-Macrophage-Colony Stimulating Factor (GM-CSF) and upregulation of Tumour Growth Factor-Beta (TGF-β) in filarial positive, compared to filarial negative diabetic subjects [9]. Interestingly, the immunomodulatory effect of helminth infection was seen only inT1DM and T2DM subjects but not among the coronary artery disease (CAD) patients [10]. Even though these were cross-sectional studies, they indicate probable immune-mediated protection against both T1DM and T2DM by prior filarial infection. This also indicates some degree of overlap in the disease pathology between these two seemingly different forms of diabetes, which the helminth infection is able to target [3, 11]. If this is true, the decreasing incidence of filariasis (due to mass drug administration programs) which is being carried globally, can fuel diabetic pandemic in future [3, 11]. Thus, childhood infection can either have a beneficial or harmful role in determining the susceptibility to T2DM depending upon the nature of immune training-induced [3, 11].

2. Role of innate immune cells in insulin resistance and immunomodulation

Traditionally monocytes/macrophages, dendritic cells, Natural killer (NK) cells and granulocytes (neutrophils, eosinophils and basophils) together form the cellular arm of innate immunity, since they recognize the pathogen and damage-associated molecular patterns (PAMPs and DAMPs) [2]. T and B lymphocytes together form the cellular arm of the adaptive immunity, since they recognize antigens/epitopes and have immunological memory [2]. During an immune response, cells of innate immunity recognize PAMPs and DAMPs through various innate immune receptors like Toll-like Receptors (TLRs), NOD-Like Receptors (NLRs), RIG-1 Like Receptors (RLRs) and C-Type Lectin Like Receptors (CLRs), etc. and get activated. Most of these cells take up the cargo, process them and present them to the T cells within the context of MHC [12]. B cells on the other hand take up antigens by antibody-mediated endocytosis, process them and present them to the T cells [12]. The T cells which recognize these MHC: epitope complexes through their T Cell Receptors (TCRs), get activated and secrete cytokines and chemokines [12]. These cytokines and chemokines in turn activate and attract more number of antigen-presenting cells (APCs), completing the positive feedback loop [12]. Thus, antigen processing and presentation and subsequent secretion of cytokines and chemokines establish the cross-talks between innate and adaptive immune responses, which finally determine the magnitude and nature of the immune response [12]. Next, we will look at the role played by specific cell-types in IR and immunomodulation.

2.1 Macrophages in insulin resistance and immunomodulation

Out of several immune cell types, macrophages were the earliest to be associated with IR [13]. Macrophages are phagocytic cells that serve as the first line of defence mechanism against infections [14]. They are of two types: M1 (classically activated) and M2 (alternatively activated), which differ in their cytokine secretion and functions [14]. The infiltration of macrophages into adipose tissue under conditions of obesity-associated IR was reported as early as 1976 [13]. Classically activated or $CD11c^{+}CD206^{-}$ M1 macrophages were found to be elevated in visceral adipose tissue (VAT) of diet-induced obese (DIO) mice which secrete increased levels of pro-inflammatory cytokines like TNF-α, IL-1β and IL-6 (**Figure 1**) [15]. Transcriptional profiling of adipose tissue from leptin knock-out mice revealed the upregulation of 1,304 genes which showed a strong correlation with the body mass index. Of the top 100 genes which were differentially expressed, 30% were specific for macrophages [16]. Resident macrophages in lean mice expressed Macrophage Galactose-binding C-type lectin (MGL-1) along with other genes associated with M2 macrophages

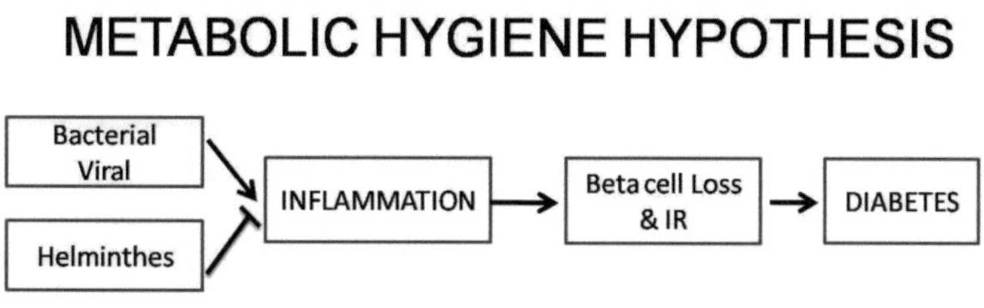

Figure 1.
Model explaining "Metabolic Hygiene Hypothesis". Chronic inflammation serves as a link between infections and type-2 diabetes. During early stages of the disease, the inflammation is more tissue restricted and primarily affects pancreas and target organs of insulin namely skeletal muscle, adipose tissue and liver. This in turn leads to pancreatic beta cell loss and insulin resistance, respectively. During latter stages, the inflammation becomes more systemic and affects the blood vessels leading to vasculopathies. If small blood vessels are affected, it results in microvasculopathies. If larger blood vessels are affected it results to macrovasculopathies. While most viral and bacterial infections, can trigger chronic inflammation, helminth infections are unique in attenuating inflammation, by means of immunomodulation. Thus, a drastic decrease in helminth infections due to mass drug administration can fuel epidemic increase in metabolic diseases.

($Ym1^+$, $CCR2^-$, $Arg\text{-}1^+$ and IL-10, 15, 16]. With diet-induced obesity, a new population of $Ym1^-$, $MGL\text{-}1^-$, $CCR2^+$, $iNOS^+$ M1 macrophages were recruited which cluster around the necrotic adipocytes forming crown-like structures. While the M1 macrophages are associated with IR, M2 is more associated with insulin sensitivity (**Figure 1**) [15–17]. In general, peripheral macrophages in newly diagnosed diabetic patients are hyporesponsive to inflammatory signals due to the downregulation of TLRs [18]. In contrast, macrophages from chronic diabetic patients show chronic activation due to constitutive upregulation of B7–1 molecules [19].

With respect to helminth infection, despite the central role played by lymphocytes and dendritic cells, the role played by macrophages in both pathology and protection cannot be undermined [20]. Helminth products are known to polarize macrophages into M2 phenotype which orchestrate fibrosis and wound healing [21]. Helminth infected macrophages are also termed as nematode-elicited macrophages that express a peculiar M2 phenotype [21]. The master cytokines involved in M2 polarization are IL-4 and IL-13. The macrophages which are polarized by helminth infection express YM1, YM2, Resistin-Like Molecule alpha (RELMα) and other markers of M2 phenotype and produce IL-10 [21]. Diet-induced obese mice treated with *Litomosoides sigmodontis* (Ls) antigen showed an increased number of M2 macrophages in the epididymal adipose tissue (EAT) inducing a type-2 immune response which improved glucose tolerance (**Table 1**) [22]. Recently, *Heligmosomoides polygyrus* infected high-fat diet mice showed M2 polarization of adipose macrophages which reduced IR [27]. Mice injected with *Schistosoma mansoni* antigens showed significant improvement of metabolic control and increased frequency of M2 in HFD mice [28]. HFD mice infected with *Nippostrongylus brasiliensis*had decreased weight gain and improved glucose tolerance which was largely due to the polarization of adipose macrophages into the M2 phenotype (**Table 1**) [23].

2.2 Dendritic cells in insulin resistance and immunomodulation

While macrophages are major phagocytic cells, Dendritic cells (DCs) are the major antigen-presenting cells that play a crucial role in linking innate and adaptive immunity. DCs can interact with both T cells and B cells. Animal studies looking at the role of DCs in IR are limited. The $CD11c^+$ myeloid DCs were significantly increased in the adipose tissue of obese mice [29]. This suggests that DCs might be involved in T cell polarization and activation of macrophages thereby playing an important role in adipose inflammation and IR [29]. In the adipose tissue of obese mice, there was a substantial increase in the percentage of DCs which was associated with crown-like structures [30]. Mice lacking DCs (Flt3−/−) had reduced number of adipose and liver macrophage content, whereas DC replacement in DC-null mice increased liver and adipose macrophage infiltration and IR [30]. Both myeloid DCs and plasmacytoid DCs from chronic diabetic patients show upregulation of lineage markers due to high levels of circulating GM-CSF [31].

In helminth infections, DCs are arrested in an immature state characterized by an absence/moderate expression of co-stimulatory molecules along with reduced pro-inflammatory cytokine secretion [32]. This feature might presumably induce the development of a Th2 immune response [33]. While Toll-Like Receptor-mediated activation brings about DC maturation in general, helminth products have evolved alternate pathways of activation which can induce an anti-inflammatory response [34]. Helminth antigen treated dendritic cells produced increased levels of IL-4 and IL-10 [35]. Also, human monocyte-derived dendritic cells (mhDCs) when infected with live *Brugia malayi* microfilariae showed downregulation of TLR3 and TLR4 expression and diminished production of pro-inflammatory

DOI: http://dx.doi.org/10.5772/intechopen.98230

S. No	Filarial antigen	Organism/ species	Disease condition	Immune cells involved	Mechanisms	Outcome	Ref.
1	*Litomosoides sigmodontis* (L.s) antigens	C57BL/6 J DIO mice and C57BL/6 J DEREG mice	Diet induced obesity and glucose intolerance	Eosinophils, macrophages, innate lymphoid cells	Increased number of eosinophils, M2 macrophages, ILC-2 and Tregs in AT	Increased insulin sensitivity and glucose tolerance	[22]
2	*Nippostrongylus brasiliensis* (L3)	C57BL/6 J mice	Diet induced obesity and glucose intolerance	Macrophages	Increased M2 macrophages and increased expression of IL-13.	Reduced body weight and improved glucose metabolism	[23]
3	*Brugiamalayi* adult soluble (Bm A S) or microfilarial excretory-secretory (Bm mf ES) or microfilarial soluble (Bm mf S) antigens	BALB/c mice	STZ induced T1D	Antibodies	Increased IgE levels and sub-isotype switch of anti-insulin antibodies from IgG2a to IgG.	Improvement in glucose metabolism	[24]
4	Filarial proteins rWbL2(recombinant *Wuchereriabanc rofti*l.2) or rBmALT-2 (recombinant *B. malayi*abundant larval transcript 2)	Female Balb/c mice	STZ induced T1D	Antibodies	Inhibition of TNF-α and IFN-γ secretion and augmentation of IL-4, IL-5 and IL-10 secretion. Production of insulin specific IgG1 and antigen-specific IgE antibodies	Improvement in glucose metabolism	[25]
5	rDiAg (Recombinant *Dirofilaria immitis* antigen)	NOD/shi female mice	Autoimmune T1D	Antibodies	Reduced level of anti insulin autoantibodies. Th1 to Th2 shify. Elevated IgE levels	Prevention of insulitis	[26]

Table 1.
Effect of filarial antigen treatment on glucose metabolism and insulin sensitivity in Type-2 diabetic mice models.

cytokines following TLR challenge [36]. Recent research shows that priming of DCs with helminth products brings about Th-2 polarization and improves metabolic dysregulation [37].

2.3 Neutrophils in insulin resistance and immunomodulation

Neutrophils are microphages which are short-lived phagocytic cells that remove and destroy invading microorganisms and also cellular debris [38, 39]. In diet-induced obese mice, increased infiltration of neutrophil into adipose tissue was reported during weight gain and was associated with IR. In addition to host defence, neutrophil-derived serine proteases, such as neutrophil elastase, have been implicated in sterile inflammation [40]. Treatment of hepatocytes with neutrophil elastase-induced IR (by IRS-1 degradation) while deletion of neutrophil elastase in obese mice restored insulin sensitivity [40]. Taken together, neutrophils can be added to the extensive repertoire of immune cells that participate in inflammation-induced IR.

Compared to macrophages the role played by neutrophils in helminth infection is well studied [41]. In recent times, like macrophages, neutrophils were shown to get polarized either towards classically activated (N1) or alternatively activated (N2) phenotypes, following bacterial infections [42]. Whether such polarization takes place during helminth infections is not clearly known. Neutrophils were found to provide resistance to *H. polygyrus* infection *in vivo* and were able to kill the worm under *in vitro* conditions [43]. More recent reports indicate an important role for neutrophils in killing the larval stages of *Strongyloides stercoralis* [44]. Thus there is a possibility of neutrophils polarization during helminth infection which might aid host metabolism. *Haemonchus contortus,* a gastric parasite, secretes a 55 kDa secretory glycoprotein (gp55) which binds to CD11b/CD18 integrin present on neutrophils and inhibits its action [45].

2.4 Eosinophils in insulin resistance and immunomodulation

Eosinophils are generally associated with allergic responses as seen in parasitic infections [46]. While IL-5 serves as the main growth factor for eosinophil development, eotaxins (CCL11, CLL24 and CCL26) serve as its major chemotactic factors [46]. Activation of eosinophils results in its degranulation on to the target cells [46]. They carry eosinophilic granules which are rich in cytotoxic cationic proteins including major basic protein (MBP), eosinophil peroxidase (EPO), eosinophilic cationic protein (ECP) and eosinophil-derived neurotoxin (EDN) [46]. Adipose tissue eosinophils are needed for metabolic homeostasis and are involved in the maintenance of alternatively activated macrophages (AAMs) (**Figure 1**) [47]. They serve as the major source of IL-4 which polarizes the macrophages into the M2 phenotype. Absence of eosinophils can lead to adiposity and systemic IR in obese mice [47]. In these animals, IL-5 deficiency leads to loss of eosinophil accumulation in the adipose and increased IR [48].

Clinically, helminth infections are the most common cause of persistent eosinophilia, wherein they play a vital role in parasitic killing and elimination [49]. Ligation of parasite-specific Ig to Fc receptors or direct binding of helminth products to TLRs leads to eosinophil activation and degranulation [49]. Activated eosinophils bring about worm expulsion in two ways: 1. Direct killing of the worm by depositing cytotoxic granules along with reactive oxygen species on to the worm membrane and 2. Expulsion/encystment of the dead worm, by coordinating with other immune and non-immune cells [49]. However, recent evidence has indicated eosinophil activation during helminths infection is an immune evasive strategy favouring the parasite [50]. Eosinophils may influence the immune response in a manner that would sustain chronic infection and ensure worm survival [50]. Recently, in a high-fat diet mice model, animals infected with *Nippostrongylus brasiliensis* showed sustained metabolic control characterized by decreased fasting glucose and improved insulin sensitivity, which was associated with increased eosinophil content in the adipose tissue (**Figure 1**) [51]. Obese mice injected with *Litomosoides sigmodontis* (Ls) antigen showed an increased number of eosinophils in the epididymal adipose tissue which normalized glucose intolerance (**Table 1**) [22].

2.5 Basophils and mast cells in insulin resistance and immunomodulation

Basophils and mast cells are known for their involvement in allergies and airway inflammation [52]. Both cell lineages share a common ancestry: while basophils circulate; mast cells remain resident in tissues under normal conditions [52, 53]. As like other immune cells, recent studies have implicated them in glucose homeostasis and adipogenesis [54]. VAT from obese mice as well as humans contained a significant amount of mast cells [54]. Mast cell-deficient mice showed better glucose homeostasis with increased metabolic rate [55]. Leptin deficient Ob/Ob mice have an increased mast cell content in their adipose tissue and were found to secrete an increased amount of TNF-α [56].

Like eosinophils, basophils also serve in the first line of defence mechanism against helminth infection [57]. However recently, this concept has been challenged for certain helminth infections [58]. The cross-linking of surface IgE on basophils by helminth antigens induced IL-4 secretion [59]. Thus, the anti-inflammatory Th-2 response is augmented by basophils and mast cells [60]. During helminth infections, eosinophils, neutrophils and basophils directly participate in the parasite killing and expulsion [61]. Basophil deficient mice, infected with L3 larvae of *Brugia malayi* showed decreased eosinophil count, decreased titers of parasite-specific IgE, reduced $CD4^+$ T cell proliferation and decreased antigen-specific IL-4 production demonstrating the importance of basophils in the amplification of type-2 immune response [62]. Helminth infected mice have an increased number of basophils which were capable of priming of Th-2 response [63].

2.6 NK and NKT cells in insulin resistance and immunomodulation

Natural killer (NK) cells are an important component of the innate immune response to viral infections and tumours [64]. They have the ability to provide an early source of both innate (IL-6 and TNF-α) and adaptive (IFN-γ, IL-4, IL-5 and IL-13) immune cytokines and can also lyse the target cells through perforin-granzyme-mediated cytolytic pathway [64]. Natural Killer T (NKT) cells are sub-population of lymphocytes that serve as a link between the innate and adaptive immunity [65]. They are a heterogeneous group of lymphocytes that share the properties of both T cells and NK cells. Many of these cells recognize self and foreign lipids and glycolipids bound to the non-polymorphic CD1d molecule [65]. Very little is known about the role played by NK and NKT cells in metabolic homeostasis [66]. VAT obtained from obese subjects was found to have an increased frequency of IFN-γ expressing NK cells [67]. The role of iNKT cells in the regulation of metabolism is just emerging. Previously, it was found that adipose tissues and liver of both mice and humans contain a population of iNKT cells, which decreased with increasing adiposity and IR (**Figure 2**) [68]. In fact, this coincides with the infiltration of macrophages and T cells into the adipose tissue.

Compared to other cell types, the role played by NK cells in helminth mediated immunomodulation is intriguing. NK cells were found to express IL-4 and IL-13

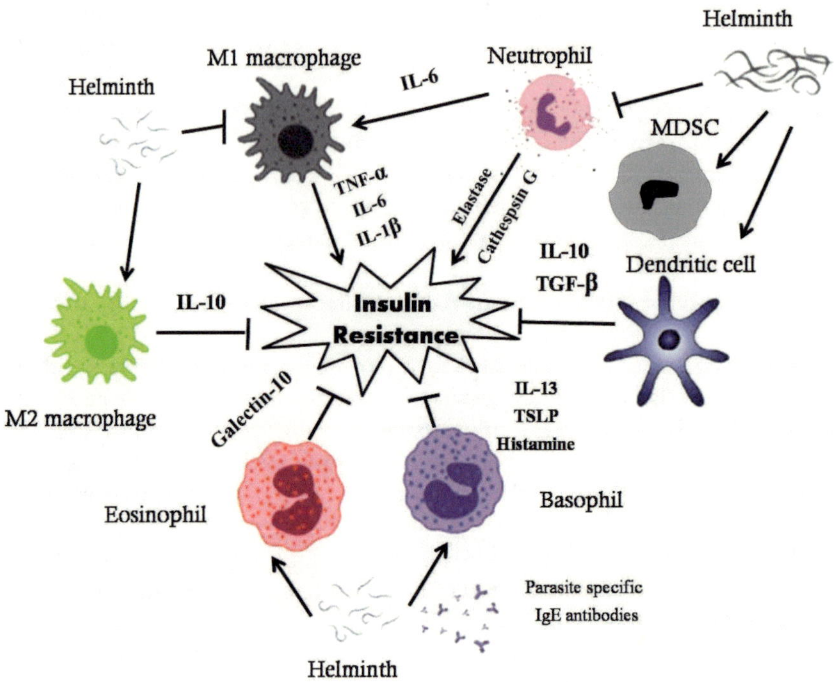

Figure 2.
Myeloid cell network in Insulin Resistance (IR) and immunomodulation. Helminth infections can bring about macrophage polarization from the pro-inflammatory M1 phenotype to anti-inflammatory M2 phenotype. They also polarize neutrophils from pro to anti-inflammatory phenotype. They augment both eosinophils and basophils which attenuate IR. They induce tolerogenic dendritic cells and myeloid derived suppressor cells which inhibit Th1 immunity.

in response to microfilaremia but not L3 infection [69]. The early activation of NK cells led to apoptosis in response to live L3 exposure, but not to live microfilaremia infection [69]. Impairment of NK cell function had a profound effect on worm burden and delays the clearance of the parasite. Infection of BALB/c mice with *L. sigmodontis* was shown to suppress the activation of inhibitory receptors but promoted the induction of activating receptor on NK cells [70]. NKT cells during helminth infections were shown to produce IL-4 as an immunoregulatory cytokine when exposed to the nematode glycolipids [71]. Helminths activate both iNKT and non-iNKT cells *in vivo*, enabling them to differentially influence the Th1/Th2 balance [71]. NKT cells were known to be the early source of IL-4, in the spleen, within 24 h of L3 *B. phangi* infection in mice [71].

2.7 Other innate immune cells in insulin resistance and immunomodulation

Myeloid-Derived Suppressor Cells (MDSCs) are heterogenous immature myeloid cells which were first discovered in the tumour stroma wherein they were found to suppress anti-tumour immune response [72]. Recently, MDSCs were shown to alleviate insulin resistance and confer protection against diabetes [73]. Adoptive transfer of MDSC cells into HFD mice showed better glucose tolerance [74]. Loss of these cells in obese animals aggravated IR [74]. Within the adipose tissue milieu, these cells were found to suppress Th1 activation [74]. During helminth infection, anti-proliferative MDSCs emerge which inhibit T cell proliferation using eicosanoids generated through 12/15 lipoxygenase pathway [75]. Similarly, *Schistomes* soluble egg antigens were shown to prime MDSC cells which strongly inhibited T cell activation [76].

Nuocytes or Innate lymphoid cells (ILC) are recently discovered innate lymphoid cells capable of augmenting other immune cells like helper T cells [77]. ILCs are primarily tissue-resident lymphocytes, found in both lymphoid (immune-associated), and non-lymphoid tissues, and rarely in the peripheral blood (<1%) [77, 78]. They are particularly abundant at mucosal surfaces controlling mucosal immunity and homeostasis [77, 79]. They differ from other immune cells by the absence of regular lymphoid morphology, TCR and BCR rearranged, and expression of myeloid-specific CD markers [77]. Based on the difference in developmental pathways, phenotype, and cytokine secretion, in 2013, ILCs were divided into three groups: 1. ILC-1 cells upon priming with IL-12, IL-15 and IL-18 secrete IFN-γ and TNF-α; 2. ILC-2 cells upon priming with TSLP, IL-25 and IL-33 a secrete IL-4, IL-5 and IL-13; 3. ILC-3 cells upon priming with IL-1β, IL-23 and IL-6, secrete IL-17 and IL-22 [77]. ILC-1 recruitment into the adipose tissue is directly linked to fat accumulation and exacerbates IR [80], while ILC-2 cells are involved in browning of visceral adipose tissue [81]. During helminth infection, the early source of IL-13 was from nuocytes, through IL-25 and IL-33 dependant priming [82]. Administration of *Schistosoma mansoni* egg-derived ω1 antigen into diabetic mice induced Th-2 response, which correlated with increased frequency of ICL-2 in adipose tissue, which in turn increased the metabolic homeostasis [83].

3. Adaptive immune cells in insulin resistance and immunomodulation

The adaptive immune cells include T cells and B cells which play an important role in both IR and immunomodulation.

3.1 T-helper cells in insulin resistance and immunomodulation

T cells are lymphocytes which mature from the thymus (and hence the name) and are the major components of the adaptive immune system [84]. They perform three major functions: 1. Helper T cells (Th) activate B cells, macrophages, DCs, other T cells and other immune cells, 2. Cytotoxic T cells (Tc) directly kill tumour cells and pathogen-infected cells and 3. Regulatory T cells (Tregs) maintain immune homeostasis [84]. The Th cells are distinguished by their CD4+ phenotype and are further classified based on their cytokine profile as 1.Th1 (IFN-γ, IL-2, and TNF-β), Th2 (IL-4, IL-5 and IL-13), 3. Th17 (IL-17 and IL-17F), 4.Th9 (IL-9 and IL-10), 5.Th22 (IL-22), etc. [84]. T cells in coordination with macrophages and DCs fuel VAT inflammation [85]. Both pro-inflammatory cytotoxic T cells (CTLs) and interferon-γ (IFN-γ)-producing Th-1 cells contribute to inflammation (**Figure 2**) [86]. On the contrary, VAT-resident Tregs and Th2 cells tend to suppress inflammation (**Figure 2**) [87]. Obese IFN-γ-knockout animals, compared with obese wild-type mice, showed modest improvements in insulin sensitivity, decreased adipocyte size, and an M2-macrophage phenotype and cytokine expression [88]. Genetic ablation of IL-13 in mice resulted in hyperglycemia, which progressed to hepatic IR and systemic metabolic dysfunction [89]. However, studies conducted in our lab on serum cytokine profiles in subjects with metabolic syndrome (MS) showed a mixed Th1-Th2 response with increased levels of IL-12, IFN-γ, IL-4, IL-5 and IL-13 in the serum of subjects with metabolic syndrome (a precondition of diabetes, if not already present) [90]. The role of recently discovered Th17 in VAT inflammation is still an enigma. Some studies have shown strong pro-inflammatory phenotype for these cells inducing IR [91], while our study showed a decline in serum IL-17 levels in subjects with MS (**Figure 2**) [92]. The Tregs in VAT has a unique function of maintaining immune-homeostasis and improving insulin signalling by PPAR-g activation [93]. The role of other recently identified Th cell subtypes like Th22 and Th9 in IR is not clearly known. In general, type-2 diabetic subjects show a mixed Th1-Th2 response which becomes more Th1 polarized as the diabetic subjects develop microvascular [94] and macrovascular complications [95]. Serum IL-17 levels are generally low in patients with diabetic nephropathy [96].

T cell-mediated immune responses during filarial infection depend on the phase of the infection: 1.The acute phase is skewed towards Th2 (IL-4, IL-5 and IL-13) response, 2. The chronic phase is skewed towards "modified Th2 response", with Tregs playing a more prominent compared to Th2 cells and 3. The third phase is chronic pathology phase, which is characterized by a drastic shift from "modified Th2" response to Th1/Th17 (IFN-γ, IL-2 and IL-17) response, which happens only in those who develop lymphatic pathology [97]. Thus, the differential immune response seen during various phases of the filarial infection is paralleled by the life cycle of the parasite: 1. Microfilaremic stage-predominant Th2 response, 2. Adult worm stage- modified Th2-Treg response and 3.Chronic pathology stage- Th1/Th17 response [97]. Infection of HFD induced obese mice with *Heligmosomoides polygyrus*, an intestinal nematode parasite, resulted in significantly attenuated obesity with marked upregulation of uncoupling protein 1 (UCP1), a key protein involved in energy expenditure in adipose tissue [98]. Further suppression of glucose and triglyceride levels and alteration in the expression of key genes in the liver involved in lipid metabolism were also seen [98]. An augmented helminth induced Th2/Treg response and M2 macrophage polarization was characteristic of this attenuated obesity [98].

3.2 Cytotoxic T cells (CTLs) in insulin resistance and immunomodulation

Cytotoxic (CD8+) T cells are one of the effector cells in T-cell mediated immunity which directly kills the target cells (virus or bacteria-infected cells and tumour cells). CD8+ T cells were found to migrate into the adipose tissue much before the accumulation of macrophage in obese mice [99]. IFN-γ produced by CTLs promotes the recruitment and polarization of M1 macrophages (**Figure 1**) [99]. This results in adipose tissue inflammation and IR [99]. In the obese mice, increased infiltration of CTLs into the adipose tissue around 22nd week after the initiation of a high-fat diet was seen [99]. Antibody-mediated or genetic depletion of CTLs lowered macrophage infiltration and adipose inflammation, ameliorating IR [99].

When compared to T-helper cells, the amount of literature available on the role of CTLs in helminth infection is limited. Atleast in mice, there is evidence to show that CTL population is dispensable for anti-helminth immunity [100]. In clinical studies, LF infection was shown to upregulate HLA-A thereby activating CTLs [101]. However, these activated CTLs showed poor proliferative response under *in vitro* conditions [101]. The CTL activity was largely seen during lymphedema development, rather than acute/modified immune response to helminths [101]. Further, these activated CTLs were largely immunomodulatory rather than pro-inflammatory in nature [101]. It would be interesting to see whether these activated immunosuppressive cells are in fact the recently discovered CD8(+) Tregs population (**Figure 3**).

3.3 B cells in insulin resistance and immunomodulation

B cells form a major component of adaptive immunity and perform two vital functions namely: 1. Antigen presentation to T cells which links innate and adaptive arms of the immune response and 2. Production of antibodies which perform the effector functions. In obese mice, B cells were found to migrate into the adipose

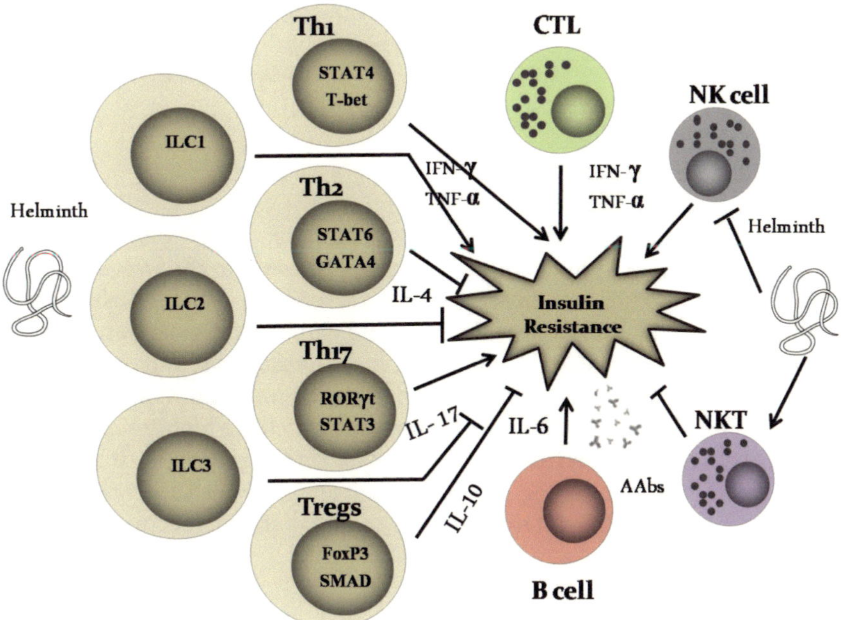

Figure 3.
Lymphoid cell network in Insulin Resistance (IR) and immunomodulation. Helminth infections can bring about T cell polarization from the pro-inflammatory Th1 and Th17 phenotype to anti-inflammatory Th2 phenotype. They also induce proinflammatory ILC-1 and -3 and induce anti-inflammatory ILC-2 cells. They augment both Tregs and iNKT cells which attenuate IR. They inhibit pro-inflammatory CTLs and NK cells.

tissue shortly after the initiation of a high-fat diet [102]. The initial signal for B cell activation is provided by the stressed adipocytes by releasing the self-antigens [102]. The activated B cells then induce the activation of pro-inflammatory macrophages and T cells and the production of auto-antibodies [102]. Correspondingly, increased IgG production (predominantly of IgG2c subtype) and increased IgG+ B cells were seen in the VAT of obese mice [102, 103]. B cell null mice showed reduced immune cell activation and IR in VAT and transfer of IgG antibodies from obese wild type mice to B cell null obese mice worsened glucose tolerance [102]. The IgG antibodies, apart from promoting B cell-mediated adipose inflammation, can also bind to Fc receptors present on macrophages, NK cells, neutrophils and eosinophils, and can bring about cellular activation augmenting inflammation [102, 104]. However, recently ZnT8 specific naturally occurring autoantibodies were found to be significantly reduced in type-2 diabetes, indicating a beneficial effect for these antibodies in reducing IR [26].

The function of B cells in helminth infection is largely restricted to the protective Th2 response [97]. IL-4 mediated activation, class switching and affinity maturation of B cells are responsible for the elevated levels of IgE antibodies in infected individuals [97]. In streptozotocin-induced diabetic mice, treatment with *Brugia malayi* adult soluble antigen (Bm AS) or microfilarial excretory-secretory antigen (Bm mf ES) decreased pancreatic beta-cell destruction [24]. This was due to class switching of anti-insulin autoantibodies from IgG2a to IgG1 subtype (**Table 1**). In the same mice model, treatment of diabetic animals with two filarial proteins namely recombinant *Wuchereria bancrofti* L2 (rWbL2) and *Brugia malayi* abundant larval transcript 2 (rBmALT-2), resulted in the augmentation of insulin specific IgG1 autoantibodies and normalization of glucose metabolism (**Table 1**) [25, 105]. IL-10-producing B cells also termed as regulatory B cells (Bregs) can dampen inflammation under certain conditions [105]. Thus B cells play contrasting roles in IR and helminth infections; in the context of helminth infections, they orchestrate regulatory immune responses via IL-10, whereas in IR they induce adipose inflammation via autoantibodies.

4. Conclusion and future directions

A decrease in helminth infections (like lymphatic filariasis) could potentially account for the increased prevalence of metabolic diseases in the western world. The same immunomodulatory effect can have an impact on type-2 diabetes, as was seen in tropical countries. Recently, several helminth antigens were shown to confer significant protection against obesity, insulin resistance and diabetes, in animal models. The implications of helminth induced immunomodulation are thus twofold: Mass drug administration in populations which are highly susceptible to type-2 diabetes has to be carried out with care; Secondly, more research is needed in identifying and characterizing novel helminth antigens with a strong immunomodulatory effect which can later be developed into diabetes vaccines.

Author details

Vivekanandhan Aravindhan* and Sibi Joy Manohar
Department of Genetics, Dr. ALM PG IBMS, University of Madras, Chennai, India

*Address all correspondence to: cvaravindhan@gmail.com

References

[1] Hotamisligil GS. Inflammation and metabolic disorders. Nature. 2006; 444: 860-867.

[2] Aravindhan V, Madhumitha H. Metainflammation in Diabetic Coronary Artery Disease: Emerging Role of Innate and Adaptive Immune Responses. J Diabetes Res. 2016; 2016:6264149.

[3] Aravindhan V, Anand G. Cell Type-Specific Immunomodulation Induced by Helminthes: Effect on Metainflammation, Insulin Resistance and Type-2 Diabetes. Am J Trop Med Hyg. 2017;97:1650-1661.

[4] Strachan DP. Hay fever, hygiene, and household size. BMJ. 1989;299:1259-1260.

[5] Alexandre-Silva GM, Brito-Souza PA, Oliveira ACS, Cerni FA, Zottich U, Pucca MB. The hygiene hypothesis at a glance: Early exposures, immune mechanism and novel therapies. Acta Trop. 2018;188:16-26.

[6] Gao S, Wang S, Song Y. Novel immunomodulatory drugs and neo-substrates. Biomark Res. 2020;8:2.

[7] Caraballo L. The tropics, helminth infections and hygiene hypotheses. Expert Rev Clin Immunol. 2018;14:99-102.

[8] Aravindhan V, Mohan V, Surendar J, Rao MM, Ranjani H, Kumaraswami V, et al. Decreased prevalence of lymphatic filariasis among subjects with type-1 diabetes. Am J Trop Med Hyg. 2010;83:1336-1339.

[9] Aravindhan V, Mohan V, Surendar J, Muralidhara Rao M, Pavankumar N, Deepa M, et al. Decreased prevalence of lymphatic filariasis among diabetic subjects associated with a diminished pro-inflammatory cytokine response (CURES 83). PLoS Negl Trop Dis. 2010;4:e707.

[10] Aravindhan V, Mohan V, Surendar J, Rao MM, Anuradha R, Deepa M, et al. Effect of filarial infection on serum inflammatory and atherogenic biomarkers in coronary artery disease (CURES-121). Am J Trop Med Hyg. 2012;86:828-833.

[11] de Ruiter K, Tahapary DL, Sartono E, Soewondo P, Supali T, Smit JWA, et al. Helminths, hygiene hypothesis and type 2 diabetes. Parasite Immunol. 2017;39.

[12] Shanker A, Thounaojam MC, Mishra MK, Dikov MM. Innate-Adaptive Immune Crosstalk 2016. J Immunol Res. 2017;2017:3503207.

[13] Tsuji T. Subcutaneous fat necrosis of the newborn: Light and electron microscopic studies. Br J Dermatol. 1976;95:407-416.

[14] Oishi Y, Manabe I. Macrophages in inflammation, repair and regeneration. Int Immunol. 2018;30:511-528.

[15] Russo L, Lumeng CN. Properties and functions of adipose tissue macrophages in obesity. Immunology. 2018;155:407-417.

[16] Buechler C, Schaffler A. Does global gene expression analysis in type 2 diabetes provide an opportunity to identify highly promising drug targets? Endocr Metab Immune Disord Drug Targets. 2007;7:250-258.

[17] Kumar V. Macrophages: The Potent Immunoregulatory Innate Immune Cells. In: Bhat KH, editor. Macrophage Activation Biology and Disease: IntechOpen; 2020.

[18] Madhumitha H, Mohan V, Babu S, Aravindhan V. TLR-induced secretion

of novel cytokine IL-27 is defective in newly diagnosed type-2 diabetic subjects. Cytokine. 2018;104:65-71.

[19] Madhumitha H, Mohan V, Kumar NP, Pradeepa R, Babu S, Aravindhan V. Impaired toll-like receptor signalling in peripheral B cells from newly diagnosed type-2 diabetic subjects. Cytokine. 2015;76:253-259.

[20] Faz-Lopez B, Morales-Montor J, Terrazas LI. Role of Macrophages in the Repair Process during the Tissue Migrating and Resident Helminth Infections. Biomed Res Int. 2016;2016:8634603.

[21] Smith H, Forman R, Mair I, Else KJ. Interactions of helminths with macrophages: therapeutic potential for inflammatory intestinal disease. Expert Rev Gastroenterol Hepatol. 2018;12:997-1006.

[22] Berbudi A, Surendar J, Ajendra J, Gondorf F, Schmidt D, Neumann AL, et al. Filarial Infection or Antigen Administration Improves Glucose Tolerance in Diet-Induced Obese Mice. J Innate Immun. 2016;8:601-616.

[23] Yang Z, Grinchuk V, Smith A, Qin B, Bohl JA, Sun R, et al. Parasitic nematode-induced modulation of body weight and associated metabolic dysfunction in mouse models of obesity. Infect Immun. 2013;81:1905-1914.

[24] Amdare N, Khatri V, Yadav RS, Tarnekar A, Goswami K, Reddy MV. Brugia malayi soluble and excretory-secretory proteins attenuate development of streptozotocin-induced type 1 diabetes in mice. Parasite Immunol. 2015;37:624-634.

[25] Amdare NP, Khatri VK, Yadav RSP, Tarnekar A, Goswami K, Reddy MVR. Therapeutic potential of the immunomodulatory proteins Wuchereria bancrofti L2 and Brugia malayi abundant larval transcript 2 against streptozotocin-induced type 1 diabetes in mice. J Helminthol. 2017;91:539-548.

[26] Imai S, Tezuka H, Fujita K. A factor of inducing IgE from a filarial parasite prevents insulin-dependent diabetes mellitus in nonobese diabetic mice. Biochem Biophys Res Commun. 2001;286:1051-8.

[27] Morimoto M, Azuma N, Kadowaki H, Abe T, Suto Y. Regulation of type 2 diabetes by helminth-induced Th2 immune response. J Vet Med Sci. 2017;78:1855-1864.

[28] Hussaarts L, Garcia-Tardon N, van Beek L, Heemskerk MM, Haeberlein S, van der Zon GC, et al. Chronic helminth infection and helminth-derived egg antigens promote adipose tissue M2 macrophages and improve insulin sensitivity in obese mice. FASEB J. 2015;29:3027-3039.

[29] Sundara Rajan S, Longhi MP. Dendritic cells and adipose tissue. Immunology. 2016;149:353-361.

[30] Stefanovic-Racic M, Yang X, Turner MS, Mantell BS, Stolz DB, Sumpter TL, et al. Dendritic cells promote macrophage infiltration and comprise a substantial proportion of obesity-associated increases in CD11c+ cells in adipose tissue and liver. Diabetes. 2012;61:2330-2339.

[31] Surendar J, Mohan V, Pavankumar N, Babu S, Aravindhan V. Increased levels of serum granulocyte-macrophage colony-stimulating factor is associated with activated peripheral dendritic cells in type 2 diabetes subjects (CURES-99). Diabetes Technol Ther. 2012;14:344-349.

[32] Motran CC, Ambrosio LF, Volpini X, Celias DP, Cervi L. Dendritic cells and parasites: from recognition and activation to immune response instruction. Semin Immunopathol. 2017;39:199-213.

[33] Schuijs MJ, Hammad H, Lambrecht BN. Professional and 'Amateur' Antigen-Presenting Cells In Type 2 Immunity. Trends Immunol. 2019;40:22-34.

[34] Kane CM, Jung E, Pearce EJ. Schistosoma mansoni egg antigen-mediated modulation of Toll-like receptor (TLR)-induced activation occurs independently of TLR2, TLR4, and MyD88. Infect Immun. 2008;76:5754-5759.

[35] Goodridge HS, Marshall FA, Wilson EH, Houston KM, Liew FY, Harnett MM, et al. In vivo exposure of murine dendritic cell and macrophage bone marrow progenitors to the phosphorylcholine-containing filarial nematode glycoprotein ES-62 polarizes their differentiation to an anti-inflammatory phenotype. Immunology. 2004;113:491-498.

[36] Sharma A, Sharma P, Vishwakarma AL, Srivastava M. Functional Impairment of Murine Dendritic Cell Subsets following Infection with Infective Larval Stage 3 of Brugia malayi. Infect Immun. 2017;85.

[37] Hussaarts L, Yazdanbakhsh M, Guigas B. Priming dendritic cells for th2 polarization: lessons learned from helminths and implications for metabolic disorders. Front Immunol. 2014;5:499.

[38] Mantovani A, Cassatella MA, Costantini C, Jaillon S. Neutrophils in the activation and regulation of innate and adaptive immunity. Nat Rev Immunol. 2011;11:519-531.

[39] Kumar V, Sharma A. Neutrophils: Cinderella of innate immune system. Int Immunopharmacol. 2010;10:1325-1334.

[40] Talukdar S, Oh DY, Bandyopadhyay G, Li D, Xu J, McNelis J, et al. Neutrophils mediate insulin resistance in mice fed a high-fat diet through secreted elastase. Nat Med. 2012;18:1407-1412.

[41] Allen JE, Sutherland TE, Ruckerl D. IL-17 and neutrophils: unexpected players in the type 2 immune response. Curr Opin Immunol. 2015;34:99-106.

[42] Deniset JF, Kubes P. Neutrophil heterogeneity: Bona fide subsets or polarization states? J Leukoc Biol. 2018;103:829-838.

[43] Kannan Y, Entwistle LJ, Pelly VS, Perez-Lloret J, Walker AW, Ley SC, et al. TPL-2 restricts Ccl24-dependent immunity to Heligmosomoides polygyrus. PLoS Pathog. 2017;13:e1006536.

[44] O'Connell AE, Hess JA, Santiago GA, Nolan TJ, Lok JB, Lee JJ, et al. Major basic protein from eosinophils and myeloperoxidase from neutrophils are required for protective immunity to Strongyloides stercoralis in mice. Infect Immun. 2011;79:2770-2778.

[45] Anbu KA, Joshi P. Identification of a 55 kDa Haemonchus contortus excretory/secretory glycoprotein as a neutrophil inhibitory factor. Parasite Immunol. 2008;30:23-30.

[46] Rothenberg ME, Hogan SP. The eosinophil. Annu Rev Immunol. 2006;24:147-174.

[47] Wu D, Molofsky AB, Liang HE, Ricardo-Gonzalez RR, Jouihan HA, Bando JK, et al. Eosinophils sustain adipose alternatively activated macrophages associated with glucose homeostasis. Science. 2011;332:243-247.

[48] Rozenberg P, Reichman H, Zab-Bar I, Itan M, Pasmanik-Chor M, Bouffi C, et al. CD300f:IL-5 cross-talk inhibits adipose tissue eosinophil homing and subsequent IL-4 production. Sci Rep. 2017;7:5922.

[49] Strandmark J, Rausch S, Hartmann S. Eosinophils in Homeostasis and Their Contrasting Roles during Inflammation and Helminth Infections. Crit Rev Immunol. 2016;36:193-238.

[50] Gebreselassie NG, Moorhead AR, Fabre V, Gagliardo LF, Lee NA, Lee JJ, et al. Eosinophils preserve parasitic nematode larvae by regulating local immunity. J Immunol. 2012;188:417-425.

[51] Guigas B, Molofsky AB. A worm of one's own: how helminths modulate host adipose tissue function and metabolism. Trends Parasitol. 2015;31:435-441.

[52] Varricchi G, Raap U, Rivellese F, Marone G, Gibbs BF. Human mast cells and basophils-How are they similar how are they different? Immunol Rev. 2018;282:8-34.

[53] Kumar V, Sharma A. Mast cells: emerging sentinel innate immune cells with diverse role in immunity. Mol Immunol. 2010;48:14-25.

[54] Altintas MM, Azad A, Nayer B, Contreras G, Zaias J, Faul C, et al. Mast cells, macrophages, and crown-like structures distinguish subcutaneous from visceral fat in mice. J Lipid Res. 2011;52:480-488.

[55] Liu J, Divoux A, Sun J, Zhang J, Clement K, Glickman JN, et al. Genetic deficiency and pharmacological stabilization of mast cells reduce diet-induced obesity and diabetes in mice. Nat Med. 2009;15:940-945.

[56] Wang J, Shi GP. Mast cell stabilization: novel medication for obesity and diabetes. Diabetes Metab Res Rev. 2011;27:919-924.

[57] Mitre E, Nutman TB. Basophils, basophilia and helminth infections. Chem Immunol Allergy. 2006;90: 141-156.

[58] Hartmann W, Linnemann LC, Reitz M, Specht S, Voehringer D, Breloer M. Basophils Are Dispensable for the Control of a Filarial Infection. Immunohorizons. 2018;2:296-304.

[59] Mitre E, Taylor RT, Kubofcik J, Nutman TB. Parasite antigen-driven basophils are a major source of IL-4 in human filarial infections. J Immunol. 2004;172:2439-2445.

[60] Saini SS, Klion AD, Holland SM, Hamilton RG, Bochner BS, Macglashan DW, Jr. The relationship between serum IgE and surface levels of FcepsilonR on human leukocytes in various diseases: correlation of expression with FcepsilonRI on basophils but not on monocytes or eosinophils. J Allergy Clin Immunol. 2000;106:514-520.

[61] Makepeace BL, Martin C, Turner JD, Specht S. Granulocytes in helminth infection -- who is calling the shots? Curr Med Chem. 2012;19: 1567-1586.

[62] Spencer LA, Porte P, Zetoff C, Rajan TV. Mice genetically deficient in immunoglobulin E are more permissive hosts than wild-type mice to a primary, but not secondary, infection with the filarial nematode Brugia malayi. Infect Immun. 2003;71:2462-2467.

[63] Min B. Basophils induce Th2 immunity: is this final answer? Virulence. 2010;1:399-401.

[64] Abel AM, Yang C, Thakar MS, Malarkannan S. Natural Killer Cells: Development, Maturation, and Clinical Utilization. Front Immunol. 2018;9:1869.

[65] Godfrey DI, Hammond KJ, Poulton LD, Smyth MJ, Baxter AG.

NKT cells: facts, functions and fallacies. Immunol Today. 2000;21:573-583.

[66] Bonamichi B, Lee J. Unusual Suspects in the Development of Obesity-Induced Inflammation and Insulin Resistance: NK cells, iNKT cells, and ILCs. Diabetes Metab J. 2017;41:229-250.

[67] O'Rourke RW, Metcalf MD, White AE, Madala A, Winters BR, Maizlin, II, et al. Depot-specific differences in inflammatory mediators and a role for NK cells and IFN-gamma in inflammation in human adipose tissue. Int J Obes (Lond). 2009;33:978-990.

[68] Lynch L, Nowak M, Varghese B, Clark J, Hogan AE, Toxavidis V, et al. Adipose tissue invariant NKT cells protect against diet-induced obesity and metabolic disorder through regulatory cytokine production. Immunity. 2012;37:574-587.

[69] Babu S, Blauvelt CP, Nutman TB. Filarial parasites induce NK cell activation, type 1 and type 2 cytokine secretion, and subsequent apoptotic cell death. J Immunol. 2007;179:2445-2456.

[70] Korten S, Volkmann L, Saeftel M, Fischer K, Taniguchi M, Fleischer B, et al. Expansion of NK cells with reduction of their inhibitory Ly-49A, Ly-49C, and Ly-49G2 receptor-expressing subsets in a murine helminth infection: contribution to parasite control. J Immunol. 2002;168:5199-5206.

[71] Faveeuw C, Mallevaey T, Trottein F. Role of natural killer T lymphocytes during helminthic infection. Parasite. 2008;15:384-388.

[72] Gabrilovich DI, Nagaraj S. Myeloid-derived suppressor cells as regulators of the immune system. Nat Rev Immunol. 2009;9:162-174.

[73] Wang T, Wen Y, Fan X. Myeloid-derived suppressor cells suppress CD4+ T cell activity and prevent the development of type 2 diabetes. Acta Biochim Biophys Sin (Shanghai). 2018;50:362-9.

[74] Xia S, Sha H, Yang L, Ji Y, Ostrand-Rosenberg S, Qi L. Gr-1+ CD11b+ myeloid-derived suppressor cells suppress inflammation and promote insulin sensitivity in obesity. J Biol Chem. 2011;286:23591-23599.

[75] Brys L, Beschin A, Raes G, Ghassabeh GH, Noel W, Brandt J, et al. Reactive oxygen species and 12/15-lipoxygenase contribute to the antiproliferative capacity of alternatively activated myeloid cells elicited during helminth infection. J Immunol. 2005;174:6095-6104.

[76] Yang Q, Qiu H, Xie H, Qi Y, Cha H, Qu J, et al. A Schistosoma japonicum Infection Promotes the Expansion of Myeloid-Derived Suppressor Cells by Activating the JAK/STAT3 Pathway. J Immunol. 2017;198:4716-4727.

[77] Vivier E, Artis D, Colonna M, Diefenbach A, Di Santo JP, Eberl G, et al. Innate Lymphoid Cells: 10 Years On. Cell. 2018;174:1054-1066.

[78] Kumar V. Innate lymphoid cells: new paradigm in immunology of inflammation. Immunol Lett. 2014;157:23-37.

[79] Kumar V. Innate Lymphoid Cells: Immunoregulatory Cells of Mucosal Inflammation. European Journal of Inflammation. 2014;12:11-20.

[80] O'Sullivan TE, Rapp M, Fan X, Weizman OE, Bhardwaj P, Adams NM, et al. Adipose-Resident Group 1 Innate Lymphoid Cells Promote Obesity-Associated Insulin Resistance. Immunity. 2016;45:428-441.

[81] Brestoff JR, Kim BS, Saenz SA, Stine RR, Monticelli LA, Sonnenberg GF, et al. Group 2 innate lymphoid cells promote beiging of white adipose tissue and limit obesity. Nature. 2015;519:242-246.

[82] Loser S, Smith KA, Maizels RM. Innate Lymphoid Cells in Helminth Infections-Obligatory or Accessory? Front Immunol. 2019;10:620.

[83] Hams E, Bermingham R, Wurlod FA, Hogan AE, O'Shea D, Preston RJ, et al. The helminth T2 RNase omega1 promotes metabolic homeostasis in an IL-33- and group 2 innate lymphoid cell-dependent mechanism. FASEB J. 2016;30:824-835.

[84] Kumar BV, Connors TJ, Farber DL. Human T Cell Development, Localization, and Function throughout Life. Immunity. 2018;48:202-213.

[85] Wang Q, Wu H. T Cells in Adipose Tissue: Critical Players in Immunometabolism. Front Immunol. 2018;9:2509.

[86] Winer S, Chan Y, Paltser G, Truong D, Tsui H, Bahrami J, et al. Normalization of obesity-associated insulin resistance through immunotherapy. Nat Med. 2009;15:921-929.

[87] Feuerer M, Herrero L, Cipolletta D, Naaz A, Wong J, Nayer A, et al. Lean, but not obese, fat is enriched for a unique population of regulatory T cells that affect metabolic parameters. Nat Med. 2009;15:930-939.

[88] O'Rourke RW, White AE, Metcalf MD, Winters BR, Diggs BS, Zhu X, et al. Systemic inflammation and insulin sensitivity in obese IFN-gamma knockout mice. Metabolism. 2012;61:1152-1161.

[89] Stanya KJ, Jacobi D, Liu S, Bhargava P, Dai L, Gangl MR, et al. Direct control of hepatic glucose production by interleukin-13 in mice. J Clin Invest. 2013;123:261-271.

[90] Surendar J, Mohan V, Rao MM, Babu S, Aravindhan V. Increased levels of both Th1 and Th2 cytokines in subjects with metabolic syndrome (CURES-103). Diabetes Technol Ther. 2011;13:477-482.

[91] Tao L, Liu H, Gong Y. Role and mechanism of the Th17/Treg cell balance in the development and progression of insulin resistance. Mol Cell Biochem. 2019;459:183-188.

[92] Surendar J, Aravindhan V, Rao MM, Ganesan A, Mohan V. Decreased serum interleukin-17 and increased transforming growth factor-beta levels in subjects with metabolic syndrome (Chennai Urban Rural Epidemiology Study-95). Metabolism. 2011;60:586-590.

[93] Cipolletta D, Feuerer M, Li A, Kamei N, Lee J, Shoelson SE, et al. PPAR-gamma is a major driver of the accumulation and phenotype of adipose tissue Treg cells. Nature. 2012;486:549-553.

[94] Anand G, Vasanthakumar R, Mohan V, Babu S, Aravindhan V. Increased IL-12 and decreased IL-33 serum levels are associated with increased Th1 and suppressed Th2 cytokine profile in patients with diabetic nephropathy (CURES-134). Int J Clin Exp Pathol. 2014;7:8008-8015.

[95] Madhumitha H, Mohan V, Deepa M, Babu S, Aravindhan V. Increased Th1 and suppressed Th2 serum cytokine levels in subjects with diabetic coronary artery disease. Cardiovasc Diabetol. 2014;13:1.

[96] Vasanthakumar R, Mohan V, Anand G, Deepa M, Babu S, Aravindhan V. Serum IL-9, IL-17, and TGF-beta levels in subjects with

diabetic kidney disease (CURES-134). Cytokine. 2015;72:109-112.

[97] Babu S, Nutman TB. Immunology of lymphatic filariasis. Parasite Immunol. 2014;36:338-346.

[98] Su CW, Chen CY, Li Y, Long SR, Massey W, Kumar DV, et al. Helminth infection protects against high fat diet-induced obesity via induction of alternatively activated macrophages. Sci Rep. 2018;8:4607.

[99] Nishimura S, Manabe I, Nagasaki M, Eto K, Yamashita H, Ohsugi M, et al. CD8+ effector T cells contribute to macrophage recruitment and adipose tissue inflammation in obesity. Nat Med. 2009;15:914-920.

[100] Rajan TV, Nelson FK, Shultz LD, Koller BH, Greiner DL. CD8+ T lymphocytes are not required for murine resistance to human filarial parasites. J Parasitol. 1992;78:744-746.

[101] Kalinkovich A, Weisman Z, Greenberg Z, Nahmias J, Eitan S, Stein M, et al. Decreased CD4 and increased CD8 counts with T cell activation is associated with chronic helminth infection. Clin Exp Immunol. 1998;114:414-421.

[102] Winer DA, Winer S, Shen L, Wadia PP, Yantha J, Paltser G, et al. B cells promote insulin resistance through modulation of T cells and production of pathogenic IgG antibodies. Nat Med. 2011;17:610-617.

[103] Mallat Z. The B-side story in insulin resistance. Nat Med.17:539-40.

[104] Nokoff NJ, Rewers M, Cree Green M. The interplay of autoimmunity and insulin resistance in type 1 diabetes. Discov Med. 2012;13:115-122.

[105] Hussaarts L, van der Vlugt LE, Yazdanbakhsh M, Smits HH. Regulatory B-cell induction by helminths: implications for allergic disease. J Allergy Clin Immunol. 2011;128:733-739.